The Incidence and Economic Costs of Major Health Impairments

The Incidence and Economic Costs of Major Health Impairments

A Comparative Analysis of Cancer, Motor Vehicle Injuries, Coronary Heart Disease, and Stroke

Nelson S. Hartunian
Charles N. Smart
Mark S. Thompson

An Insurance Institute for Highway Safety Book

LexingtonBooks
D.C. Heath and Company
Lexington, Massachusetts
Toronto

Library of Congress Cataloging in Publication Data

Hartunian, Nelson S
    The incidence and economic costs of major health impairments.

    Bibliography: p.
    Includes index.
    1. Coronary heart disease—Economic aspects—United States. 2. Coronary heart disease—United States—Statistics. 3. Cerebrovascular disease—Economic aspects—United States. 4. Cerebrovascular disease—United States—Statistics. 5. Cancer—Economic aspects—United States. 6. Cancer—United States—Statistics. 7. Crash injuries—Economic aspects—United States. 8. Crash injuries—United States—Statistics. I. Smart, Charles N., joint author. II. Thompson, Mark, joint author. III. Title. [DNLM: 1. Economics, Medical—United States. 2. Costs and cost analysis. 3. Neoplasms—Occurrence—United States. 4. Accidents, Traffic—Economics—United States. 5. Wounds and injuries—Occurrence —United States. 6. Coronary disease—Occurrence—United States. 7. Cerebrovascular disorders—Occurrence—United States. W 74 H336i]
RA410.53.H373   362.1'0422   80-27943
ISBN 0-669-03975-6

Published simultaneously in Canada.

Printed in the United States of America.

International Standard Book Number: 0-669-03975-6

Library of Congress Catalog Card Number: 80-27943

Contents

List of Figures

List of Tables

Foreword

This book reports the results of several years' work to estimate the costs, both direct and indirect, of coronary heart disease, stroke, cancer, and motor vehicle crash injuries that occurred in one calendar year in the United States. Supported by the Insurance Institute for Highway Safety, the work was conducted independently by an expert group of health economics analysts.

The results show that the economic losses being sustained by the people of the United States from *each* of these four kinds of damage to the body are huge, with the costs of cancer leading the rest. In fact, the magnitudes of the costs of coronary heart disease, stroke, and cancer more than justify the present great scientific efforts and expenditures directed at reducing our nation's morbidity and mortality from them and call emphatically for far better application of what is already known.

The major surprise for most readers will probably be the astounding costs of motor vehicle injuries. These equal the costs of coronary heart disease and exceed those of stroke by more than two to one. Yet, unlike society's response to coronary heart disease, stroke, and cancer, there is no great scientific effort to reduce damage to people sustained on the highway. Moreover, lifesaving motor vehicle crash packaging and other technology and important scientific knowledge to reduce motor vehicle crash injuries remain unused many years after their development.

Viewed somewhat differently, society's economic and institutional response varies hugely with the kind of bodily damage involved. Or, to paraphrase George Orwell, some kinds of morbidity and mortality are more equal than others.

Surely it is rational and sensible for private and public decisionmakers to pay attention to both the absolute and relative economic losses that result from different kinds of damage to the bodies of Americans. In this light, and aside from its considerable contribution to the methodology of economic analysis, one of the most important contributions of this work is its finding that motor vehicle injuries are one of the leading causes of health-related expenditures by the people of the United States. It is tragic and illogical that such injuries are not receiving commensurate attention in government and private research and control activities.

William Haddon, Jr., M.D., M.P.H.
President, Insurance Institute for
Highway Safety

Preface
and Acknowledgments

The enormity of the economic impact of disease and injury during the last fifteen years has become increasingly a matter of concern for our nation's policymakers and a quandary for the allocators of resources for health care. How can, or must, the limited funds available for prevention, research, and delivery of health services be appropriated equitably among the various causes of health impairment? Gratefully, the final responsibility for this task has not fallen to us. What we have attempted to present in this book is a starting point for the colloquy of scientists and decisionmakers—a method of most clearly estimating the real direct and indirect costs of illness and injury to our society, by the use of an *incidence-based* cost-analysis methodology. To underscore the relevance and value of this methodology, we have applied it to measure the costs associated with four major health impairments in the United States in 1975.

The study on which this book is based was supported primarily by a contract from the Insurance Institute for Highway Safety, Washington, D.C. The encouragement and professional support and advice provided by the Insurance Institute's President, William Haddon, Jr., M.D., and its Vice President for Research, Brian O'Neill, were critical to the initiation and successful completion of the study. We are indebted to them both for their great assistance. Additionally, certain aspects of our research were refined under Contract No. 233-79-2048 from the National Center for Health Statistics of the U.S. Department of Health and Human Services, and also through grants from the Robert Wood Johnson Foundation and the Commonwealth Fund to the Center for the Analysis of Health Practices at the Harvard School of Public Health. However, the contents of this book do not necessarily reflect either the views or policy of the Insurance Institute, the USDHHS, or the aforementioned foundations.

Much of the research which led to this book was performed at Policy Analysis Inc., Brookline, Massachusetts, and we wish to recognize the assistance of our former colleagues. In particular, the significant contribution of Elizabeth Mills to the research on stroke must be cited; the work of Nancy Gad on coronary heart disease and that of James R. Kanak on cancer are also gratefully acknowledged. We must also include our appreciation of the painstaking efforts of research assistants Joan L. Sizer and Louise Sawyer. Finally, we thank Ralph E. Berry, Jr., President, for his insightful comments and generous support over the duration of our work at Policy Analysis.

Because support in obtaining necessary data and information is crucial to the successful outcome of any analysis, it is appropriate that we acknowledge, with thanks, the contributions of those who assisted us in this regard:

JoAnn K. Wells of the Insurance Institute and James Hedlund of the National Highway Traffic Safety Administration, for motor vehicle crash injury data; William Castelli, M.D., and Patricia McNamara of the Framingham Heart Study, on coronary heart disease and stroke; and Fred Vanderschmidt of Abt Associates and John Young of the National Cancer Institute, on cancer. Although too numerous to mention here, we are indebted to many other individuals who contributed much to this study in a variety of ways.

Brian O'Neill, William Haddon, Jr., M.D., Thomas Willemain, and Thomas Hodgson read and reviewed earlier versions of the manuscript and provided important suggestions for revisions. In this regard we would also like to take this opportunity to mention the assistance of Alfred Yankauer, M.D., editor, who oversaw the earlier publication of the summarized results of our work in the *American Journal of Public Health*.

Special acknowledgment must be made of the extraordinary competence of our primary editor, Elizabeth Thompson, and also of the extensive editorial assistance of Paul Hood of the Insurance Institute, and of Alma Nahigian. The twelfth-hour research efforts of Helena Reilly of Smart and Hartunian were most appreciated. Finally, the enormous contribution of Karen Whibley of the Insurance Institute on typing and typographical revisions, and typists Dorothy Linick, Elizabeth Gulezian, and Joanne Hartunian of Smart and Hartunian must, we feel, rival any wonder of the modern world.

We have attempted to present the concepts inherent in our analysis in such a way that they might unfold as clearly for the lay person, or policymaker, as for the technical economist. Only the reader can gauge the degree of our success in this endeavor. Any errors in the manuscript, of course, are our own.

The Incidence and
Economic Costs of
Major Health
Impairments

1 Introduction

The economic explosion in the health-care sector is a well-documented, widely recognized phenomenon. Over the last 15 years, national health expenditures in the United States have risen from $43 billion in 1965, to $75 billion in 1970, to $132 billion in 1975, and to $192 billion in 1978. while the gross national product (GNP) has been increasing at an average annual rate of 9 percent during that period, health expenditures have more than quadrupled, with an average annual increase of more than 12 percent. As a percentage of GNP, the expenditures on health-related goods and services have grown from a moderate 6 percent in 1965 to over 9 percent in 1978—a startling almost 50 percent relative increase in less than 15 years.[1]

The reasons for such unusual growth in health-care expenditures are many: changes in medical technology, especially those which apply to hospital care; population growth; changing demographic trends that have led to an ever-increasing proportion of the population being over 65 years of age and thus more in need of medical care; increased per capita use of certain medical services; and an inflation rate for health-care costs that has eclipsed in the past the inflation rate in other sectors of the economy. One of the aftereffects of this surge in health-related costs has been a realization among policymakers that the resources necessary to meet the demands for health care are becoming more limited. There is now a growing consensus that the United States, like other Western, industrialized countries, will have to plan carefully its policies for resource allocation for health care.

As Birnbaum (1978) argues, the finiteness of resources in our economy suggests that certain decisions must be made concerning the share that can be allocated to health problems. We also must decide how our expenditures are to be spent within the health sector, for the list of alternatives is extensive. It includes, among others, medical research, health-education programs, public health activities aimed at disease prevention and diagnostic screening, and the direct provision of health care for both acute and chronic conditions.[2] The vast array of alternatives and the need to select logically from among them brings us to the rationale behind the study of the economic costs of illness presented in this book.

Study Rationale

During the time that the economy has experienced soaring levels of national health expenditures, there also have been numerous advances in the ways to

1

prevent and treat major diseases and injuries. These advances provide virtually unlimited claims for resources to extend lives, to enhance health status, and to reduce existing health costs. To aid public-spending decisions, methods of assigning priorities to alternative prevention and amelioration programs are necessary. We feel that one important tool—and the basis for most methods—is the calculation of the economic costs of illness.

It is virtually undisputed that economic costs, or more precisely, quantifiable economic costs, cannot alone uniquely guide public health choices. Too many other factors are of concern. In particular, such noneconomic costs as the intangible aspects of disability, the pain and suffering, the psychic harm done family and friends are of unquestioned importance. Ironically, however, these costs normally are not included with more conventional economic costs in policy analysis because of the great difficulty in properly specifying and measuring them.

Notwithstanding this drawback, the pertinence of economic costs—as one important criterion among others—for many public health decisions is equally undisputed. In allocating research moneys to study different health impairments, it is important to know the economic burdens they pose. To justify certain prevention and amelioration programs in light of other programs competing for the same, limited funds—perhaps through benefit-cost or cost-effectiveness analysis—requires knowledge of the potential economic impact. The design of strategies for cost containment and for allocation of funds requires an understanding of economic costs, broken down by impairment and expenditure subcategory.

For all these reasons, the past 20 years have seen dramatically increased attention given to measuring the economic costs of disease and injury. Important ground-breaking works of the late 1950s and early 1960s were Fein's analysis of mental illness, the general methodologies of Weisbrod and of Mushkin and Collings, and Klarman's study of syphilis.[3] These works addressed a number of important methodological questions, among them the appropriate ways for dealing with discounting, employment rates, the presence of multiple diseases, transfer payments, and the value of household labor. Collectively, they set the stage for Dorothy Rice's landmark study of 1966, which presented and applied a methodology for estimating the costs of major disease categories.[4] An updated version of Rice's work by Cooper and Rice appeared in 1976 and is the current reference point for researchers in this field.[5] The 1970s saw a number of papers measuring the economic costs of specific activities, diseases, and conditions. These include studies by Acton on heart attacks, by Berry and Boland on alcohol abuse, by Conley and Milunsky on genetic diseases, by Luce and Schweitzer on smoking, by Mills and Thompson on stroke, by Rufener on drug abuse, by Smart and Sanders on spinal cord injury, and by Weisbrod on polio.[6]

This book reports the results of a three-year study measuring the economic costs associated with the incidence of four major illnesses in the United States in 1975. The four that have been investigated represent major causes of death in that year and account for substantially greater reductions in life expectancy than most other health conditions.[7] They are cancer, coronary heart disease, stroke, and motor vehicle injuries—with motor vehicle injuries representing an extension of the conventional definition of illness to include injuries as well as disease states. Although Cooper and Rice examined each of these health conditions, their approach differs from ours in two aspects: the degree of disaggregation and the analytical approach.

Disaggregation and Analytical Approach

Disaggregation

Cooper and Rice presented a comprehensive picture of the economic costs of illness. The comprehensiveness, however, resulted in disaggregation only by cost component and by sixteen major disease categories. We have focused on only four conditions and consequently have been able to break them down by subconditions—for example, cancers of different sites—and by age and sex groups as well as by cost components.

Analytical Approach

Cooper and Rice—as well as most of the other authors cited earlier—followed the *prevalence* approach in measuring costs. By far the most common analytical strategy, this approach, for any given disease or injury and year, (1) identifies all health-care costs and productivity losses owing to sickness that accrued during that year to persons suffering from the condition and (2) calculates the lost expected future earnings of persons dying of the condition in that year. The *incidence* approach, which is followed in this book, instead focuses only on costs associated with those disease or injury histories incident in the year in question. However, for those incidence cases, it estimates a *present-value equivalent* (to be explained later) for both health-care expenditures and lost productivity regardless of when that expenditure or loss might occur, be it during that year or during some year in the future.

Prevalence. Since the conceptual differences between the prevalence and incidence approaches are significant, they deserve further explanation. *Prevalence*, by definition, is either the number of cases of a specific disorder existing at a specified time or the average number of cases existing during some specified time interval, normally a calendar year. The economic cost of disease prevalence is measured by the value to society of all resources consumed as a result of the diagnosis, treatment, and repercussions of the particular disorder during the time period in question and by the value of lost productivity resulting from morbidity and premature mortality caused by the disorder during the same period. Prevalence analyses, therefore, are primarily concerned with costs occurring in the fixed period under examination or with costs otherwise attributable to that period.

Incidence. *Incidence*, however, is the estimated number of new cases of a disorder that have their onset during a specified time interval, again normally a calendar year. The economic cost associated with incidence, like that of prevalence, has both health-care-expenditure and lost-productivity components. Unlike prevalence analyses, however, incidence-cost analyses must examine the total lifetime costs of a disorder from onset until cure or death. They must therefore include not only the present value of future productivity losses owing to premature mortality (as in prevalence studies), but also the present value of future productivity losses owing to morbidity and the health-care costs for the treatment of the disorder both now *and* in the future. Only this dual time perspective, which consolidates costs occurring in the future as well as costs occurring during the period immediately following disease onset, will permit an accurate assessment of the total economic burden associated with the incidence of disease. Notice, however, that for illness that is acute and transient (for example, less than 1 year's duration), the prevalence-based cost estimates and the corresponding incidence-based cost estimates will be substantially the same.

A brief example may help to illustrate the difference between the two approaches. Consider a person with coronary heart disease incident in 1975, who, over the next 4 years, pays for medical care for the disease and misses some work, and who dies in 1979. The *prevalence* approach assigns the medical expenses and the missed work to the years in which they occurred and the lost future earnings owing to premature death to 1979. The *incidence* approach present-values and assigns all costs associated with the disease—from onset to eventual death—to the year of incidence, 1975. Many persons with coronary heart disease incident in 1975 are still alive, implying that estimation of costs owing to 1975 incidence must be partially based on epidemiological projections of the disease course. Such projections inevitably entail uncertainty. An unanticipated technological breakthrough that, starting in 1982, would affect costs and survival would not be reflected in current incidence-based estimates of economic costs. At the same time, the prevalence-based approach has a comparable drawback since future expected earnings also might be altered by unpredictable factors. The two approaches enjoy a certain similarity in this regard. They also tend to benefit from the same general "solution" to the problem, for such contingencies—be they incidence- or prevalence-specific—are usually best handled by using *sensitivity analysis* to show the expected effect on economic cost of uncertainty in other variables. (The concept and application of sensitivity analysis in cost-of-illness studies is considered more fully in chapter 2.)

Whether the incidence or the prevalence approach is the more useful depends on the policy issues at stake. For policymakers concerned with controlling current medical costs and absenteeism, the prevalence approach is superior. For policymakers evaluating preventive programs or programs aimed at immediate rehabilitation and the arresting of illness progression, the prevalence approach is misleading, inasmuch as it largely focuses on the current costs of conditions that commenced in the past and that present programs cannot affect. For conditions such as cardiovascular disorders whose incidence has changed significantly over recent years, the prevalence approach is even less useful. Much more relevant in such cases are economic costs accounted for by incidence. These provide best estimates of the costs that may be averted and, hence, of the economic benefits that may be gained by programs aimed at altering disease incidence. Precisely because neither the prevalence nor the incidence approach is in all circumstances the superior methodology, each provides a useful basis for comparison and an alternative perspective that aids interpretation of the other.

Some Basic Economic Concepts

Since economic analysis will be the frame of reference used throughout this book, it may be useful, especially to the noneconomist, to digress briefly and to consider the basic concepts of economic cost as they relate to health problems. These include the following topics: economic scarcity and opportunity costs, direct versus indirect economic costs, present-value analysis and the selection of discount rates, and the identification of transfer payments as distinguished from true economic costs. These concepts encompass many of the major issues that analysts and policymakers must consider if they intend to evaluate comprehensively the various costs associated with illness.

Economic Scarcity and Opportunity Costs

Economics is, in simplest terms, the science of scarcity. When, therefore, we examine the cost of a disease or injury from an economic perspective, we must deal invariably with the limits of our resources. The productive resources available to treat diseases, conduct medical research, and satisfy a host of other needs are extremely scarce, while, on the other hand, the wants of individuals and society both in a health- and non-health-related context are virtually unlimited. Every society, even the most affluent, faces the basic problem of how best to allocate finite resources. Questions such as what goods and services should be produced and which members of society should receive these goods and services demand answers. Consequently, a society must concern itself with how much it receives from depleting scarce resources and, more important, how to distribute those resources so that it receives the maximum from them in terms of the satisfaction of its constituent wants.

Whenever a specific good or service is produced to satisfy a particular want, some of the scarce resources are used up. The increased production of one good thus implies that less of some other goods can be produced, since the resources used for the one are not available for the other. As a result, the cost of any good or service derives from the forgone opportunity of using the resources employed to produce something else and, hence, is appropriately described as its *opportunity cost*.

When we estimate the economic costs of a disease or injury, we must measure the opportunity costs society incurs as a result of that condition. Economic costs may accrue in either of two general forms. On the one hand, a health impairment, such as stroke, for example, may lower productivity through the illness, incapacitation, or death of workers. On the other hand, it may be necessary to produce certain goods and services to cope with the effects of stroke. Either of these two sets of consequences reduces the amount of goods and services available for other purposes. The former set, indirect costs, lowers the overall production of goods and services; the latter set, direct costs, diverts to specific health-related services resources that might have served other ends.

The crux of the problem, then, is to identify the consequences of a health impairment that result in lost production and forgone alternatives. By identifying and quantifying the various opportunity costs associated with the adverse consequences of a health impairment, we can estimate both the economic costs per case and the total costs associated with the incidence of that impairment.

Direct versus Indirect Economic Costs

The costs associated with a disease or injury can be classified into two principal categories: direct costs and indirect costs. *Direct costs* represent the value of resources used to prevent, detect, treat, and rehabilitate the health impairment or its effects. They include, within the health sector, expenditures for emergency assistance, hospitalization, physicians' and surgeons' services, special paramedical services, outpatient clinical care, nursing home care, drugs, medical appliances, and the like. In addition, there are often non-health-sector direct costs borne both by the patient and others. These can run the spectrum from expenses for structural modifications to a patient's home necessitated by his or her condition and extra expenditures for household help to institutional costs, such as the administration expenses incurred by insurance companies and government agencies in funding illness expenditures and the legal and court costs of litigation that may relate to the illness. If we were to extend the definition of direct costs even further, we also might include the costs of government public health activities, research programs, and medical facilities construction. However, these last categories of cost are frequently difficult to allocate by health condition, and even when that is possible, it is virtually impossible to disaggregate them into exclusively incidence-oriented as opposed to non-incidence-oriented activities. For this reason, they have not been included in our analysis.

Indirect costs, however, bear a more implicit relationship to the health impairment. They are not expenditures directly tied to the treatment of the impairment or unambiguous expenses necessitated by impairment sequelae. Instead, the primary component of indirect costs is the lost or forgone output of patients suffering premature death or disability. This is normally measured in terms of the wages that would have been earned by these individuals if they had not had the illness. Output losses also extend to the imputed market value of unperformed housekeeping services. It is extremely important to include the value of housekeeping services, since its omission may result in a serious underestimate of the indirect costs of illness, especially when the health condition in question has a disproportionate effect on women.

We also should mention that output losses may be generated not only by patients, but also by family members, friends, and co-workers. It is possible for these individuals either to lose time from work or homemaking activities or to suffer reductions in their productivity because of the patient's condition. This can happen in the case of family members and friends when someone must remain at home to care for an ill person. Hodgson and Meiners (1979), among others, have hypothesized that it also can happen in the workplace when the productivity of another worker suffers because of the patient's diminished performance at work or absence from the workplace. Output losses of this sort constitute a secondary component of indirect costs. However, although their potential magnitudes may be significant for certain illnesses, the empirical difficulties associated with data collection and, in certain instances, attribution of cause virtually always prevent their estimation.

A similar estimation problem obtains for the noneconomic costs of disease and injury. The pain and emotional deprivation experienced by the patient, his or her family, and his or her friends because of a health impairment—including the possible reduction in self-esteem, the increase in anxiety and dependency, and the other reductions in the quality of life that often accompany a debilitating condition—are real social costs. They constitute an important and potentially large component of total costs, but unfortunately, such social costs resist quantification. Construction of quality-of-life indicators that accurately reflect pain and suffering is not easy. The task is further hindered by the procedural problems of data collection and by the difficulty in integrating basically nonmonetary information on quality of life with the dollar estimates of direct and indirect costs.

Present-Value Analysis and Selection of Discount Rates

Not all costs of a health impairment occur simultaneously. In the case of incidence-based analyses, some costs occur in the present during the year of onset of the impairment but many more accrue in future years.

Economists achieve comparability among future and present cost flows by converting future flows to their present values by using an appropriate discount rate. Discounting takes into account the fact that a given amount of dollars today is worth more than that same amount of dollars in the future. This is reasonable, since a sum of dollars not spent now can be invested to yield a larger number of dollars in the future. As an example, if we assume an annual rate of return of 8 percent, it follows that $\$Y$ in costs or benefits accruing n years hence should be worth $\$Y/(1.08)^n$ today, because this amount of money invested at 8 percent would yield $\$Y$ in n years. Therefore, this is the *present value* of $\$Y$ accruing n years in the future at a discount rate of 8 percent.

What is an appropriate value to use for the discount rate? There is no clear-cut "right" answer to this question. Although economists agree on the necessity to discount future costs, there is no corresponding consensus as to the level at which the discount rate should be set. Differences of opinion are due, in large measure, to the variations among the rates of return and interest rates observed in our economy, which, in turn, indicate differences between the productive potential of investment capital and the preferences of individuals for present versus future consumption of goods and services. Some economists have argued that the discount rate used in public investment decisions, such as those for health care, should reflect the opportunity cost of public capital in other ventures, including investment alternatives in the private sector. This would recommend the use of a high discount rate, probably close to the market rates of return observed in the private sector. Others have suggested a lower rate, reflecting what they believe to be a "social" rate of time preference. This would represent society's rate of tradeoff between present and future consumption. The lower rate would give more weight to costs occurring in the future and, presumably, would give more recognition to the welfare of future generations bearing those costs.

In our analyses, three discount rates have been used: 10 percent, 6 percent, and 2 percent. Currently, 10 percent is the rate recommended by the United States Office of Management and Budget to evaluate federal investment decisions.[8] It is considered to approximate closely the opportunity cost of public capital, if that capital were invested in the private sector. It represents the government's current estimate of the average pretax rate of return on private investment, after correcting for inflation. However, 6 percent and 2 percent are values that undoubtedly come closer to capturing the idea of a "social" discount rate. Using each rate, all future costs and forgone earnings are discounted back to the present, here taken to be the year of onset of the disease or injury.

The use of three rates provides a valuable indicator of just how sensitive the present value of future costs is to changes in the discount rate, with the higher rates obviously producing the lower present values for any one health impairment. It also will show how the relative importance (in terms of present-valued costs) of several impairments may change depending on the discount rate used. This information may aid the decisions of policymakers who must select from among alternate programs designed to reduce the incidence of different impairments or to ameliorate their consequences.

Transfer Payments

Transfer payments, such as welfare, unemployment, or public-assistance payments, do not represent true economic costs of illness and therefore should not be included in the total for direct and indirect costs. While direct and indirect costs clearly reflect resource losses that would not happen if a disease or injury were eradicated or its incidence reduced, transfers represent only a shift in the burden of these costs from one portion of society to another. They do not represent additional economic costs, but only a "transfer" of part of the cost from one individual to another.

The nature of transfer payments and their significance can perhaps be best understood by considering an income-maintenance payment made to an individual who has been so incapacitated by illness that he can no longer work. If his salary was $15,000 a year, the annual output loss sustained by society is approximated by his $15,000 loss in earned income. If the government awards him $6500 per year from public-assistance funds, the recipient's net share of the $15,000 loss is $8500. The $6500 that is taken from general taxes represents a transfer of part of the burden of the loss from the afflicted individual to the taxpaying public; it becomes the taxpayers' share. Although a transfer of this sort represents an expense to the taxpayers in the form of a reduction in their after-tax incomes, the taxpayers' loss is another's gain, and the net cost to society resulting from this transaction in terms of resources used is zero (with the possible exception of those costs which may be incurred in operating the public-assistance program providing the transfer). The total economic cost is the value of the lost production, $15,000, *not* $15,000 plus the $6500 value of the transfer payment.

Medical-expense payments made by third-party reimbursement agencies, such as Medicare, Medicaid, or private insurance companies, are also transfers. They, like income-maintenance payments, should not be added to the total of economic costs. In a similar vein, lost income taxes will already have been included in the estimate of lost production and thus already expressed in total indirect costs. To add them again would result in a double count of that portion of indirect costs.

While the value of transfer payments per se is not an economic cost, we, like others, recognize that transfers may have significant influence on the quality of life. As Hodgson and Meiners (1979) suggest, it might be valuable from a welfare standpoint to investigate transfers owing to illness, focusing on their magnitude and on the resulting redistribution of income that occurs. This is, however, beyond the scope of our study. Even if it were possible, Hodgson and Meiners recommend that the results of such an investigation be reported independently and not confused with the estimates of the total cost of illness. The inability to differentiate and isolate transfer payments from economic costs may lead to a significant upward bias in those costs.

Study Scope and Objectives

This study seeks to evaluate and to compare the economic costs borne by society as a result of the annual incidence of (1) coronary heart disease, (2) cerebrovascular disease (stroke), (3) cancer, and (4) motor vehicle injuries. The computation and breakdown of such costs will, we believe, assist social policymakers in allocating available resources to those alternative employments where the potential benefits are the greatest. One might look askance at the temerity of balancing, for example, motor vehicle crash costs—predominantly incident on a younger and fitter population—with those of stroke—a disease of the elderly. In the former case, the impact is relatively less visible, for it centers on the economic and social loss resulting from the death or permanent disability of people who do not live to accomplish what they might otherwise have done. In the case of stroke, costs are more visible: They are heavily concentrated on direct expenditures for medical care, rehabilitation, and long-term nursing.

Yet further reflection shows that society implicitly must make such comparisons. Each of these four afflictions competes for scarce economic and social resources. An additional dollar budgeted for the management of coronary heart disease may well be a dollar taken away from cancer research or treatment. Consequently, in this study we hope to make these implicit comparisons—inherent in every budget of every government—explicit.

The two most formidable aspects of our investigations are (1) the weighing of direct costs, which represent resources used primarily for the treatment of a disease or injury, against indirect costs, which reflect productivity losses sustained because an otherwise healthy individual dies prematurely or is disabled, and (2) the contrasting of present, near-term future, and long-term future costs. The resolution of these two problems has required an extension and refinement of the still evolving incidence approach to analyzing the cost of illness. We have built on the seminal work of two studies mentioned earlier (Smart and Sanders, 1976; and Mills and Thompson, 1978) to develop what we feel is a state-of-the-art methodology. Using this methodology, we have addressed the problem of measuring indirect costs by employing variants of existing economic models of forgone productivity in an attempt to evaluate the economic product lost owing to permanent disability as well as that owing to premature death and transient disability. Virtually every current study that seeks to place a quantified value on extending or saving lives uses forgone productivity as a measure. We recognize, nevertheless, that forgone productivity is but an imperfect surrogate for the high value that society places on the life of an individual. The amount of wages an individual would have earned if not disabled or killed can hardly be accepted as a complete measure of the life-joy he or she loses when crippled or of the family's pain when he or she dies. Forgone productivity is a purely tangible economic measure of loss that we take as a conservative indicator of true dysbenefit. We fully realize that we thereby miss a significant portion of the personal and social dimensions of the tragedy caused by a disease or injury.

The second problem—that of comparing costs incurred at different points in time—has ramifications for the calculation of both direct and indirect costs in incidence analysis. In each case, the comparison of intertemporal cost flows is handled by the method of time discounting. Although we have acknowledged that discounting is a controversial issue in applied analysis, we also know that the current disagreements tend to center on appropriate rates for discounting and not on the validity of the procedure itself. Reflecting the lack of complete agreement on discount rates, we have prepared alternative results discounted at three separate, but commonly applied rates.

The end products of our analysis are numerical comparisons of the economic burdens placed on society by heart disease, stroke, cancer, and motor vehicle crashes. They may be taken conversely as potential economic benefits to be achieved with the removal for 1 year (taken to be 1975) of each source of death or impairment. One must, in this light, bear in mind the differential feasibility of ameliorating each of the conditions. This normally involves identifying alternative disease- and injury-control programs and estimating the likely impacts of those programs as measured in terms of a reduction in the number of incidence cases and/or the amelioration of the consequences of incidence cases that still occur. Estimates of the costs of such programs are also important, especially if a meaningful comparison is to be made between the expected benefits of any one program and the expected resources that must be sacrificed to make it work. These requirements are not easy for the economist alone to fill. They go beyond the standard fields of economic expertise—even health economic expertise—to encompass areas more familiar to the epidemiologist and to others trained in the theory of illness occurrence, containment, and prevention. Therefore, we have not attempted to tackle the epidemiological aspects of disease and injury control. Rather, we have chosen to concentrate our efforts on providing best estimates of the economic benefits that are possible, if and when new control programs are enacted, and, in the absence of such programs, the economic costs society currently endures because of these four health conditions.

Traditionally, the more salient conditions—those with greater impact on direct costs—have absorbed more of society's attention and resources. A primary goal of this study is, therefore, to place indirect costs on a par with direct costs. This examination of unseen and frequently unmeasured social drains should enable wiser allocations of resources across major target areas of health policy (even though the intangible dimensions of loss must still, and with inevitable subjectivity, be acknowledged.) In particular, this analysis suggests that with full recognition of all economic costs, motor vehicle crash injuries may not have received the attention they deserve as a health problem.

The study further breaks down costs into a number of subcategories, including the components of direct costs and per-capita and total-cost displays for different age, sex, and diagnostic subgroups. This is intended to make clear just where the moneys are going and where loss is suffered. We hope that such breakdowns will help to illuminate any possible discrepancies between the social value derived from various activities and the funds devoted to them. Perhaps more important, however, is the analytic philosophy underlying our explicit breakdowns. We believe that analysis becomes more credible just as it exposes its own workings and thus leaves itself open to possible challenges. To this end, we have not only itemized costs into many subcategories, but we also have made explicit all working assumptions and explained all computations.

Outline and Overview

This book provides a profile of the incidence and costs of four major health conditions in the United States. Chapter 2 provides a comprehensive discussion of the study methodology. There we develop general techniques used (1) to estimate the annual incidence of disease and injuries, (2) to project mortality and survival rates for individuals suffering from particular health conditions, and (3) to calculate direct and indirect costs. Also presented are discussions on sensitivity analysis, the numerical differences between the prevalence and incidence approaches, and the data bases used in the study. In chapter 3, the methodology is applied to evaluate the annual consequences of coronary heart disease. Incidence, survival rates, direct and indirect costs are all estimated and a sensitivity analysis is performed to determine the effect on total costs of particular assumptions and uncertain parameter values. Chapters 4, 5, and 6 describe similar applications of the methodology to stroke, cancer, and motor vehicle injuries, respectively. In chapter 7, we summarize the results of the four illness analyses and offer opinions on their comparative significance.

While we believe that the cost estimates presented in this book will be of special interest to policymakers concerned with public health problems, their potential value to other individuals and organizations should not be overlooked. Insurance carriers and health-maintenance organizations often must know the expected levels of both short- and long-term treatment costs for people suffering from these conditions and in what proportions these costs accrue to the various age, sex, and diagnostic subgroups. Lawyers engaged in tort action proceedings may find the methodology discussion on forgone productivity especially valuable. The estimates offered for lost earnings resulting from motor vehicle injuries provide good examples of the methodology's application in a personal-injury setting. Even medical practitioners and health-care administrators who do not have specific responsibility for the funding of illness-related costs or for the implementation of disease-control programs may gain useful insights. Indeed, the comparison of the costs attributable to these four major impairment groups has relevance for those who see their relative economic magnitudes as at least a partial indicator of their relative societal impacts.

Although we feel that these estimates of incidence, survival rates, and costs are reasonably accurate and represent the best data available, they are only estimates. Data available for use in health economic analysis have always left something to be desired and probably always will. The information used in this book is no exception. To a certain degree, we have been able to test the significance of specific data imperfections through sensitivity analysis, and we recommend that the interested reader pay special attention to the sensitivity-analysis discussions. We freely acknowledge that more work can, and probably should, be done to refine these estimates. However, given the resource constraints on the study and the nascent state of the art of incidence-based investigations, we nevertheless view our results as necessary and valuable first-order estimates.

Notes

1. Developed from data in U.S. Department of Commerce, Bureau of the Census, *Statistical Abstract of the United States, 1979* (Washington: U.S. Government Printing Office, 1979), tables 143 and 714, pp. 100 and 435.

2. Howard Birnbaum, *The Cost of Catastrophic Illness* (Lexington, Mass.: Lexington Books, D.C. Heath, 1978), pp. 1–2.

3. Rashi Fein, *Economics of Mental Illness* (New York: Basic Books, 1958); Burton A. Weisbrod, *Economics of Public Health* (Philadelphia: Univ. of Pennsylvania Press, 1961); Selma J. Mushkin and Edward A. Collings, Economic costs of disease and injury, *Public Health Reports* 74(a):795–809, 1959; and Herbert E. Klarman, Syphilis control programs, in Robert Dorfman (ed.), *Measuring the Benefits of Government Investments* (Washington: Brookings Institution, 1965), pp. 367–414.

4. Dorothy P. Rice, *Estimating the Cost of Illness*, Health Economics Series, No. 6, PHS Publication No. 947-6 (Washington: U.S. Government Printing Office, May 1966).

5. Barbara S. Cooper and Dorothy P. Rice, The economic cost of illness revisited, *Social Security Bulletin* 39(2):21–36, 1976.

6. Jan P. Acton, *Evaluating Public Programs to Save Lives: The Case of Heart Attacks* (Santa Monica, Calif.: Rand Corporation, 1973); Ralph E. Berry and James P. Boland, *The Economic Cost of Alcohol Abuse* (New York: Free Press, 1977); R. Conley and A. Milunsky, The economics of prenatal genetic diagnosis, in A. Milunsky (ed.), *The Prevention of Genetic Disease and Mental Retardation* (Philadelphia: Saunders, 1975); B.R. Luce and S.O. Schweitzer, Smoking and alcohol abuse: A comparison of their economic consequences, *New England Journal of Medicine* 238:569–571, 1978; Elizabeth Mills and Mark S. Thompson, The economic costs of stroke in Massachusetts, *New England Journal of Medicine* 299:415–418, 1978; B.L. Rufener, J.V. Rachal, and A.M. Cruze, Management effectiveness measure for NIDA drug abuse treatment programs, in *Cost to Society of Drug Abuse*, vol. 2 (1976), pp. 271, and 975–1016; Charles N. Smart and Claudia R. Sanders, *The Costs of Motor Vehicle Related Spinal Cord Injuries* (Washington: Insurance Institute for Highway Safety, 1976); and

Burton A. Weisbrod, Costs and benefits of medical research: A case study of poliomyelitis, *Journal of Political Economy* 79(3):527–544, 1971.

7. U.S. Department of Health, Education and Welfare, Health Resources Administration, National Center for Health Statistics, Final mortality statistics, 1975, *Monthly Vital Statistics Reports* 25(11), (suppl.) 1977.

8. U.S. Executive Office of the President, Office of Management and Budget, *Circular No. A-94 (Revised)*, Washington, March 27, 1972.

2 Methodology

In this chapter, we build on the work of Smart and Sanders (1976), Mills and Thompson (1978), and others to develop a state-of-the-art methodology for *incidence-based analyses* of the cost of illness. The discussion here is analogous to similar discussions on the methodology of *prevalence-based analyses* presented first by Rice (1966) and extended later by Cooper and Rice (1976). Although the two methodological approaches utilize many of the same economic concepts, they are fundamentally different in their perspectives. The underlying rationale of the prevalence approach is that disease and injury costs should be assigned to the years in which they are borne or are directly associated. Under this approach, direct costs and productivity losses resulting from disease or injury are assigned to the years in which they occur and lost expected future earnings resulting from premature mortality are assigned to the year of death. During any one year, the focus is on the prevalence population of afflicted individuals accounting for such costs. In contrast, the incidence approach is based on the principle that the stream of costs associated with an illness should be assigned to the year in which the stream begins. All costs, both direct costs and productivity losses owing to morbidity and mortality, are present-valued and assigned to the year in which the disease or injury case first appears. Under this approach, the focus is on the incidence population—not the prevalence population—generating these costs.

The difference in perspective between the two approaches has led to major differences in the data requirements and in the level of disaggregation of the cost results. For instance, Cooper and Rice's application of the prevalence approach resulted in a comprehensive picture of the economic costs of illness in the United States in 1972. Their analysis made use of preexisting estimates for that year of total annual direct costs by cost component for the entire ill population (that is, total expenditures for hospital care, physician services, drugs, and so forth) and of similar, though less complete, estimates of illness-related productivity losses. The comprehensiveness of their work, however, resulted in disaggregation of their final figures only by cost component and by sixteen major illness categories.

Had the incidence approach been followed in the Cooper and Rice study, the data requirements would have been more extensive and the level of disaggregation of the data and cost results, more pronounced. Even if but one of the sixteen illness categories, such as cancer, had been studied, it would have been necessary to determine the costs incurred at each stage in the course of that illness. Such data normally cannot be collected in any reasonable sense at an organ-system level representing "all cancers." Instead, the cancer-incidence population must be disaggregated at least into cancers of different anatomic sites and, for each site, into patient cohorts of different age and sex. As chapter 5 will explain more fully, resource utilization costs vary significantly among different types of cancers and even among different age and sex groups within the same type; furthermore, for each cancer subcategory, a typical patient's treatment requirements and costs are normally greater during the first year past onset of the disease than during subsequent years. Any assumption that all cancer patients face similar treatment and costs or, for that matter, that an individual cancer patient's costs in the first year are necessarily indicative of his or her costs in other years would be unfounded. The end result is that for cancer and, as we shall show, for other types of disease and injury, the incidence approach requires that the analysis be performed "from the bottom up," totaling the lifetime costs of many distinct subcategories of illness. This, in turn, requires that input data be gathered at a level of disaggregation commensurate with that of the illness subcategories. It also permits an estimation and display of economic costs at the same level of disaggregation. This contrasts with the traditional prevalence approach employed by Cooper and Rice, where, in general, the analysis is performed "from the top down," allocating portions of a known total expenditure to each of several broad disease and injury categories.

This chapter lays the technical foundation for the incidence-based methodology applied in succeeding chapters. We outline here the general methods of approach used to estimate the annual incidence of diseases and injuries by age, sex, and subcondition; to project mortality and survival rates for individuals in different illness subcategories; to calculate direct and indirect costs for individuals in each subcategory; and to test the sensitivity of our cost results to data imperfections and certain key assumptions. In addition, we present a numerical example that compares further the differences between the incidence and prevalence approaches, and we offer some brief comments on the types of data bases used in this study.

In applying the methodology to coronary heart disease, stroke, cancer, and motor vehicle injuries, we have selected 1975 as the reference year. This has been done for two reasons. First, and most important, 1975 represents the most recent year for which satisfactory data were available for all four conditions. Second, it is a convenient coincidence that this year also has significance as the three-quarter mark of the twentieth century.

Incidence Estimates

Disaggregation by Age, Sex, and Subcondition

The annual incidence models employed in the different parts of the study exhibit a common approach in disaggregating by age and sex the populations experiencing first or "new" occurrences of a health impairment. These impairment populations have been broken down by sex and by eight age groupings: 0 to 14 years, 15 to 24 years, 25 to 34 years, 35 to 44 years, 45 to 54 years, 55 to 64 years, 65 to 74 years, and 75 years or over. (In the case of stroke, which has a significant incidence among those over 85 years of age, we deviate slightly from this format to include an extra interval, 75 to 84 years, at the end of the age spectrum.) Much of the data in the literature follows this breakdown. In cases where specific year-by-year statistics are required—such as in estimating annual mortality rates or in projecting future cost streams—we assume that persons of midpoint ages (8, 20, 30, 40, 50, 60, 70 and 80) are generally representative of their respective age groups. To facilitate computations, we also have assumed that no one lives beyond the age of 99. Sensitivity analysis (to be discussed later) shows that little imprecision is introduced into our cost results because of these simplifying assumptions.

In addition to disaggregation by age and sex, we also have distinguished among specific subconditions within the four major impairments studied. Distinction has been made among the various subgroups both to discriminate among those with different impacts on costs and to take advantage of existing data. Our breakdown of coronary heart disease, for instance, recognizes four disease subcategories: sudden death, other myocardial infarction (MI), coronary insufficiency (CI), and angina pectoris uncomplicated (APU). For strokes, we have distinguished among hemorrhagic and infarctive completed strokes and transient ischemic attacks (TIAs). For cancer, our categorization scheme by tumor type and by anatomic site excluded all carcinoma in situ (tumors that normally grow to the size of a pinhead but no larger and that do not penetrate surrounding tissues) and any nonmalignant tumors. The nine major diagnostic groups for our disaggregation are cancers of the digestive, nervous, reproductive, respiratory, and urinary systems; cancers of the buccal cavity; leukemias; lymphomas; and cancers of other sites. In addition to anatomic site, each cancer is described in terms of one of three possible stages of disease development or spread: local, regional, or distant. Motor vehicle injuries are first subdivided into fatalities and nonfatalities. Fatalities include all injury-induced deaths occurring within 1 year of the motor vehicle crash. Nonfatalities are ranked according to severity levels.

The rationale for these various dimensions of disaggregation can be seen in their consequences. Different age levels, both sexes, and diverse impairment categories have substantially different rates of incidence, patterns of recurrence, mortality rates, and per-patient costs. Productivity losses, for example, depend critically on age, sex, and impairment level. Only by breaking the incidence population down into these subgroups do we capture those significantly different components of cost.

For both direct and indirect costs and for each incidence subcategory, average per-patient costs and total costs are presented. These breakdowns should be of use to the policymaker concerned with targeting public moneys to particular population segments and to specific disease and injury subcategories where they would provide the greatest benefits.

Recurrences

The estimation of disease incidence in a given year, such as 1975, raises an important issue: the possibility of future disease recurrences among that incidence population and the specific consequentiality of those recurrences. Consider, for example, the case of an individual who has a first stroke in 1975 and a second stroke 4 years later in 1979. A number of reasonable hypotheses are possible: (1) the second stroke may be caused by the first in the sense that it would not have occurred in the absence of the first or its likelihood of occurrence would have been much lower; (2) the two strokes may be linked in the sense that a common aggravating condition—for instance, hypertension—was implicated in both; or (3) the two strokes are causally unrelated (if the first were avoided, the occurrence of the second would not be affected). In the first case, averting the earlier stroke eliminates the latter or makes it far less likely. In the second case, affecting the underlying factors has impact on both strokes. For these cases, a prospective analytical approach that looks forward from the first incidence of stroke to include subsequent recurrences seems most appropriate. It best presents to a policymaker concerned with prevention the totality of possible effects of his or her current actions.

In the third case, it might be convenient to ascribe the costs of the later stroke to the year of its incidence rather than to the year of the earlier stroke. Were it possible to distinguish causally related and independent recurrences, that method of accounting might be used. Since, however, for heart disease, cancer, and stroke, recurrences are known to be largely related to first incidence, we have adopted the prospective mode of accounting. Because recurrences and incidence may be due to common underlying factors or may (more rarely) be causally independent, we should avoid the language of causation. In this study, we are not measuring the costs of all 1975 incidence and all *consequent* recurrences, but rather the costs of 1975 incidence and all *associated* recurrences (those afflicting the same individual).

Mortality Rates and Survival Probabilities

The role of mortality rates and survival probabilities is critical in deriving the economic costs of illness on an incidence basis. Using the incidence approach, we estimate both present and future direct costs generated by the incidence population of diseased and injured individuals and the lost earnings resulting from disability and premature mortality of this same population. The more accurately we can estimate the probabilities of their survival to generate future direct costs and to recoup earnings that would otherwise be lost, the more accurate will be our calculations of both the direct and indirect costs of illness.

In this section we define survival probabilities; show how they may be estimated using standard life table methods, relative survival rates, or relative mortality rates; and explain how they may be summed to yield life expectancies. In subsequent sections of this and other chapters, we will illustrate how survival probabilities are used to help determine the present value of future direct and indirect costs.

Concept of Probability of Survival

Each individual alive today has a certain likelihood of surviving to some future time. For a person of sex s whose age in years is l, this likelihood can be expressed as the probability that he or she will survive n additional years to age $l + n$. For people in the general population, this probability can be determined from general life tables, such as those published by the U.S. government,[1] and it is equal to the ratio of the number of persons in a specific sample alive at age $l + n$ to the number of persons alive at age l. If $P_{l,s}(l + n)$ represents the probability that a person of age l and sex s in the general population will survive to age $l + n$, then it follows that:

$$P_{l,s}(l + n) = \frac{\text{number of persons of sex } s \text{ in sample alive at age } l + n}{\text{number of persons of sex } s \text{ in sample alive at age } l}$$

(In constructing general life tables, one could theoretically start out with a sample of people born at the same time and follow this sample until all members have died, recording the number of survivors each year after birth. This would represent a prospective form of analysis. In practice, a cross-sectional rather than a prospective approach is used to project the number of survivors. This makes use of demographically matched groups of people of different ages whose survival experience is tracked over the same fixed-time interval, normally 5 or 10 years.)

It is possible to condition the value of the survival probability on other parameters in addition to sex and current age (for example, race, ethnic group, or health impairment). This level of specificity is only occasionally necessary in analyses limited to the general population. In an analysis such as ours, however, which considers the various consequences of different health impairments, it is important to condition the value of the survival probability on a particular impairment being present or not. Accordingly, we define $P_{l,s}^i(n)$ as the probability that a person of sex s who acquires impairment i at age l will survive to age $l + n$. If this impairment has a mortality rate greater than or equal to that of the general population, we would expect that the likelihood of a patient with the impairment surviving to some future time is less than or, at best, equal to the corresponding likelihood of an age- and sex-matched peer in the general population. This relationship can be expressed as

$$P_{l,s}^i(l + n) \leq P_{l,s}(l + n) \qquad \text{for } n > 0$$

In order to estimate $P_{l,s}(l + n)$ for persons in the general population, we often make use of the probabilities of survival over a series of subintervals (often taken as 1 year each). We define this *annual probability of survival* as the probability that an individual of age m and sex s alive at the beginning of the year in question survives to the end of the year. We have, therefore,

$P_{m,s}(m + 1) =$ annual probability of survival of a person of age m and sex s

The cumulative probability of survival from age l to age $l + n$ several years in the future can be represented as the product of the annual probabilities of survival from age l to age $l + n$:

$$P_{l,s}(l + n) = [P_{l,s}(l + 1)] \cdot [P_{l+1,s}(l + 2)] \cdots [P_{l+n-1,s}(l + n)]$$

As an example, consider a man aged 55 in the general population. From the life tables,[2] he has a cumulative probability of surviving to age 65 of 0.8197, which may be expressed as

$$\begin{aligned}
P_{55,M}(65) &= (0.9874) \cdot (0.9863) \cdot (0.9851) \cdot (0.9835) \cdot (0.9817) \cdot \\
&\quad (0.9797) \cdot (0.9777) \cdot (0.9757) \cdot (0.9739) \cdot (0.9722) \\
&= 0.8197
\end{aligned}$$

where M indicates male sex, 0.9874 is the probability of surviving from 55 to 56, 0.9863 is the probability of surviving from 56 to 57, and so on.

This procedure also applies in the case of a person with impairment i. We can define the annual probability of survival for such an individual as

$P^i_{l+j,s}(l + j + 1) =$ annual probability of survival of a person of sex s who acquired impairment i at age l and has already survived j years past diagnosis

As for the general population, if we know the annual probabilities of survival for impairment i, we may find the cumulative probability of survival from age l to age $l + n$ by multiplying these annual survival probabilities:

$$P^i_{l,s}(l + n) = [P^i_{l,s}(l + 1)] \cdot [P^i_{l+1,s}(l + 2)] \cdots [P^i_{l+n-1,s}(l + n)]$$

If the same 55-year-old man were to contract impairment i, and if the annual probability of survival during the first year past onset was, for instance, 0.80 followed by successive annual probabilities of 0.90, 0.85, 0.80, 0.75, and so forth, then his cumulative probability of surviving to age 65 would be

$$P^i_{55,M}(65) = (0.80) \cdot (0.90) \cdot (0.85) \cdot (0.80) \cdot (0.75) \cdot (0.70) \cdot (0.65)$$
$$\cdot (0.60) \cdot (0.55) \cdot (0.50) = 0.0300$$

For certain health impairments, however, it is entirely possible that k years after initial diagnosis, the surviving patients may once again experience the same mortality rates as those of their counterparts in the general population. For some value of k, we thus may have

$$P^i_{l+k,s}(l + n) = P_{l+k,s}(l + n) \qquad n > k \qquad (1)$$

This relationship implies that a patient with impairment i who contracted the condition at age l and survived k years can from that point in time expect to have the same probability of surviving to age $l + n$ as his age- and sex-matched peer in the general population. By definition, his probability of surviving to age $l + n$ equals the product of his probability of surviving to age $l + k$ and his subsequent probability of surviving to age $l + n$:

$$P^i_{l,s}(l + n) = P^i_{l,s}(l + k) \cdot P^i_{l+k,s}(l + n) \qquad n > k$$

Since his probability of surviving from age $l + k$ to age $l + n$ is equivalent to that of an individual in the general population, then, using the relationship stated in equation (2.1), we have

$$P^i_{l,s}(l + n) = P^i_{l,s}(l + k) \cdot P_{l+k,s}(l + n)$$

This relationship provides a straightforward procedure for estimating a patient's probability of surviving to any age $l + n$, where $l + n$ is greater than $l + k$, if we know (or assume) that k years after diagnosis his mortality rate reverts to that of demographically matched individuals in the general population. For instance, if our 55-year-old man with impairment i survives 5 years past diagnosis and then has the same expected mortality rate (or equivalently, the same annual probabilities of survival) as his peers in the general population, his probability of surviving from age 55 to age 65 becomes

$$P^i_{55,M}(65) = P^i_{55,M}(60) \cdot P_{60,M}(65)$$

Since, from previous information, we calculate that

$$P^i_{55,M}(60) = (0.80) \cdot (0.90) \cdot (0.85) \cdot (0.80) \cdot (0.75) = 0.3700$$

and

$$P_{60,M}(65) = (0.9797) \cdot (0.9777) \cdot (0.9757) \cdot (0.9739) \cdot (0.9722)$$
$$= 0.8849$$

then

$$P^i_{55,M}(65) = (0.3700) \cdot (0.8849) = 0.3274$$

While considerably less than 0.8197 (the probability of a 55-year-old man in the general population surviving to age 65), this value is still a factor of 10 greater than the corresponding survival probability (0.0300) estimated when mortality rates were not expected to revert after 5 years to those of the general population.

The "Selection" Effect

After a sufficiently long time, it is theoretically possible that the annual survival rates for the surviving members of a diseased or injured population may exceed those for demographically matched individuals in the general population. That is,

$$P^i_{l+k,s}(l + n) \geq P_{l+k,s}(l + n) \qquad n > k$$

Shepard and Zeckhauser (1980) considered this paradoxical "selection" effect (which has not yet been documented fully for any health impairment) a possible consequence of demographic heterogeneity. As an example, consider two populations, one with impairment i and the other consisting of a matched cohort of people free of the impairment. Suppose that within each of these populations there exist two subcategories of individuals, the first being at a relatively high risk of death and the other at a lower risk of death. Suppose, also, that there is no appreciable difference in mortality rates between corresponding low-risk individuals in the two populations but that there is a significant difference for high-risk individuals, with members of the impaired population having uniformly larger mortality rates. If both populations initially contain the same proportion of high- and low-risk individuals, it can be shown that as the populations age, the impaired group will contain a progressively smaller proportion of high-risk persons than the matched, impairment-free group. After a sufficiently long time, the surviving members of the impaired population may be collectively stronger and exhibit a smaller *average* annual mortality rate (and thus a larger *average* annual survival rate) than surviving members of the impairment-free population. This effect would be observed even though the impairment continues to extract a greater mortality among high-risk individuals.

Since the selection effect is a result of the underlying heterogeneity present in any population, this study attempted to minimize the selection effect by partitioning the population into subpopulations that were as homogeneous as the data allowed, recognizing that invariably there will be demographic differences that can lead to differences in the mortality risks experienced by members of the supposed homogeneous subpopulation. The selection effects are still active within the subpopulation, but they act with less force.

Estimating Survival Probabilities of Subpopulations

Using Life Tables. A *life table* describes the rates of death and survival among a given population over a specific time period. This population is generally homogeneous. However, even within a relatively homogeneous population sample, individuals will differ. The most reasonable procedure is to partition a population into subpopulations that have as many common attributes as possible besides the usual sex, age, and illness characteristics. Unfortunately, this is not always practicable.

The ideal life table would begin with a sample of people who are followed from their birth, with the number of survivors recorded each year after birth, until they all die. Or, a sample could begin at any other desired age after birth and be followed into the future. The resulting life tables would give unbiased estimates of the mortality experience of the population under study. This method of constructing life tables, while ideal, is generally impractical. The usual procedure is to examine present mortality on a cross-sectional basis rather than using the prospective forms of analysis. It is then assumed that without any further medical advances, this cross-sectional mortality experience will persist over time. Thus, a 20-year-old today is assumed to face the mortality rate at age 50 that today's 50-year-old faces at present.

Current improvements in health care, however, may lead to reductions in current mortality rates and eventually to systematic understimates of the mortality rates far in the future. This phenomenon already has contributed to reductions in the cross-sectional mortality rates observed today for young people: the rates are lower, for instance, than those the present 50-year-old faced at equivalent ages. This means that the 50-year-old population of today undoubtedly has a lower proportion of high-risk individuals than will the 50-year-old population of 25 or 30 years in the future. This is a direct result of the selection effect described by Shepard and Zeckhauser (1980). If one uses cross-sectional analysis to construct life tables, this situation could lead to underestimates of future mortality rates. However, we note that if health progress is made in the future to reduce mortality at older ages, as well as at younger ages, the total bias in the estimated mortality rates would be reduced, since such progress would tend to counteract the selection effect.

To calculate probabilities of survival $P_{l,s}^i(n)$ for myocardial infarction (MI) patients, for example, we constructed life tables using data from the Framingham Heart Study (FHS) on survival after first MI.[3] Owing to small sample sizes, these data were aggregated into five age-sex cohorts: male, 35 to 54; male, 55 to 64; male, 65 and older; female, less than 65; and female, 65 and older. The data appropriate for males 65 years and older are given in table 2–1 using standard life table terminology (that is, I represents the time after onset, L represents the number alive at the beginning of an interval, D the number of persons who died within the interval, and W the number withdrawn from the sample during the interval).

To calculate indirect and direct costs, we extended these survival probabilities to age 99 (the cutoff age). In the absence of disease-specific data and after discussion with medical experts, this can be accomplished by assuming that the patients who survived for 6 years after disease onset follow the conditional probabilities of survival for the U.S. general population. (Empirical data beyond 6 years were available for the other cohorts. For male patients from age 35 to 54, for example, probability of survival data were available for 13 years.)

Using Relative Survival Rates. Mortality data are often available in the literature in the form of relative survival rates (RSR). The relative survival rate can be defined in two equivalent ways: (1) given two samples of equal size—one consisting of individuals of a specific age and sex having impairment type i, the second consisting of the first sample's age- and sex-matched peers in the general population—the RSR is the ratio of the number of persons in the first sample alive n years later divided by the number of persons in the second sample alive n years later; or (2) the RSR is measured as the cumulative probability of a person with impairment i surviving n years divided by the cumulative probability of his age- and sex-matched peer in the general population surviving the same n years. Using the second formulation, let $\sigma^i_{l,s}(t)$ be the ratio of the probability of a person of sex s and age l with impairment i surviving to age $l + t$ (where l is age at diagnosis and t is the number of years following diagnosis) to the probability of a similar person of sex s and age l in the general population surviving to age $l + t$. We express this as

$$\sigma^i_{l,s}(t) = \frac{P^i_{l,s}(l + t)}{P_{l,s}(l + t)}$$

The RSR approach is comparable to the life table method described earlier and is, in certain cases, a more efficient method for computing streams of survival probabilities; in the case of cancer, for example, mortality data are often given in the form of relative survival rates. Under this approach, it can be shown that if the value of the relative survival rate $\sigma^i_{l,s}(t)$ becomes a constant k years after diagnosis, then a patient initially diagnosed at age l with disease i will have the same annual survival rate as his peer in the

Table 2–1
Life Table for Male Myocardial Infarction Patients 65 Years of Age and Older

I	L	D	W	L^a_{ADJ}	Q^b	P^c	CP^d
0–30 days	60	16	0	60	0.2667	0.7333	0.7333
30 days–1 year	44	3	1	43.5	0.0690	0.9310	0.6828
1–2 years	40	3	3	38.5	0.0779	0.9221	0.6289
2–3 years	34	3	6	31	0.0968	0.9032	0.5680
3–4 years	25	4	3	23.5	0.1702	0.8298	0.4713
4–5 years	18	0	2	17	0.0000	1.0000	0.4539[e]
5–6 years	16	1	5	13.5	0.0741	0.9259	0.4364

[a]Adjusted number at risk $= L - W/2$.
[b]Probability of dying during interval $= D/L_{ADJ}$.
[c]Probability of surviving interval $= 1 - Q$.
[d]Cumulative probability of survival $CP_h = P_1 \cdot P_2 \cdots P_h$.
[e]Derived by linear interpolation between the values 0.4713 and 0.4364.

general population from age $l + k$ onward. Recall that if a patient experiences the same survival rate as his peer in the general population after k years, then

$$P^i_{l+k,s}(l + n) = P_{l+k,s}(l + n) \qquad n > k$$

The converse is also true: a similarity in annual survival rates between the diseased and general population k years after diagnosis implies a constant RSR.

Hence, if we assume that after k years the population with disease or injury i has approximately the same mortality and survival experience as its respective age and sex cohorts in the general population, then we may estimate the cumulative probability of a person with the condition surviving $n > k$ years following diagnosis. We multiply the probability of survival for a member of the general population, $P_{l,s}(l + n)$, by the patient's relative survival rate k years out, $\sigma^i_{l,s}(k)$. That is,

$$P^i_{l,s}(l + n) = \sigma^i_{l,s}(k) \cdot P_{l,s}(l + n)$$

where $n > k$ and $\sigma^i_{l,s}(k)$ is constant for $n > k$.

Consider, for example, the case of a male patient with localized lung cancer who is age 60 at diagnosis. He is assumed to have a normal mortality experience providing he survives to age 75. In that case, the probability that he will survive to age 80, given that he was diagnosed with the disease at age 60, is given by

$$P^{\text{lung, local}}_{60,\text{male}}(80) = \sigma^{\text{lung, local}}_{60,\text{male}}(15) \cdot P_{60,\text{male}}(80)$$

Using data from the END results study (Axtell, 1974), we find that

$$\sigma^{\text{lung, local}}_{60,\text{male}}(15) = 0.1500$$

and from the standard U.S. life tables, we determine that

$$P_{60,\text{male}}(80) = 0.3405$$

Therefore,

$$P^{\text{lung,local}}_{60,\text{male}}(80) = (0.1500) \times (0.3405) = 0.0511$$

When the RSR curve becomes flat (that is, when the value of the RSR becomes constant), the average annual survival rate for the diseased cohort becomes equal to the annual survival rate of the general population cohort. This does not imply necessarily that excess mortality from the disease has ceased after k years. The slope of the relative survival curve at any time depends on two effects: (1) the excess mortality in each individual resulting from the impairment being studied, and (2) the difference in selection effects owing to heterogeneity in risk among subpopulations of the diseased and comparison groups. A flat relative survival curve some time after disease onset does not necessarily indicate that the excess mortality has ceased, but only that it is offset by the selection effect. In fact, if the selection effect is stronger than the disease effect, the RSR can actually rise, which we find in the case of some cancers.

Using Relative Mortality Rates. For some conditions, mortality data are presented in the form of a relative mortality rate (RMR). The relative mortality rate is defined as the mortality rate for the impaired population divided by the mortality rate for the general population:

$$\alpha^i_{l,s}(k) \equiv \frac{\text{mortality rate of patients } k \text{ years after diagnosis,}}{\text{mortality rate of a person in general population,}} $$

$$\alpha^i_{l,s}(k) \equiv \frac{\substack{\text{mortality rate of patients } k \text{ years after diagnosis,}\\ \text{age at diagnosis } l,\text{ sex } s}}{\substack{\text{mortality rate of a person in general population,}\\ \text{age } l + k,\text{ sex } s}}$$

Using the RMRs and annual mortality rates for the general population derived from standard life tables, it is possible to estimate survival probabilities for impaired individuals of different ages and sex (Smart and Sanders, 1976) as

$$P^i_{l,s}(n) = \prod_{t=l}^{t=n-1} [1 - \alpha^i_{l,s}(t - l)Q_s(t)] \qquad \text{for } n > l$$

where $\alpha^i_{l,s}(t - l) =$ RMR for people with impairment i, $t - l$ years after diagnosis at age l

$Q_s(t) =$ probability of a person of sex s in the general population dying during the year following his t birthday, given survival to age t

(Note, for $n = l$, $P^i_{l,s}(n) = 1$ by assumption.)

This illustrates the relationship assumed between the average annual mortality rate for the impaired person and the corresponding rate for a member of the general population of a similar age and sex: impairment i mortality rate equals general population mortality rate times relative mortality rate. Given RMRs, we can model the probability of a person with impairment i surviving to a subsequent age, conditioned on impairment status, age at diagnosis, and sex.

It is theoretically possible to have different RMRs for each year after incidence. However, in the case of nonfatal motor vehicle injuries where the RMR approach is applied, data limitations have forced us to assume constant RMRs for the different injury-severity subcategories (see chapter 6). In the sensitivity-analysis section of chapter 6, we consider the possibility of the RMR shifting to 1 after a sufficient number of years elapse following injury. This assumption is equivalent to assuming that the injured person experiences a survival history from that time on that is similar to his peers in the general population.

To illustrate the use of this procedure, consider the case of a 20-year-old male with a nonfatal motor vehicle injury. Under our definition of a nonfatal injury, this person will survive at least to age 21. If the injury was to the lower spinal cord and was incomplete, the person is classified as a paraplegic incomplete. Such people can be shown to experience a RMR of 1.81 (Geisler, 1977). The following table illustrates the computed probabilities of survival of such a person compared with those of his peers in the general population. The table is carried out for 10 years in this illustration (note that the person in the general population is assumed to survive to age 21 in order to maintain consistency):

Age	General Population	Paraplegic Incomplete
20	1.0000	1.0000
21	1.0000	1.0000
22	0.9978	0.9960
23	0.9955	0.9918
24	0.9932	0.9877
25	0.9910	0.9838
26	0.9889	0.9799
27	0.9868	0.9762
28	0.9848	0.9726
29	0.9828	0.9691
30	0.9808	0.9655

Calculating Life Expectancies. The average life expectancy (ALE) for a person in a given disease or injury group i can be obtained by summing the stream of survival probabilities applicable to persons of that age in that group:

$$ALE_{l,s}^{i} = \sum_{n=l+1}^{99} P_{l,s}^{i}(n)$$

As an example, suppose a person with a critical disease has the following probabilities of survival:

Time after Onset	Probability of Survival
0	1.00
1	0.70
2	0.50
3	0.35
4	0.25
5	0.10
6	0

Then this person's life expectancy is 1.90 years (that is, $0.7 + 0.5 + 0.35 + 0.25 + 0.1$).

The "Illness-Free" Group. An impaired person's forgone earnings—the difference in earnings between a person free of impairment i in the incidence year and a person with impairment i—is a function of the probability of survival free of the impairment $P_{l,s}^{free}(n)$ and with the impairment $P_{l,s}^{i}(n)$. (It is also a function of various other parameters, all of which will be extensively discussed in the indirect-cost section of this chapter.) The term $P_{l,s}^{free}(n)$ is not necessarily equal to the probability of survival of a person (age l, sex s) in the general population $P_{l,s}(n)$. In fact, we expect that $P_{l,s}^{free}(n) > P_{l,s}(n)$, since the general population contains persons with impairment i. However, for our purposes, the person need only be free of impairment i in the incidence year. If $P_{l,s}(n)$ were used as a surrogate for $P_{l,s}^{free}(n)$, we might slightly underestimate the latter parameter and therefore underestimate forgone earnings. The degree of underestimation would not be significant, however, since the incidence of any disease or injury is only a tiny subpopulation of the general population. In any case, it can be shown that, because of the presence of the selection effect, $P_{l,s}^{free}(n)$ approaches $P_{l,s}(n)$ as n increases. We assume, therefore, that $P_{l,s}(n)$ is a good approximation of $P_{l,s}^{free}(n)$.

Duration of Impairment and Double Counting of Mortality Effects

Duration of Impairment. Incidence analysis attempts to ascertain the lifetime cost associated with a given health impairment. If an impairment has long-term sequelae, it is assumed that costs would be generated until the patient dies. This model should be used cautiously, however, since some conditions, although long-term, may not always be lifelong conditions, and duration of the condition also may be a function of general health and other attributes. For these reasons, it may be desirable to obtain age- and sex-specific tables of impairment duration. These do not appear to be readily available (although there may be isolated data on specific conditions), nor can they be calculated from existing life tables.

For the conditions considered in this study, survival probabilities are a good estimate of duration, since life expectancy and expected duration are close to each other in value. For conditions with short-term sequelae, for example, less severe motor vehicle injuries, the question of duration is not a problem. In these cases, the cost streams have been cut off early to account for the short duration of injury-induced effects.

Double Counting of Mortality Effects. Some double counting of mortality effects is unavoidable in an incidence analysis. A person with coronary heart disease may at the same time be at high risk of a stroke, and the increased mortality owing to the two conditions is counted separately for each condition. Because mortality may or may not result from some common underlying factor, in this study any increase observed in the mortality rates is *associated* with the condition and is not to be viewed necessarily as a *consequence* of the condition. The result of this analytical choice is that certain incidence costs may be slightly overestimated. A person who develops both coronary heart disease and stroke and who dies young, for example, would have his full forgone earnings assigned to both conditions.

Direct Costs

Direct costs represent the value of goods and services actually used to diagnose, treat, or otherwise accommodate the disease or injury in question. They typically include expenditures on emergency services, hospitalization and outpatient treatment, drugs, medical applicances, home modifications, paramedical expenses (for example, special diets, clothing, transportation), nursing home care, and rehabilitation services. In addition, direct costs include the administration costs incurred by insurance companies and government agencies in funding disease and injury expenses. For certain conditions, such as motor vehicle injuries, legal and court costs resulting from related litigation are also included as direct costs. Direct costs are the most apparent and, for some individuals, the most significant economic costs associated with their health condition.

We present in this section a general model that may be used to estimate total direct costs, incorporating the many different components of those costs. The cost components that will be evaluated include:

Emergency assistance

Initial inpatient hospital care

Physician and surgeon services (rendered on an inpatient basis)

Vocational and physical rehabilitation

Nursing home and home attendant care

Drugs, medical supplies, and appliances

Outpatient medical and surgical care

Rehospitalization (owing to recurrences)

Home modifications

Paramedical and miscellaneous expenses

Insurance administration

Legal and court expenses

The Direct-Cost Model

General Framework. For each health condition, we estimate all the relevant categories of direct costs just listed as well as their patterns of occurrence following incidence. To illustrate the analytical techniques used to evaluate these costs and to explain the technical relationship between cost components and other variables, the present-value model of the costs accruing to a representative patient is described in the following paragraphs.

Numerically, the present value of expected direct costs PVC for any individual of given sex, impairment category, and age at onset of impairment may be expressed as

$$PVC = \sum_{n=l}^{99} \frac{P_{l,s}^{i}(n) \cdot DC_{l,s}^{i}(n - l + 1)}{(1 + r)^{n-l}}$$

where n = the various ages of the individual
l = the age at impairment onset
$P_{l,s}^{i}(n)$ = the probability that a person of sex s who acquires condition i at age l will survive to age n
$DC_{l,s}^{i}(n - l + 1)$ = the dollar value of the average annual direct costs

generated by such persons during year $n - l + 1$
following impairment onset
$r =$ the discount rate

The present value of an individual's expected direct costs PVC is modeled as a function of (1) the discount rate; (2) the survival probabilities applicable to the individual, which, in the case of a health condition with long-term sequelae, serve as our best estimates of the condition's likely duration; and (3) the average annual direct costs generated by condition survivors during each year past onset. The average annual direct costs in each year are obtained by summing the average values for each cost component that accrues. In the first year past onset, for instance, the predominant cost components are those associated with treating the initial episode of the condition. This normally includes the costs of emergency services, initial hospitalization, inpatient physician and surgeon services, and occasionally nursing home or home attendant care. Although nursing home care may continue in subsequent years (especially for diseases such as stroke and cancer), the direct costs in those years are, in general, more heavily weighted toward continuing outpatient care and rehabilitation, drugs, and medical appliances, and in the case of recurrent illness episodes, re-hospitalizations and attendant inpatient care.

The values estimated for the cost components reflect our assumption that individuals suffering a particular type of condition (or particular subcategory of that condition) may, as a group, generate average values for each of those components that differ from corresponding values generated by individuals suffering other conditions. Although our model can in theory accommodate separate cost-component values for people of different ages and sexes with the same health impairment, little attempt has been made to do this in practice because of data limitations. In a few instances, however, data were available that allowed partial disaggregation by age—primarily into two groups: those under 65 years of age and those 65 years of age and older. Disaggregation by sex usually was either impossible, unwarranted, or both. (An exception is the analysis of the direct costs of motor vehicle fatalities in chapter 6.) While the cost-component values are normally conditioned only upon the individual's impairment, the set of survival probabilities for the individual depends also, as we have seen earlier in this chapter, on his or her sex and age at onset. Consequently, for a given discount rate, different estimates of the present value of a person's overall direct costs are possible for individuals of different ages or sexes suffering from the same impairment, especially if that impairment is characterized by long-term sequelae.

Because health-resource needs are often a function of disease or injury stage and, hence, of time past onset of the condition, any model of incidence-related direct costs should contain a provision for different levels of average costs during each year past onset. A provision of this sort is contained in our model through the cost parameter $DC^i_{l,s}(n - l + 1)$, which could conceivably take on different values for each year past onset. However, because of data limitations, we have been forced again to deviate from the theoretical ideal in performing the actual analyses. For the most part, values for the annual cost components have been separated into a maximum of three intertemporal groups: those costs generated by an individual during the first year following onset of the disease or injury; unique or unusual costs occurring during the second year; and for those conditions with long-term consequences, follow-on care costs starting normally at the beginning of the second year (third year for cancer patients) and accruing annually over the individual's lifetime.

Costs during the first year past onset are primarily determined by the value of resources needed to treat the initial episode of the disease or injury. As indicated earlier, these may include the costs of emergency services, initial hospitalization, inpatient physician and surgeon services, and nursing home or home attendant care. In addition, expenses for home modifications necessitated by the condition and incipient expenses for outpatient care, drugs, medical appliances, and so forth are not uncommon.

Unique or unusual costs occurring during the second year include the costs of physical and vocational rehabilitation programs *following hospital discharge* for severely injured motor vehicle nonfatalities. For computational purposes, these programs are assumed to start no earlier than 1 year after injury occurrence, although some start before this. With the exception of selected vocational programs requiring formal education or continued counseling that may extend beyond the end of that year, the average duration of a program is usually short enough that assigning all rehabilitation costs to the second year does not appreciably alter their present value. This second group of costs also encompasses extended hospitalization and physician costs for cancer patients.

The follow-on costs in the third group are generated by all incidence populations considered in this study except for case fatalities and the minor or moderately injured motor vehicle nonfatalities. This group includes the average annual costs of drugs and medical supplies, medical appliances, outpatient medical and surgical care, nursing home and home attendant care, rehospitalization (owing to recurrences and relapses), and other miscellaneous expenses necessitated by the condition. In our model, the present value of future follow-on costs is a strong function of the combined effect of two factors: (1) the probability of the impaired person surviving to each successive year beyond the year of incidence, and (2) the discounting multiplier applicable to that future year. Since persons suffering from conditions considered in this study have noticeably higher mortality rates than individuals in the general population and thus lower survival probabilities and life expectancies, the reduction in present value caused by multiplying costs times survival probabilities is significant. Similarly, as the time from onset of injury increases, the values of the annual discounting multiplier decrease, thereby causing progressively greater reductions in the effective present value of costs assigned to distant future years. However, despite the influence of both these factors, it is interesting to note that the present value of follow-on costs accounts for a significant fraction of the aggregate value of all direct costs measured in our analyses.

In applying the direct cost model to each of the four health impairments, only certain types of costs are relevant for individuals with certain subconditions. In the case of motor vehicle injuries, for instance, the treatment costs of fatalities are limited to emergency services, some initial hospitalization care, and some related inpatient physician and surgeon services. In contrast, the treatment costs of nonfatal, but permanently impairing spinal cord injuries include not only the expenses of emergency services and initial hospitalization, but also home-modification costs, rehabilitation charges, and large, long-term expenditures for follow-on care.

Incidence-related estimates of present-valued direct costs pose the risk entailed in any extrapolation of current treatment practices into the future. Innovation in medical technology and changes in the future course of various illnesses may have significant effects on the real value of future follow-on costs of individual illness entities and thus on the present economic value of those costs. In addition to shifts in the pattern of health-resource utilization in the future, which are virtually impossible to predict with any accuracy, we also must consider the question of the relative present and future valuation of specific health resources. Inflation aside, a given resource, such as certain classes of medical personnel, may become relatively scarce and hence more valuable in the future, while another resource may increase in supply such that its relative value declines over time. Two approaches are possible to this problem. One is to project incidence-year resource-cost relationships into the future, on the assumption that the relative value of medical-care resources will not change substantially, and the other is to adjust incidence-year costs by the ratio of expected changes in the medical-care component of the consumer price index (CPI) to expected changes in the overall CPI.

We have concluded that the first approach is the proper one in trying to estimate the value of direct costs accruing in years past disease or injury onset. All costs are evaluated according to the base year's (1975) price levels. In particular, the annual values estimated for an individual's follow-on costs are formulated using these price levels and are then assumed constant over time in the cost model. Because the discount rate used in the model is *real* rather than *nominal* (which reflects inflation), the effects of inflation may be neglected. Although it is possible to build into the model an adjustment for potential increases or decreases in the *real* values of these costs after the base year, the lack of an adjustment factor reflects our belief that while medical-sector prices have risen more rapidly than the general price level in the last few years, it is not at all certain that such price relationships will be maintained into the long-run future. Of course, if the increase in real costs experienced in the health sector during the immediate past is a reliable indicator of future *short-run* trends, then the real costs of health services and supplies may be expected to increase during the immediate future. As a result, the present value of follow-on costs based on 1975 price levels may, *ceteris paribus*, represent a slight underestimation of the true present value of these costs. (Notice that if, for some reason, we desire to estimate the effect of an anticipated real increase in medical-sector prices, we could do so by discounting future costs at a smaller rate. For example, if we feel that the general price level will, on average, continue to inflate at 8 percent but medical-sector prices will continue to increase at 12 percent—a roughly 4 percent real differential—then discounting future follow-on costs at 2 percent instead of 6 percent would reflect this real increase in medical-sector prices.)

Determining the present value of *total* direct costs for an entire incidence population is a straightforward calculation once estimates of the present value of expected direct costs per person have been determined for each incidence (age, sex, and subcondition) subcategory. It follows that the present value of total expected direct costs will equal the products of the present value of those costs per person multiplied by the number of people in each incidence subcategory summed over all subcategories.

Estimation of Treatment-Related Costs

The details of estimating treatment-related costs are covered in the forth-coming chapters on coronary heart disease, stroke, cancer, and motor vehicle injuries. Although the specific approaches often differ to accommodate available data, a general procedure is normally followed in estimating the values of cost components accruing in a given year. It involves estimating for each cost component the average resource utilization per person Q_j, and multiplying that by the estimated price per unit P_j to yield the average cost per person $P_j \cdot Q_j$ of the component. If these results are added across cost components, this will yield the dollar value of the average annual treatment costs per person generated by individuals in the particular incidence sub-category.

As an example, consider the case of a 30-year-old man who suffers a serious, but non-life-threatening motor vehicle injury, such as a multiple rib fracture. He generates emergency services, initial hospitalization, inpatient physician services, and outpatient medical care costs in the first year past onset of injury. Although there is no reduction in his life expectancy, some expenses for outpatient care are expected in the second year past onset.

The average costs for emergency services for patients with his injury are known to be approximately $200 (in 1975 dollars). Initial hospitalization costs, however, are estimated from the average number of inpatient days necessary to care for that type of injury, 15, multiplied by the average cost per day, $136, to yield average hospitalization costs of $2040. Inpatient physician charges are estimated by taking the average number of inpatient visits—approximately equal in number to the length of hospital stay—and multiplying by the average cost per visit, $25. This individual also undergoes surgery that results in $1000 in professional charges. The end result is $1375 in inpatient physician and surgeon costs. At the time of injury, the expectation is that he will require about four outpatient physician visits in both the first and second year past injury at $20 per visit; the average cost for outpatient care in each year, therefore, will be $80.

Totaling up the emergency services, initial hospitalization, inpatient physician and surgeon, and first-year outpatient costs, we have an average first-year cost of $3695. The expected second-year cost is $80. Using a discount rate of 6 percent and noting that the annual probability of survival of a 30-year-old male in the general population is 0.9981, we find the present value of average direct costs in 1975 dollars to be

$$PVC = \text{first-year costs} + \frac{\text{probability of survival to age 31} \cdot \text{second-year costs}}{1.06}$$

$$= 3695 + \frac{(0.9981) \cdot (80)}{1.06}$$

$$= \$3770.$$

Estimation of Other Direct-Cost Components

Insurance Administration Costs. According to a study by Mueller and Gibson (1976) published by the Social Security Administration, U.S. expenditures on personal health care in fiscal year 1975 amounted to approximately $103.2 billion.[4] These included expenditures for hospital care, physician services, drugs and sundries, medical appliances, nursing home care, and other miscellaneous health services. Of the total spent, close to $69.6 billion, or 67.4 percent, was financed by either private third-party payers such as insurance companies and philanthropic organizations or by public payment programs such as Medicare and Medicaid.[5] In health-care cost reimbursement, both public and private agencies incur significant administrative expenses. These expenses, commonly referred to as *insurance administration costs*, include all overhead costs for personnel and facilities as well as any return on investments for the private agencies. The magnitude of insurance administration costs in private insurance companies is determined by the difference between premiums collected and money returned to policyholders in the form of payments on claims. In public agencies, the cost of administration is equal to the difference between department budgets and the total funds allocated for the provision of medical services to aid recipients.

Exact data are not available on the proportions of the expenditures for cancer, stroke, coronary heart disease, and motor vehicle injury treatment financed by public and private third-party payers. However, information developed in our study on the percentage distribution of treatment costs for each of these conditions by health-service category (that is, costs of hospital care, physician services, drugs, and so forth) suggests that these cost distributions are roughly similar in each instance to that of overall U.S. health expenditures. Of particular import is the fact that for each condition, hospital care and physician services costs constitute the bulk of all treatment costs. This is also the case for the United States as a whole, where hospital care and physician services costs constitute aproximately 60 percent of total health-care costs.[6] Nationally, about 84 percent of the costs in these two categories are financed by third-party payments, and over 82 percent of all third-party payments are allocated to expenditures for these two types of services.[7] Since the vast majority of all third-party payments are now made for hospital care and physician services, and since the experience for each condition relative to these two types of costs seems to parallel the overall national experience, it may be reasonable to assume that the proportion of all expenditures financed by third-party payers is roughly the same for each of the four conditions as for the United States as a whole. This would suggest that expenditures for each condition, like overall U.S. health expenditures, are financed primarily by third-party payers.

In the extreme short run, insurance administration costs incurred by agencies funding the treatment of cancer, stroke, coronary heart disease, or motor vehicle injuries are unlikely to be significantly affected by a change in the incident level of any one of these impairments. Over a longer period, however, a reduction in incidence should bring decreased insurance administration costs. The variable components of insurance administration, such as supplies and extra personnel, should be lowered in direct proportion to the reduction in incidence. Because of the relatively large incidence of each condition, a partial lowering of the fixed expenses for plant facilities and core personnel also should accompany a significant incidence reduction. For the purposes of this study, however, we are estimating only the economic cost associated with the incidence in 1975. We are not considering the extended situation in which incidence of the disease or injury is permanently lowered in the future. It is then unrealistic to assume that the fixed component of insurance administration costs would change by a significant amount. We therefore attempt to ascertain the variable component of insurance administration costs alone.

In order to measure this cost, we would ideally determine first the total administrative costs associated with financing the care of each disease or injury and, second, the percentage of this total that represented variable costs. Given the current paucity of data on insurance administration costs, this approach is not possible for each of the conditions on an individual basis. However, it is possible to make a more global, although admittedly less precise, analysis of the costs associated with the reimbursement of total U.S. health expenditures.

The study by Mueller and Gibson mentioned earlier presents a national estimate of insurance prepayment and administrative expenses in fiscal year 1975 of approximately $4.6 billion. Of this, roughly $3.4 billion was generated by private third-party payers and $1.2 billion by public agencies. A subsequent study by Mueller (1975) of the costs generated in 1975 by private health insurance organizations alone estimated total insurance administration costs for those organizations at $4.7 billion.[8] The discrepancy in the 1975 cost estimates for the private agencies ($3.4 billion versus $4.7 billion) suggests that the former set of estimates may include primarily variable costs with perhaps some limited fixed costs, while the latter set presents total fixed and variable costs together. If this is true, then during 1975 the variable administrative expenses for both private and public third-party payers were approximately 4.5 percent (4.6/103.2 × 100 percent) of all other costs for national health services and supplies.

A study of the cost of health insurance administration by Blair and Vogel (1975) estimated that the cost of health administration in 1971 was $4.1 billion. In that same year, they estimated that other national health expenditures totaled $75 billion.[9] Therefore, health administration costs represented 5.8 percent of all other health expenditures in 1971. Blair and Vogel noted that the $4.1 billion administration cost included fixed costs, and therefore, the variable component is clearly less than 5.8 percent.

For the purpose of our analysis, we assume that for each health condition, the ratio of relevant administrative expenses to other direct costs is roughly the same as the ratio determined for national administrative expenses to other national health expenditures for fiscal year 1975. It is also assumed that this ratio will remain constant over time. Hence the present value of administrative costs accruing to members of a 1975 incidence sample over their lifetimes may be estimated at 4.5 percent of their total treatment-related expenditures. This means that for each $1000 of treatment costs an estimated $45 in insurance administration expenses may be assumed to have been generated.

Legal and Court Costs. For motor vehicle injuries, we have included the legal and court costs of injury-related litigation. These costs have both criminal- and civil-action components and transcend the litigation costs already included in the administrative overhead for health insurance. The calculation of these costs is covered in chapter 6.

We have not specifically estimated and included comparable costs for the three diseases studied. A case could be made for separately calculating such charges as litigation costs involved in workmen's compensation proceedings for people with cancer. We have not done so for three main reasons. First, data are sparse; second, what data that exist indicate the relative insignifiance of these costs; and third, many of these costs—unlike those computed for motor vehicle injuries—are included as part of health insurance administration expenses.

Indirect Costs

The *indirect costs* calculated in this study derive from the forgone economic productivity of injured and diseased individuals. The magnitude of indirect costs makes their contribution to total economic costs extremely significant. We shall show in later chapters that over 70 percent of the total costs in 1975 of the four conditions considered in this study was indirect. Incidence analysis incorporates the value of all impairment-related productivity losses occurring over an affected individual's lifetime. These losses include diminution in productivity because of morbidity and disability as well as productivity losses resulting from an impairment-induced reduction in life expectancy.

Methods of Evaluating Indirect Costs

The importance of deaths has been gauged by economists in two major ways: the *human-capital approach* and the *willingness-to-pay approach*. A major cost of death or extended disability is the forgone productivity of individuals. The quantity, and hence the value, of available goods and services is reduced by the individual's incapacities. This reduction in output eventually leads to economic losses felt not only by the individuals and their families, but also by society in general. Economists have relied primarily on the human-capital approach for valuing this productivity loss. The human-capital approach is based on the use of a person's expected lifetime earnings, discounted back to the year of incidence, as a surrogate measure of his future productive worth if the disease or injury had not occurred. This approach would be entirely appropriate if humans were considered simply as productive machines. The fact that societies value the very young and the elderly as well as the middle-aged signifies that attributes other than a person's level of production (as measured by his present-value earnings) are important to human values. In order to capture better these aspects of lives, the willingness-to-pay approach is thought by some economists to be the more appropriate from a theoretical standpoint, although it has major problems in implementation. However, it should be kept in mind that the purpose of our study is to ascertain the *economic* costs of disease and injury. That purpose is best met by defining a conceptually straightforward procedure that both captures economic considerations and is empirically tractable. The human-capital approach, when its limitations are recognized, is such a procedure.

Weisbrod (1961) and Rice (1966) have written important seminal works developing the principles and techniques involved in measuring future productivity. Many applied studies have used the human-capital approach for such diverse conditions as alcohol abuse (Berry and Boland, 1977), genetic disease (Conley and Milunsky, 1975), hypertension (Weinstein and Stason, 1976), smoking (Luce and Schweitzer, 1978), and spinal cord injury (Smart and Sanders, 1976). Hodgson and Meiners (1979) have recently reaffirmed the appropriateness of this approach in cost-of-illness studies peformed by the U.S. Public Health Service.

In addition to the general recognition that the human-capital approach considers only one aspect of human value, there are a number of questions raised and measurement problems associated with the methodology. These include (1) whether a person's market earnings, used to quantify productivity, exactly mirror economic product created; (2) what value should be placed on nonmarket labor, such as household or volunteer work; (3) what is the appropriate rate to use to account for secular growth in a person's productivity; (4) what is the best method to forecast future employment levels; and (5) what is the appropriate discount rate to apply to future earnings?

Alternatives to the Human-Capital Approach

The discounted-future-earnings figure generally underestimates the total perceived loss to the individual. Alternatives to the human-capital approach that attempt to measure total societal value for life have been developed. Most fall under the heading *willingness to pay*. What would we be willing to pay to extend our life or reduce the risk of death for ourselves or our loved ones? As Rhoads (1978) argues, the sum of each person's willingness to pay for reduced risk for all those affected reflects their collective preferences. This aggregate willingness to pay is divided by the number of deaths that might be prevented to determine what the government might justifiably spend to save a life in the program under consideration. An extension of this approach is presented by Thompson (1980).

Although proponents of willingness to pay agree that consumer preferences are the best guide for public policy, they disagree about the best means to determine its value. Schelling (1966) stresses the statistical nature of the decision that determines how much we are willing to spend to reduce the *probability* of death or severe disability. On an individual, de facto basis, he readily admits that the resources we might spend are limitless. We are not rational in our judgments in this situation because we identify with the specific individual and feel unusual responsibility for his or her welfare. However, marginal changes in mortality statistics for the population at large do not evoke these same sentiments.

Schelling feels that discounted future earnings have limited validity in measuring what it is worth to someone to increase the likelihood of survival. These earnings are simply part of the income and wealth data that go into the decisions. Economic losses to society may be approximated by lost productivity, but these market criteria may only be within a factor of 2 or 3 (perhaps 5 or 10) of what a person and/or his family feels they actually lose if a death or catastrophic, disabling condition occurs.

Schelling's model distinguishes between life and livelihood. Livelihood, that is, earnings, can be insured. Assessing the value of life to an individual or to another party who is willing to pay to prolong that life is not as easy. One way of doing this is the use of a price system to see what people are willing to pay. However, market evidence is scarce, very likely biased, and no doubt unrepresentative.

Mishan (1971) bases his willingness-to-pay methodology for life valuation on the criterion of a potential Pareto improvement. This requires that the loss of a person's life be referenced by the minimum amount he is prepared to accept in exchange for surrender or, conversely, in the case of lifesaving, by the maximum amount he is prepared to pay to prevent its loss. (In the vast majority of cases, the overall chances of death or disability are unknown. Thus the appropriate figure to ascertain becomes the amount that would compensate each individual for the extra or marginal risk of death or disability to which he would be exposed or the amount that he would be willing to pay to avoid that additional risk.) Mishan accepts the commonly used, if unproven, economic dictum that the individual knows his own preferences best. All social gains or losses are evaluated solely on the basis of individuals' own perceptions of the relevant effects on their welfare, given the information they have at the time the decision is made. If it is not possible to make the members of a community better off in a collective sense by a redistribution of net gains from a proposed project, a potential Pareto improvement cannot be achieved and any such project should not be undertaken.

This method bases public policy solely on individuals' preferences. It takes consistently into account the preferences of those who might paradoxically feel *worse* as more lives are saved, for the possibility does exist that costs could conceivably exceed benefits of a life saved. Thus personal preferences become the driving force in determining and evaluating societal welfare.

Since the ultimate criterion in determining benefits in willingness-to-pay decision-making approaches is the individual's estimate of what a program is worth to him at the time the valuation is made, these methodologies often favor the well-to-do, because they have more wealth and thus are willing to pay more. Under this system, public money would tend to follow private donations (or at least, private evaluations), and certain welfare inequities might result. Mishan addresses this issue and its possible resolution in light of a proposed lifesaving program. The preferences of all concerned would be added to determine a composite value for the program. As long as some of the nonpoor are willing to pay to help the poor achieve a minimum standard of safety and medical care, the combined values, he feels, would justify the implementation of the program. If this is not the case, costs would outweigh benefits and such a program would be canceled.

There are problems with both the human-capital and the willingness-to-pay methodologies. Discounted future earnings rely on projections based on current earnings data, current mortality and survival statistics, and uncertain estimates of productivity increases and decreases in the future. Men are consistently valued at a higher level than women, owing to inequities in salary levels and a past preponderance of men in the marketplace. There is also disagreement as to the appropriate discount rate to be used. The utility of a person to his family and friends beyond that of earnings power is ignored. However, with all its problems, the value of discounted future earnings is, at a first pass, measurable and, in a sense, relatively unambiguous in nature. Willingness-to-pay is not so easy to quantify. People have a hard time conceptualizing probabilities of death or anxiety and suffering. Stated preferences and actual behaviors often differ. Decisions that individuals will make when their lives are actually at risk may be very different from those made when asked about statistical probabilities of life-threatening situations. As a result, we expect that until such time as anxiety can be quantified, researchers and policymakers confronted with actual decisions will continue to use discounted future earnings as a best approximation of at least the productive value of a human life.

Issues Related to the Human-Capital Approach

If lifetime earnings are used as a basis for evaluating forgone productivity and those earnings are estimated in terms of average wages prevailing in the marketplace, several important conceptual problems remain. Several of these have been touched on earlier. One concerns the validity of the tacit assumption that earnings expressed in terms of average market wages are, in fact, a reasonable approximation of the market value of an individual's productivity. Another deals with the issue of whether or not to deduct personal consumption in computing an individual's net contribution to total output. Still another centers on how to evaluate nonmarket productivity, in particular the productivity of a homemaker.

Valuation of Productivity. The validity of estimating the market value of forgone productivity resulting from a disease or injury by estimating the amount of reduced earnings of workers who die or are disabled because of the condition depends critically on whether or not people are paid according to the value of their contribution to output. Technically, forgone productivity or, equivalently, lost production could be valued by earnings if and only if workers were paid the value of their marginal product. Practically, however, the application of this evaluation methodology requires only that, on the average, earnings reflect economic productivity. If average earnings as measured in terms of average market wages tend to reflect productivity—as they do generally in most Western industrialized countries—then lost earnings will be a reasonable approximation of the value of lost production.

Deduction of Personal Consumption or Not. In estimating the total value of lost production, many health economists (Rice, 1966; Fein, 1958; and Prest and Turvey, 1965) agree that no adjustment need be made for the personal consumption of individuals. If the loss resulting from forgone productivity is evaluated in terms of total societal loss, it becomes clear that what individuals happen to consume out of their total production is no less a part of societal welfare than what someone else happens to consume as a result of those individuals' productive labors. Society as a whole is interested in changes in the level of total output, and the personal consumption of individuals represents a significant portion of that output.

Valuation of Nonmarket Productivity. One concern with the development of estimates of lost productivity is that they tend to understate the effect of disease and injury on women if household productivity losses are not somehow included. Studies such as Mushkin (1962) considered only wages and salaries earned in the marketplace. Household services were not valued because they were not considered paid contributions to production. Studies that do incorporate an estimate for household services, along with direct costs and marketplace productivity losses, are reflecting the total "opportunity loss" of illness rather than simply the loss to the market economy.

The problem of appropriately valuing work performed in the home has continually plagued analysts. The lack of an existing wage rate in the labor market for homemakers' services has made it difficult to place an economic value on their work. Although their direct wages are zero, their actual productivity is normally quite high and their responsibilities span a variety of important tasks. Several attempts have been made in the past to establish surrogate market values for homemakers' work by pricing the alternative services of a domestic servant or housekeeper. In Rice's earlier study, (1966), homemakers' labor was valued using wages paid a domestic servant. Cooper and Rice (1976) considered this to be an underestimate, since homemakers' labor includes many additional tasks over and above the work performed by a domestic servant. Cooper and Rice used a more refined technique, the *market-value, or market-cost, approach* [based on Brody (1975)]. This approach uses estimates based on the market wages for each of the individual services a homemaker performs. The rationale here is the desire to achieve consistency with other direct- and indirect-cost estimates that are based on market values (that is, prices and wages).

An alternative to the market-value approach is the *opportunity-cost approach*. It has been suggested by Prest and Turvey (1965) that the value of homemakers' work be equated with their opportunity cost in the marketplace or, in other words, what they could earn at paid jobs. While this approach has significant intellectual appeal, there are several practical problems associated with it. The most important among these is the problem of imputing the correct earnings level. Another factor is the effect on existing wages if a large proportion of homemakers simultaneously entered the labor markets.

We have chosen to follow the lead of Cooper and Rice and to incorporate a household-labor component. In our base-case analyses, we valued this household labor at its market-value equivalent as proposed by Brody. (The opportunity-cost approach was utilized in the sensitivity analyses.) Following the example of Parringer and Berk (1977), we also have incorporated a household-labor component for persons already employed either full or part time in the marketplace.

Productivity Losses Not Estimated. No attempt has been made to estimate the productivity losses that may be sustained by the family, friends, or co-workers of impaired people. Empirical difficulties associated with data collection prevented their estimation. Consequently, our estimates of total productivity losses should be interpreted as representing the primary component of those losses—that resulting from the impaired population—but, unfortunately, none of the secondary components that might exist.

Estimation of Forgone Productivity

Forgone Productivity of Case Fatalities. To calculate the forgone productivity of an individual who dies shortly after the onset of his condition, such as a motor vehicle fatality or a coronary heart disease sudden death, a number of simplifying assumptions must be made. It is assumed that

1. If the disease or injury had not occurred, an individual would have followed the pattern of life expectancy for people of equivalent age and sex in the illness-free population (as approximated by life-expectancy patterns for the general population reported in the 1977 edition of the U.S. life tables).

2. Barring disease or injury, an individual would have worked in the labor force or engaged in housekeeping tasks over his or her lifetime in accordance with the current patterns of labor-force participation and housekeeping involvement for people of equivalent age and sex. Data available from the Department of Labor on employment and housekeeping rates effective in 1970 and 1975 are the primary source of information for labor-force participation patterns.[10] Use of the numbers employed in 1970 would assume conditions of full employment (approximately 5 percent of the labor force unemployed), while the 1975 conditions represent a situation of less than full employment (approximately 8.5 percent of the labor force unemployed because the country was recovering from the 1974 recession). The 1970 and 1975 data on employment and housekeeping rates were averaged to provide representative estimates of future labor-force participation patterns.

3. Mean earnings for workers (and mean household labor values for homemakers) are the proper surrogate measure to use in evaluating forgone productivity. Furthermore, the future pattern of earnings for individuals of a particular sex will remain approximately the same as that reported by the Bureau of the Census in 1975, with the exception of an annual percentage increment in earnings owing to the average annual rate of growth in the productivity of labor.[11]

4. The average annual rate of growth in the growth of the productivity of labor in the future is approximately 1 percent. (Until the early 1970s, it was an easy task to assign a value to this factor, since the annual productivity growth rate in the United States clearly averaged about 2 percent. However, because the productivity growth rate has been closer to 0 percent during much of the 1970s, we feel that 1 percent may be a more reasonable estimate of this rate in the intermediate future).

5. The present value of an individual's expected future-earnings stream

(at time of disease or injury) is an appropriate economic measure of what his or her expected lifetime productivity would have been if the disease or injury had not occurred.

Based on this set of assumptions, the present value of expected forgone earnings *PVFE* of a person of sex s who dies at age l may be modeled as

$$PVFE = \sum_{n=l}^{85} P_{l,s}(n) \cdot Y_s(n) \cdot E_s(n) \cdot \left(\frac{1 + \gamma}{1 + r}\right)^{n-l} \qquad \text{for } l \geq 16$$

(Note: For $l < 16$, start summation at $n = 16$.)

where $l =$ the age at onset (and death)
$s =$ the sex of the individual
$\gamma =$ the average annual rate of growth in labor productivity (assumed to be 1 percent)
$Y_s(n) =$ the mean annual earnings of employed people and homemakers in the general population of age n and sex s, measured at incidence-year (1975) levels
$E_s(n) =$ the proportion of the general population of age n and sex s employed in the labor force or engaged in housekeeping tasks
$P_{l,s}(n) =$ the probability of a person in the general population of age l and sex s surviving to a subsequent age n
$r =$ the discount rate

The model's framework is similar to that of analogous economic models developed by Rice (1966) and Smart and Sanders (1976) for estimating the present value of an individual's future forgone earnings. Each of these models, like our own, has as its basis a time series consisting of products of mean earnings multiplied by age- and sex-specific survival probabilities, employment and housekeeping participation rates, and labor-productivity factors; the series is summed and discounted over a time interval corresponding to the individual's remaining working lifetime.

The reader should recognize that the expected forgone earnings of a fatality resulting from disease or injury is best modeled by the earnings expectation of a demographically matched person in the *illness-free population*. (Where the illness-free population is defined as that part of the general population free of the condition in question during the incidence year.) Notice, however, that we have used the survival streams of the general population (which includes people with and without the condition in question) as an estimate of the illness-free group's survival streams. We feel that this should not appreciably bias our forgone earnings estimates. The incidence of any condition represents only a minute proportion of the general population in a given year, and therefore, it is unlikely that its eradication during that one year would have a significant influence on population survival streams. Even if the incidence of the condition were large enough to exert such an influence, it is very likely that over the long term the survival streams of the illness-free population would asymptotically approach those of the general population because of the selection-effect phenomena discussed earlier in the mortality section of this chapter.

Table 2–2 presents the employment rates and housekeeping participation rates by age and sex used in this study. As mentioned earlier, these rates are averages of the corresponding 1970 and 1975 rates published by the U.S. Department of Labor. We averaged the rates because we felt that the 1975 rates alone (1975 was a postrecession year) would probably understate average employment levels in the future. However, using the 1970 rates alone (1970) was a year of relative full employment) would undoubtedly overstate future employment levels, given the underlying unemployment problems that now seem endemic to our economy.

Mean annual productivity values, incorporating the mean earnings of people employed in the labor force and mean household-labor values, are

Table 2–2
Estimates of U.S. Employement and Housekeeping Participation Rates, by Age and Sex
(Percentages)

	Male			Female		
Age Group	Employed in Labor Force	Keeping House	Employed or Keeping House	Employed in Labor Force	Keeping House	Employed or Keeping House
16–19	49.2	0.2	49.4	38.4	10.9	49.3
20–24	76.5	0.1	76.6	54.7	29.3	84.0
25–29	89.6	0.1	89.7	47.1	45.9	93.0
30–34	92.8	0.1	92.9	44.8	48.8	93.6
35–39	93.3	0.1	93.4	48.8	45.2	94.0
40–44	92.5	0.2	92.7	52.0	42.5	94.5
45–49	91.4	0.2	91.6	52.7	41.9	94.6
50–54	88.3	0.2	88.5	51.2	43.0	94.2
55–59	83.9	0.3	84.2	46.6	47.4	94.0
60–64	67.9	0.6	68.5	33.4	58.4	91.8
65–69	34.7	1.1	35.8	15.2	73.1	88.3
70–74	16.0	1.9	17.9	5.2	72.8	78.0
75–79	7.4	1.9	9.3	1.8	72.8	74.6
80–84	3.4	1.9	5.3	0.6	72.8	73.4
85+	1.6	1.9	3.5	0.2	72.8	73.0

Source: Derived from data for 1970 and 1975 in *Employment and Earnings*, Bureau of Labor Statistics, U.S. Department of Labor, January 1971 and January 1976, and data from Parringer and Berk (1977) on employment rates for those 70 and older.

Table 2-3
Mean Annual Productivity Values, Incorporating Mean Earnings of Employed and Mean Household Labor Values (Using Market-Value Approach), by Age and Sex, United States, 1975
(Dollars)

Age Group	Males	Females
16–19	$ 4,506	4,216
20–24	9,677	7,752
25–29	13,444	9,877
30–34	16,087	10,136
35–39	17,043	9,833
40–44	17,185	10,050
45–49	17,027	9,422
50–54	16,690	9,534
55–59	14,909	7,323
60–64	13,413	5,763
65–69	8,884	3,532
70–74	6,156	2,233
75–79	4,569	1,426
80–84	2,562	808
85	1,378	452

Source: Derived from unpublished earnings data for 1975 from the U.S. Bureau of the Census; household labor values using the market-value approach from Brody (1975); and employment and housekeeping rates from table 2-2.

displayed in tables 2–3 and 2–4. The figures in table 2–3 reflect the market-value approach to evaluating household labor. These figures were derived from unpublished data on average market earnings in 1975 by age and sex from the Bureau of the Census; household-labor values estimated for 1972 by Brody (1975) and adjusted to 1975 levels; data in table 2–2 that show the distribution of those productively engaged between employment in the labor force and performance of housekeeping tasks; and data from Parringer and Berk (1977) that permitted the estimation of a part-time household-productivity component for employed people. The weighted average of earnings and housekeeping values shown in the table reflects all components of a person's productivity, both in the marketplace and at home. The somewhat larger values for mean annual productivity presented in table 2–4 reflect the opportunity-cost approach to valuing household labor. In this case, the opportunity cost imputed to homemakers' activities is the average earnings of age- and sex-matched peers employed in the labor force.

The information in tables 2–2 through 2–4 was used with the discounted-earnings model earlier to estimate the present value of average forgone earnings per fatality. The results discounted at 6 percent and disaggregated by age and sex are presented in table 2–5—using the market-value approach to evaluate household labor—and in table 2–6—using the opportunity-cost

Table 2–4
Mean Annual Productivity Values, Incorporating Mean Earnings of Employed and Mean Household Labor Values (Using Opportunity-Cost Approach), by Age and Sex, United States, 1975
(Dollars)

Age Group	Males	Females
16–19	4,481	3,479
20–24	9,797	7,311
25–29	14,054	9,971
30–34	17,204	10,194
35–39	18,449	10,130
40–44	18,697	10,376
45–59	18,756	10,418
50–54	18,449	10,816
55–59	16,732	9,720
60–64	15,689	8,769
65–69	10,886	5,587
70–74	8,052	4,375
75–79	5,998	3,580
80–84	4,411	2,989
85	2,968	2,516

Source: Derived from unpublished earnings data for 1975 from the U.S. Bureau of the Census.

approach. In both tables, the foregone earnings of males are consistently greater than those of females for people under 65 years of age. This is best explained by the large discrepancy between the sexes in mean annual productivity values. For each sex, younger and middle-aged individuals between the ages of 15 and 44 suffer the largest earnings losses per person.

The results determined using the market-value approach for household labor (table 2–5) are used in our base-case analyses. The consistently larger results using the opportunity-cost approach, which reflect the higher value ascribed to household labor under this method, are considered in the sensitivity analyses for each condition. In addition, the effect on forgone earnings of changes in the values of the discount rate and productivity growth factor are also considered therein.

Forgone Productivity of Nonfatal Cases. The lost productivity of a non-fatal patient may take either of two general forms. The first is typical of stroke or spinal cord injury patients. It is characterized by *permanent* disability that prevents individuals from performing a large portion of their work-related tasks. Lost productivity caused by permanent disability may continue for several years past onset and, without proper rehabilitation, often for the remainder of the individual's life. Even if the individual returns to work, he or she may still perform at a reduced level of efficiency and may experience

Table 2-5
Present Value of Average Forgone Earnings per Fatality (Using Market-Value Approach), by Age and Sex, United States, 1975
(Dollars)

Age Group	Males	Females
0–14	130,863	92,241
15–24	225,992	156,059
25–34	247,881	153,131
35–44	205,687	126,642
45–54	135,972	87,150
55–64	52,199	39,950
65–74	5,754	11,682
75+	533	2,556

Note: All earnings figures are in 1975 dollars, discounted at 6 percent. The market-value approach was used to evaluate household labor.

reductions in life expectancy owing to impairment-related complications. Both these outcomes manifest themselves in lost productivity. The second form of productivity loss, which is limited in nature and normally concludes during the first year following disease or injury onset, derives from absence from work or homemaking activities as a result of *temporary* disability caused by the impairment. As in the case of fatalities, both forms of forgone productivity are measured in terms of forgone earnings.

Forgone Earnings of Persons with Permanent Disabilities. Estimating the present value of forgone earnings for persons experiencing permanent disabilities and a loss of life expectancy is a complex exercise. Unlike the less

Table 2-6
Present Value of Average Forgone Earnings per Fatality (Using Opportunity-Cost Approach), by Age and Sex, United States, 1975
(Dollars)

Age Group	Males	Females
0–14	139,706	95,493
15–24	242,001	163,537
25–34	270,475	167,578
35–44	227,680	148,300
45–54	153,332	115,419
55–64	61,985	66,095
65–74	7,603	26,585
75+	928	9,786

Note: All earnings figures are in 1975 dollars, discounted at 6 percent. The opportunity-cost approach was used to evaluate household labor.

critically impaired individuals, the period of disability, and hence of forgone earnings, frequently lasts beyond the first year after condition onset. In contrast to fatalities, however, these people may return to a paid job or homemaking role. Forgone earnings per person may be calculated by subtracting the expected future earnings of a person with the condition (called the *postmorbid earnings PVPM*) from the expected future earnings of a person free of the condition of similar age and sex. The present value of forgone earnings per person may be represented algebraically as

$$PVFE = \sum_{n=l}^{85} P_{l,s}(n) \cdot E_s(n) \cdot Y_s(n) \cdot \left(\frac{1+\gamma}{1+r}\right)^{n-l}$$

$$- \sum_{n=l}^{85} P_{l,s}^i(n) \cdot E_{l,s}^i(n) \cdot Y_s(n) \cdot \left(\frac{1+\gamma}{1+r}\right)^{n-l}$$

where $P_{l,s}(n)$, $E_s(n)$, $Y_s(n)$, γ, and r have been defined in the previous section on fatalities, and $P_{l,s}^i(n)$ is the probability that a person of sex s who acquires condition i at age l will survive to a subsequent age n, and $E_{l,s}^i(n)$ is the proportion of the impaired population of sex s that is employed in the labor force or engaged in housekeeping tasks at age n, given survival to that age following condition onset at age l.

Notice that in the preceding equation the first term on the right, the expected earnings of a person in the general population (which we use to approximate the expected earnings of a person free of the condition) was derived in the earlier section on fatalities. The second term on the right side of the equation is the expected earnings of a person with the particular condition, his postmorbid earnings. This term has been reformulated in the coronary heart disease, stroke, and cancer chapters, since therein we have represented $E_{l,s}^i(n)$ as a product of two terms, the relative work rate $\beta_{l,s}^i(n)$ and the employment rate for the general population $E_s(n)$. In these cases, the postmorbid earnings term can be rewritten as

$$PVPM = \sum_{n=l}^{85} P_{l,s}^i(n) \cdot \beta_{l,s}^i(n) \cdot E_s(n) \cdot Y_s(n) \left(\frac{1+\gamma}{1+r}\right)^{n-l}$$

In the disease chapters just mentioned, however, data limitations have forced us to assign only two different values to the relative work-rate term $\beta_{l,s}^i(n)$. The first-year relative work rate was called $\alpha_{l,s}^i$, and the relative work rate appropriate for subsequent years was called $\beta_{l,s}^i$. Then the present-value postmorbid-earnings term becomes

$$PVPM = \alpha^i_{l,s} \cdot E_s(l) \cdot Y_s(l)$$

$$+ \beta^i_{l,s} \cdot \left[\sum_{n=l+1}^{85} P^i_{l,s}(n) \cdot E_s(n) \cdot Y_s(n) \cdot \left(\frac{1+\gamma}{1+r} \right)^{n-l} \right]$$

As an example of this model, let us examine the case of a 30-year-old male who acquires a disease that reduces his work efficiency to 50 percent of normal in the first year and 70 percent thereafter. The illness also causes a substantial reduction in his life expectancy. In this instance, his *PVPM* can be shown to be

$$PVPM = .5 \cdot E_M(30) \cdot Y_M(30)$$

$$+ .7 \cdot \left[\sum_{n=31}^{85} P^i_{30,M}(n) \cdot E_M(n) \cdot Y_M(n) \cdot \left(\frac{1.01}{1.06} \right)^{n-30} \right]$$

where $F_M(30) = 0.9292$

$Y_M(30) = \$16,087$

and

$$\sum_{n=31}^{85} P^i_{30,M}(n) \cdot E_M(n) \cdot Y_M(n) \cdot \left(\frac{1.01}{1.06} \right)^{n-30} = \$8645$$

Then

$$PVPM = .5 \cdot (0.9292) \cdot (16,087) + .7 \cdot (8645)$$

$$= \$13,526$$

Therefore, subtracting his postmorbid earnings from his expected earnings if he never contracted this disease, that is, $247,881, yields a present-value forgone earnings (*PVFE*) of $234,355.

Forgone Earnings of Persons with Temporary Disability. Although other indices of temporary disability exist (for example, bed-rest days, work-loss days), the most general one, and one that is frequently employed by the National Center for Health Statistics (NCHS), is the *day of restricted activity.* This is defined as a day on which a person experiences a substantial reduction in his standard activities as a result of some form of health impairment. While complete inactivity is not always assumed, a person experiencing a day of restricted activity is normally prevented from working at his job or homemaking tasks. Therefore, a rough measure of a temporarily disabled person's lost productivity may be obtained by multiplying the estimate of his average number of days of restricted activity by the average value of each of those days (measured as forgone earnings).

We estimate the value of a day of restricted activity VDR as

$$VDR = \frac{Y_s(n) \cdot E_s(n)}{365}$$

where $Y_s(n)$ and $E_s(n)$ have been defined previously.

Because it is reasonable to assume that an illness will cause restricted activity during both working and nonworking periods, we averaged the values for restricted activity days over 365 days rather than over the typical 240 to 250 days people usually work at a job (or the longer periods worked by full-time homemakers). The value of a day of restricted activity is presented in table 2–7—using the market-value approach to evaluate household labor—and in table 2–8—using the opportunity-cost approach.

To determine the average individual's forgone earnings, we multiply the estimate of the average number of days of restricted activity by the value of a day of restricted activity. As an example, note that a 30-year-old male with 10 days of restricted activity generates $370 (10 × $37) in forgone earnings using the market-value approach; if the same man is 80 years old, his forgone earnings drop to $10 (10 × $1).

Table 2–7
Value of a Day of Restricted Activity (Using Market-Value Approach), by Age and Sex, United States, 1975
(Dollars)

Age	Male	Female
0–14	0	0
15–24	14	12
25–34	37	26
35–44	44	26
45–54	42	25
55–64	30	17
65–74	6	7
75+	1	2

Source: Derived form data presented in tables 2–2 and 2–3.
Note: All earnings figures are in 1975 dollars.

Table 2–8
Value of a Day of Restricted Activity (Using Opportunity-Cost Approach), by Age and Sex, United States, 1975
(Dollars)

Age	Male	Female
0–14	0	0
15–24	14	11
25–34	39	26
35–44	47	26
45–54	46	27
55–64	34	24
65–74	8	12
75+	1	6

Source: Derived from data presented in tables 2–2 and 2–4.
Note: All earnings figures are in 1975 dollars.

Total Forgone Productivity. If the forgone-productivity estimates are multiplied by the corresponding incidence estimates and the products are summed, the result is an estimate of the present value of total expected forgone earnings. This figure represents the indirect-cost estimates for the health impairment under study. The difference between indirect and direct cost is basically one of causality. On the one hand, a health impairment may require the allocation of goods and services that exist or are being produced toward the treatment of that impairment. On the other hand, the health impairment may prevent the production of goods and services. In both cases, the amount of resources society has available for other purposes is reduced.

The human-capital approach is used to measure the amount of forgone production. It should be noted that we are ascertaining the output losses of the incidence population only; other forgone earnings, such as the productivity losses of persons associated with the patient, are not estimated. Other indirect costs, such as those pertaining to the pain and emotional deprivation experienced by patients and their families because of illness, are recognized as significant. However, these costs also are not estimated because of the current lack of information and methodology necessary to adequately measure them. Our value for indirect costs should be viewed, therefore, as a lower-bound estimate of the total indirect costs associated with the condition.

Sensitivity Analysis

Economic-cost estimates derived from models of the direct costs and productivity losses of incidence populations depend on a number of assumptions and on values determined for a variety of parameters. A parameter of particular importance, for instance, is the annual incidence of the disease or injury; an error in this variable has a significant impact on total economic costs. If the incidence estimates are in error by 25 percent across all condition subcategories, then, because of the nature of our modeling procedures, the estimate of total costs would also err by 25 percent, even if all other assumptions and parameter values underlying the models were correct. (In the case of stroke, however, this is not so for nursing home costs, which were estimated independently of the incidence estimates.) Examples of other types of parameters that may (depending on the impairment) have important, albeit less extreme, influences on total costs are the annual treatment costs during both the first and subsequent years following impairment onset, the predicted mortality patterns of impairment survivors, and the reemployment rates of those same survivors.

For each of the health conditions considered in this study, the basic analytical assumptions underlying our calculations also have significant effects on economic costs. These assumptions include estimates of the value of the societal discount rate (chosen to be 6 percent in the base case), the value of the annual productivity growth factor (estimated at 1 percent), and the specific method used to value household labor (the market-value approach). These values, however, are not to be accepted with the same faith that a physicist might accept the value of the speed of light. As we indicated in chapter 1, many economists feel that the proper discount rate to use in evaluating societal decisions is closer to 10 percent than 6 percent, and still others argue for something even less, a value closer to 2 percent. Likewise, because of the inherent uncertainty in future economic conditions, the precise value for the productivity growth factor is open to question. We feel that it is realistic to assume that this factor could range in value anywhere from 0 to 2 percent per year. Also, several economists have argued that the more appropriate method to use in evaluating the worth of household labor is to price it at its opportunity-cost equivalent rather than to use a strict market-value approach.

Precisely because the exact values of many parameters are uncertain and several of the assumptions that must be made, while reasonable, are still debatable, the prudent analyst should always anticipate the range of possible parameter values and alternative assumptions. He is then in a better position to recalculate the level of economic costs using alternative values for the parameters and different assumptions. Through this process, it becomes evident whether or not total costs associated with a particular health condition are affected appreciably by changes in specific variables. If the value of total costs is affected significantly by changes in a given variable, and if it is reasonable to believe that uncertainty exists in the variable's value, then further research to learn more about that variable may be especially valuable. Meanwhile, both the analyst and his audience are forewarned of a potential bias in total-cost results owing to uncertainty in particular parameters or possible variations in certain key assumptions.

The procedure just outlined is called *sensitivity analysis*. By this method, the most uncertain features and assumptions involved in our calculations are varied over the range of possible values—normally varying one parameter at a time, while holding the values of all other parameters fixed—to determine the effect on total economic costs. The results of sensitivity analysis may be specific to just one condition, or they may have consequences across conditions. An example of the latter situation occurs when the value of the discount rate is varied from 2 to 10 percent. As one might expect, the value of total economic costs for each of our four health conditions *is* sensitive to the value of the discount rate. Indeed, as subsequent chapters will show, the *absolute* value of total costs decreases significantly for each condition as the discount rate increases from 2 to 6 to 10 percent. In addition, the *relative* economic ordering of two of the conditions (motor vehicle injuries and coronary heart disease) changes as well.

Although the discount rate has a critical effect on the level of economic costs for all four conditions, the influence of other types of variables (for example, nursing home charges, relative mortality rates, reemployment rates) often depends on the particular condition. The behavioral and cost characteristics of the patient population, the modeling procedures necessary to capture those characteristics, and the level of uncertainty in the value of the variable all contribute to the influence on total costs. Sensitivity analysis helps to determine when a particular variable is crucial and when, perhaps surprisingly, it may not be. In this way, it helps to increase confidence in the initial cost results and, at the same time, point out areas where the data collection or analysis might be improved.

The sensitivity analyses performed for each impairment (and documented in succeeding chapters) are extensive and cover several sources of possible imprecision. These encompass the basic analytical assumptions, incidence and recurrence variables, mortality parameters, direct-cost components, and indirect-cost components. Although the variables scrutinized for each impairment are frequently the same, the results and emphases are often very different, reflecting the diversity of the four impairments studied.

The Prevalence and Incidence Approaches: A Hypothetical Example

Much has been said about the *qualitative* differences between the prevalence and incidence approaches. To illustrate the *numerical* differences between the two approaches, we consider a hypothetical example. Suppose that the incidence of a certain illness A is 400 people per year and that this illness strikes only 30-year-old men. The annual mortality rate for people with the illness is high and equal to 0.5. [Conversely, the conditional probability of survival per year for people with the illness is relatively low, but also equal to 0.5 (1 - 0.5).] Furthermore, no one who contracts the illness survives more than 5 years after onset. Under this set of circumstances, the survival pattern for an incidence cohort of 400, 30-year-old men contracting the illness in a given year is

Subsequent Age in Years	Number of People Surviving to Age
30	400
31	$200[400 \times (\frac{1}{2})]$
32	$100[400 \times (\frac{1}{2})^2]$
33	$50[400 \times (\frac{1}{2})^3]$
34	$25[400 \times (\frac{1}{2})^4]$
35	0

This means that in any given year, for instance, 1975, the prevalence population of people with the illness will total 775 (400 + 200 + 100 + 50 + 25). The age distribution of this population will be identical to the age distribution of illness survivors presented earlier.

Since the annual mortality rate is 0.5 (and no one survives more than 5 years past illness onset), 200 of the 400, 30-year-olds will die before the end of the year and 100 of the 200, 31-year-olds, 50 of the 100, 32-year-olds, 25 of the 50, 33-year-olds, and all the 25, 34-year-olds also will die before the end of the year. This mortality profile is summarized below:

Age at Death in Years	Number Dying during Year
30	200
31	100
32	50
33	25
34	25
	400

Let us further assume that annual per-person treatment costs—direct costs—are constant and equal to *ATC*. For illness survivors, the annual per-person reduction in productivity—the morbidity component of indirect costs—is also constant and equal to *ARP*. Forgone earnings owing to premature death—the mortality component of indirect costs—derive from the termination of work yielding an annual salary of *AS*. In the absence of premature death, we can assume that no one would have worked beyond a mandatory retirement age of 65. (These assumptions represent oversimplifications of what would actually occur, but they serve to simplify the numerical calculations without detracting from the example's ability to point out salient differences between the prevalence and incidence approaches.)

In the prevalence approach, the direct costs are those of the 775 persons with illness during the year: $775 \cdot ATC$. Similarly, the morbidity component of indirect costs is the productivity losses of the same 775 persons: $775 \cdot ARP$. The mortality component of indirect costs in the prevalence approach $MTC(PA)$ is the present-valued forgone earnings of the 400 people dying of the illness during the year.

For each of the 200 men dying of the illness at age 30, the present value of forgone earnings is the same as the earnings expectations of a demographically matched person in the general population. At a real discount rate of 6 percent per year, it is estimated as

$$\sum_{n=30}^{65} \frac{P_{30,M}(n) \cdot AS}{(1.06)^{n-30}} = AS \cdot \left[\sum_{n=30}^{65} \frac{P_{30,M}(n)}{(1.06)^{n-30}} \right]$$

where $P_{30,M}(n) =$ the probability of a 30-year old man in the general
population surviving to age n in the future

Since

$$\sum_{n=30}^{65} \frac{P_{30,M}(n)}{(1.06)^{n-30}} = 14.8$$

forgone earnings per person are $\sim 14.8 \cdot AS$. Total forgone earnings for this age group are thus $200 \cdot 14.8 \cdot AS = 2{,}960 \cdot AS$. When similar calculations are carried out for people dying at ages 31, 32, 33, and 34, the results are

Age at Death	Number Dying	Forgone Earnings per Person	Total Forgone Earnings
30	200	$14.80 \cdot AS$	$2960 \cdot AS$
31	100	$14.65 \cdot AS$	$1465 \cdot AS$
32	50	$14.50 \cdot AS$	$725 \cdot AS$
33	25	$14.34 \cdot AS$	$359 \cdot AS$
34	25	$14.17 \cdot AS$	$354 \cdot AS$

Total $= MTC(PA) = 5863 \cdot AS$

The incidence approach regards only the 400, 30-year-old men acquiring the illness in the year—not all those alive with it or dying as a result of it, as in the prevalence approach. The direct costs of the incidence approach $DC(IA)$ equal the present value of all current and future treatment costs for those 400 people acquiring the illness during the year. For each person, the present value of expected treatment costs may be represented as

$$DC(IA) = \sum_{n=30}^{35} \frac{P^i_{30,M}(n) \cdot ATC}{(1.06)^{n-30}} = ATC \cdot \left[\sum_{n=30}^{35} \frac{P^i_{30,M}(n)}{(1.06)^{n-30}} \right]$$

where $P^i_{30,M}(n)$ = the probability of a 30-year-old man with illness A surviving to age n in the future

Since only one-half of the original group survives at least 1 year past illness onset (to age 31), one-quarter survives at least 2 years past onset (to age 32), one-eighth survives at least 3 years past onset (to age 33), one-sixteenth survives at least 4 years past onset (to age 34), and *no one* survives more than 5 years past onset (to age 35), we have

$$DC(IA) = ATC \cdot \left[1 + \frac{\frac{1}{2}}{1.06} + \frac{\frac{1}{4}}{1.06^2} + \frac{\frac{1}{8}}{1.06^3} + \frac{\frac{1}{16}}{1.06^4} + 0 \right]$$

$$= 1.85 \cdot ATC$$

Total direct costs $DC(IA)$ are thus $400 \cdot 1.85 \cdot ATC = 740 \cdot ATC$.

The indirect costs of the incidence approach are tabulated in a different fashion than in the prevalence approach. It is not always a straightforward process to disaggregate forgone earnings into components that are exclusively morbidity- and mortality-related. Rather, we compare in the incidence approach the earnings expectation of a person just prior to illness with the earnings expectation just after contracting the illness. The difference represents the earnings forgone or lost owing to illness. In the case of a 30-year-old man, the earnings expectation prior to illness (the same as that of a matched individual in the illness-free population) was seen earlier to be $14.8 \cdot AS$. The earnings expectation after contracting the illness is

$$\sum_{n=30}^{35} \frac{P^i_{30,M}(n) \cdot (AS - ARP)}{(1.06)^{n-30}} = (AS - ARP) \cdot \left[\sum_{n=30}^{35} \frac{P^i_{30,M}(n)}{(1.06)^{n-30}} \right]$$

From our previous calculations, we have

$$\sum_{n=30}^{35} \frac{P_{30,M}^{i}(n)}{(1.06)^{n-30}} = 1.85$$

and therefore, the earnings expectation per ill person is $1.85 \cdot (AS - ARP)$. The forgone earnings per person become

$$(14.8 \cdot AS) - 1.85 \cdot (AS - ARP) = (12.95 \cdot AS) + (1.85 \cdot ARP)$$

Total forgone earnings of the 400 incidence cases are thus

$$400 \cdot [(12.95 \cdot AS) + (1.85 \cdot ARP)] = (5180 \cdot AS) + (740 \cdot ARP)$$

In summary, the economic costs of illness A using each approach are

	Prevalence Approach	*Incidence Approach*
Direct costs:	$775 \cdot ATC$	$740 \cdot ATC$
Indirect costs:	$(5863 \cdot AS) + (775 \cdot ARP)$	$(5180 \cdot AS) + (740 \cdot ARP)$
Total costs:	$(5863 \cdot AS) + 775 \cdot (ATC + ARP)$	$(5180 \cdot AS) + 740 \cdot (ATC + ARP)$

Note: Recall that ATC is the annual per-person treatment costs, ARP is the annual per-person reduction in productivity, and AS is the annual salary per person.

Comparison of Results Obtained with the Prevalance and the Incidence Approaches

From this example we can see or infer several general results from applying the two approaches to actual illness data. First, the prevalence-approach results are larger than those of the incidence approach. This will generally be the case for diseases and injuries that produce long-term sequelae, although exceptions can arise. A possible exception occurs when incidence is rising at a rate greater than the real discount rate—as perhaps occurred for chronic obstructive pulmonary disease between 1968 and 1976. The greater the discount rate used, the greater in general will be the ratio of prevalence-approach results to incidence-approach results.

Second, for conditions that do not produce long-term sequelae, there will be little difference between the prevalence and incidence approaches. Owing to the limited duration, the years in which costs are borne will typically be the years of incidence, which also will generally be the years of disease- or injury-caused death. The two approaches would thus assign all costs to the same years.

Third, the discrepancy between the prevalence and incidence approaches grows with the average duration of the condition. For instance, the ratio of direct costs between the two approaches in our example, that is,

$$\frac{775 \cdot ATC}{740 \cdot ATC} = 1.05$$

reflects the fact that some costs which are not discounted in the prevalence approach are discounted in the incidence approach.

Fourth, the discrepancies between the two approaches are larger for indirect costs (12 to 13 percent in the preceding example depending on the size of ARP) than for direct costs (5 percent). This implies that the numerical differences between the prevalence and incidence approaches will be proportionately greater for conditions with relatively large indirect costs owing to high mortality rates than for conditions with a higher proportion of direct costs and/or indirect costs owing only to short-term disability.

Fifth, the ratio of prevalence-approach costs to incidence-approach costs for a given disease or injury will generally be higher (other things being equal): (1) when incidence is declining (the prevalence approach capturing the costs of chronic disease or injury survivors from the larger incidence cohorts of earlier years); (2) when annual treatment costs and disability losses are declining over time (since the analyst should reflect this trend in calculating the future costs of present incidence cases); and (3) when annual treatment costs and disability losses rise over the course of the disease or injury (because the later, greater costs will be discounted in the incidence approach but not in the prevalence approach).

The preceding discussion may give the impression that choice between the prevalence and incidence approaches allows analysts considerable manipulative control over the numerical results. If, for instance, they wish to exaggerate the importance of a disease or injury with declining incidence, the prevalence approach serves this purpose better than the incidence approach. Yet this manipulative possibility is removed when the appropriateness of the approach is taken into account. In considering preventive measures, the prevalence approach is basically inappropriate—just as the incidence approach is unsuitable when reduction of ongoing treatment costs or amelioration of work capacity in the prevalence population is at issue.

The Data Bases: Their Scope and Limitations

For each of the four health conditions examined in this study, we sought the latest, most accurate data on incidence, recurrence, survival incapacitation, treatment costs, and indirect costs. Despite the apparent gravity of each of these illnesses, there has been limited representative data gathered; remarkably few comprehensive data sources exist. This is especially true of the more than 4 million nonfatal motor vehicle injuries suffered annually. Efforts are just now underway to systematically catalog and track those so injured.

Because of the lack of comprehensive data bases, we have relied on hundreds of sources to provide information for the analysis. In those few instances where major studies do exist that have examined the incidence or associated costs of one or more of the conditions, we have borrowed heavily from these sources. Good examples of such studies are the Framingham Heart Study (for coronary heart disease), the National Survey of Stroke (for stroke), the Third National Cancer Survey (for cancer), and the Fatal Accident Reporting System of the National Highway Traffic Safety Administration (for fatal motor vehicle injuries).[12] In addition, other objective data, where available, and judgmental assessments from experts in the health field have been incorporated. These sources include an extensive review of the pertinent literature, interviews with experts, and assorted unpublished data.

For each of the health conditions, we briefly highlight the principal data sources used, their scope, and their limitations. More complete discussions of the data bases are found in each succeeding disease and injury chapter (chapters 3 to 6).

Coronary Heart Disease

Traditionally, the analysis of the incidence of coronary heart disease (CHD) has been hampered by the sparsity of representative data. Several studies have restricted themselves to particular subsets of the population—some studies survey only white males and others have surveyed only individuals in certain limited age groups. Among studies, definitional and taxonomic idiosyncracies have occasionally led to inconsistent diagnostic terminology and to unusual variations in classification schemes. An exception to this trend is the Framingham Heart Study. Data from this study plus information from other selected sources have formed the basis for our estimates of the national incidence of coronary heart disease. The representative nature of the Framingham incidence data has been confirmed, generally, through comparisons with data in other, more limited studies. Secular changes in incidence rates were estimated by using data on declining mortality rates. In computing mortality and recurrence rates for CHD survivors, both published and unpublished data from the Framingham Heart Study were used. The mortality rates were compared with those observed in other studies and no major inconsistencies were found.

Useful information of the direct costs of coronary heart disease were obtained from a variety of sources. Among them were data from the Professional Activities Survey (PAS) and studies published in various professional journals.[13] Expert opinion from hospital administrators and clinical practitioners familiar with the treatment of coronary heart disease patients also provided valuable inputs to the cost analysis. Estimates of forgone productivity of coronary heart disease patients were derived, in part, from data in Weinblatt's study (1966) of the employment status of male heart attack survivors at different time intervals following their first attacks.

Stroke

The many epidemiological studies of stroke have used a variety of classification schemes—sometimes distinguishing embolisms from thrombosis, sometimes differentiating cerebral hemorrhage by site, often including a residual category of "unknown or other" events. Classification of strokes across studies is not consistent. Studies available that could have been used to calculate incidence and mortality were written by various authors, in particular Matsumoto (1973) and Shurtleff (1974). Unpublished data from the Framingham Heart Study also were available. Our incidence estimates were based, however, on the latest extensions of Matsumoto's work by Furlan (1979) and Garraway (1979).

Mortality estimates were based on the recent and extensive data from the National Survey of Stroke (USDHEW, 1980). The direct cost data that would have been most useful to us, but unfortunately was not made available, also would have come from the National Survey of Stroke. We fell back on the available hospitalization data from Blue Cross of Massachusetts (adjusted to national levels), nursing home cost data from the National Nursing Home Survey (NCHS, 1979), and rehabilitation costs from Emlet (1973). Estimates of vocational incapacity were derived from data in studies by Matsumoto (1973) and Gresham (1979).

Cancer

Cancer incidence rates by age and sex were abstracted from the Third National Cancer Survey (TNCS). As a consistency check, the TNCS data were compared with similar data from the California and New York state cancer registries. The ongoing SEER Program was consulted to ascertain secular changes in the *TNCS* estimates.[14] Information on mortality was based on data reported by Axtell, Cutler, and Myers (1972 and 1974).

The bulk of the information on treatment costs comes from data gathered in the TNCS. Data collected by Abt Associates and the Boston University Cancer Research Center (1976), however, were especially useful in estimating non-hospital-related treatment costs. Estimates of forgone earnings of cancer patients were derived primarily from unpublished data from the TNCS on return-to-work patterns following cancer diagnosis.

Motor Vehicle Injuries

We considered the best data on the incidence of motor vehicle fatalities to be that of the Fatal Accident Reporting System (FARS) of the National Highway Traffic Safety Administration (NHTSA) and the most comprehensive data on nonfatal motor vehicle injuries to be that of the Health Interview Survey (HIS) of the National Center for Health Statistics (NCHS).[15] To break these data down to obtain incidence estimates by age and sex and by injury severity level, we used statistics reported by thirty-two states to NHTSA and unpublished data from the National Crash Severity Study (NCSS).[16] Determining mortality rates for the initially nonfatal but nevertheless severe injuries required differentiating injuries by anatomic site or body region using unpublished data from NCSS and then applying site-specific relative mortality rates developed from data in several studies.

Studies expecially important in calculating direct costs included those by Smart and Sanders (1976), Faigin (1976), Wuerdemann and Joksch (1973), and DeLorean (1975), as well as the National Crash Severity Study and the Automobile Insurance and Compensation Study of the Department of Transportation.[17] In addition to information gathered by Smart and Sanders and the National Crash Severity Study, data presented in a study by Dresser et al. (1973) of reemployment rates for head-injured men helped to gauge work loss among crash survivors.

Closing Comments

We have mentioned earlier that certain incidence-based costs of disease or injury may be biased upward because of some double counting. Since a person with two concurrent conditions who dies prematurely will be accounted for in the incidence population of both conditions, his forgone earnings also will be counted twice, resulting in a partial overestimation of the indirect cost of illness. It is therefore inappropriate to sum the costs of the four conditions considered in this study to ascertain an estimate of the total cost of illness from the four conditions together. However, this should not imply that the costs estimated for each condition separately are not reasonable estimates of the economic implications of that condition. Recall that we are estimating *all* the economic costs *associated* with a condition. Since in general it is not possible, we are not attempting to estimate the specific costs owing to that condition alone.

We also should reemphasize that this study does not estimate the net economic effect of eliminating all motor vehicle crashes, heart disease, cancer, or stroke. Estimating the total changes brought about by the complete elimination of all cancer, for example, would require far-reaching social analysis reflecting major changes in the population-age profile and in the allocation of health-care resources. Such inquiry, however, lies outside the scope of this work. It measures instead—in order to estimate the annual costs borne by society as a result of each of the four conditions—total economic costs brought about by one year's incidence of that condition in 1975, as well as by the subsequent histories of those afflicted within the 1975 incidence population.

Notes

1. U.S.Department of Health, Education and Welfare, National Center for Health Statistics, Life tables, *Vital Statistics of the United States*, vol. 2, section 5 (Washington: U.S. Government Printing Office, 1980).

2. Ibid.

3. U.S. Department of Health, Education and Welfare, Public Health Service and National Institutes of Health. *The Framingham Study: An Epidemiological Investigation of Cardiovascular Disease*, sections 1–32 (Washington: U.S. Government Printing Office, 1977).

4. Marjorie S. Mueller and Robert M. Gibson, National health expenditure, fiscal year 1975, *Social Security Bulletin* (February 1976); derived from data in table 2, p. 7.

5. Ibid., p. 14.

6. Ibid., p. 7, table 2.

7. Ibid., p. 14.

8. Marjorie S. Mueller, Private health insurance in 1975: coverage, enrollment, and financial experience, *Social Security Bulletin* (June 1977): 18.

9. Roger D. Blair and Ronald J. Vogel, *The Cost of Health Insurance Administration*. Lexington, Mass.: Lexington Books; D.C. Heath, 1975.

10. Bureau of Labor Statistics, U.S. Department of Labor, *Employment and Earnings*, January 1971 and January 1976.

11. U.S. Department of Commerce, Bureau of the Census, *Current Population Survey*, May 1975.

12. *The Framingham Study*, section 32; U.S. Department of Health, Education and Welfare, *National Survey of Stroke*, NIH publication no. 80-

2069 (Washington: U.S. Government Printing Office, 1980); Sidney J. Cutler and John L. Young (eds.), *Third National Cancer Survey: Incidence Data*, National Cancer Institute Monograph 41, U.S. Department of Health, Education and Welfare, Public Health Service, National Institutes of Health publication no. (NIH) 75-787 (Washington: U.S. Government Printing Office, 1975); U.S. Department of Transportation, National Highway Traffic Safety Administration, *Fatal Accident Reporting Systems: 1975 Annual Report* (October 1976).

13. Commission on Professional and Hospital Activities, *Length of Stay in PAS Hospitals by Diagnosis, United States, 1975* (Ann Arbor, 1976).

14. John L. Young, Jr., Ardyce J. Asire, and Earl S. Pollack, *SEER Program: Cancer Incidence and Mortality in the United States, 1973–1976*, DHEW publication no (NIH) 78-1837 (Washington: U.S. Government Printing Office, 1978).

15. U.S. Department of Health, Education and Welfare, Health Resources Administration, National Cancer Center for Health Statistics, *Current Estimates from the Health Interview Survey, United States, 1975*, Vital and Health Statistics Series 10, No. 115 (Washington: U.S. Government Printing Office, 1977).

16. U.S. Department of Transportation, National Highway Traffic Safety Administration, National crash severity study, unpublished data on nonfatal motor vehicle injuries from May 1980 data file.

17. U.S. Department of Transportation, *Automobile Accident Litigation*, A Report of the Federal Judicial Center to the Department of Transportation (from *Automobile Insurance and Compensation Study*), April 1970.

3 Coronary Heart Disease

Types of Heart Disease

More deaths are caused each year in the United States by heart disease than by any other condition. The disease covers a broad spectrum of specific problems—classified from 390 to 429 in the eighth revision of the International Classification of Diseases, Adapted (ICDA) code. These problems range from chronic rheumatic heart disease, to hypertensive heart disease, to arrhythmias (abnormal heart beats), to bacterial and viral infections of the heart muscle, to mechanical failure of the heart as a pump, to a variety of rare syndromes.

Our focus will be one narrow segment of this spectrum: coronary heart disease (CHD)—restricted to ICDA codes 410 through 413. Alternately known as *coronary artery disease* or *ischemic heart disease*, coronary heart disease is responsible for 89 percent of all deaths ascribed to heart disease (National Center for Health Statistics, 1978). The disease can appear with varying degrees of severity and can affect different parts of the heart. Nevertheless, the same basic disease mechanism underlies these variant forms. Our study will be disaggregated according to the four major levels. CHD occurs when the supply of oxygenated blood to the muscle tissues of the heart is impaired. Such blockage generally results from atherosclerosis (hardening of the arteries) owing to the buildup of fatty deposits on the interior arterial walls. Low levels of blockage produce chest pain symptomatic of angina pectoris or of coronary insufficiency (CI). More serious blockage can cause myocardial infarction (MI) (death of heart-muscle tissue) or sudden death. The common term *heart attack* may in lay speech refer to any sudden instance of heart failure. For purposes of this study, heart attacks comprise CIs, MIs, and sudden deaths.

Risk Factors and Incidence

The precise causation of atherosclerosis in the coronary arteries is unknown. A number of risk factors important in predicting the specific occurrences of coronary heart disease have, however, been identified. These factors include such unalterable features as genetic predisposition, greater incidence in males, and increasing risk with age. Modifiable risk factors include hypertension (high blood pressure), smoking, lack of exercise, obesity, and elevated serum (blood) cholesterol. Unlike stroke, which is primarily a disease of the elderly, coronary heart disease has highest incidence in late middle age. We estimate that individuals under 65 constitute nearly 60 percent of the total disease incidence of 660,000 cases in 1975. Incidence rates are highest for persons between 55 and 64.

The United States has a relatively high death rate from coronary heart disease. Annual mortality in the United States in 1975 for men between 45 and 54 was 288 per 100,000 (Kannel, 1979). Finland (at 421 per 100,000), Northern Ireland (361), and Scotland (347) had higher rates in that year. Countries with low mortality rates from CHD include Japan (28 per 100,000 and declining), Switzerland (123), and Italy (128).

Management and Therapy

Medical management for mild coronary heart disease may take a variety of forms. Improved management of hypertension, reduced smoking, gradual increase in physical exercise, and weight loss for the obese are generally recommended. Drug therapy primarily includes the administration of nitrates (notably, nitroglycerin) and propranolol. Nitrates induce contraction of the heart—which reduces its oxygen demands—and expansion of the coronary arteries. Propranolol, a more recent drug, lowers coronary oxygen demands by slowing the heart rate and reducing the contraction speed of the heart-muscle fibers. When neither risk-factor alteration nor drug therapy are effective in controlling angina, coronary artery bypass graft (CABG) surgery may be performed. This operation entails the grafting of a section of vein from the patient's leg in such a way that blood may flow around obstructed portions of the coronary arteries. Since this technique began to be widely performed in the late 1960s, considerable controversy has arisen concerning its efficacy in prolonging life, reducing work loss, and easing pain (see, for example, Weinstein, 1977; Wisoff, 1978; and Hammermeister, 1979).

Treatment for myocardial infarction is also varied. Roughly one-quarter of all myocardial infarctions (MIs) are undetected until confirmed by later happenstance examination. At that time, management of risk factors may be indicated. The majority of acute MI survivors do not have severe impairment of heart function. For them, the main treatment modalities are pain relief (often by morphine) and bed rest. Some cardiologists have argued that hospitalization offers no advantages—as measured in terms of patient outcomes—over home care (for example, Hill, 1979). Electrocardiographic monitoring is often useful in detecting dangerous arrhythmias that may follow myocardial infarctions.

Most rapid deaths from MIs are due to the instability of the heart's electric system. Unstable rhythms may be stabilized by drugs, pacemakers, and electric shocks to the chest wall.These measures require, however, early detection and action. To enable rapid intervention, emergency-care systems have been developed for sending mobile coronary-care units—equipped to monitor and to correct electrical irregularities—to patients with suspected heart attacks. Lay persons trained in cardiopulmonary resuscitation also may revive apparently dead victims of myocardial infarctions.

Incidence

Data Limitations

Analysis of the incidence of coronary heart disease has been hampered by inadequate data. Although the national prevalence of coronary disease has been studied recently in the National Health Survey and the results were documented by Gordon and Garst (1965) and Wilder (1974), no similar nationwide examination of the incidence of the disease has been performed. What is available is a series of locally oriented studies that offer incidence figures on selected varieties of coronary heart disease.[1] The results of these studies, while pertinent to the specific regions and populations examined, are not thought representative of the nation as a whole. Several of the studies are restricted to subsets of the population (such as white males or individuals in limited age groups), and most are short-term, cross-sectional studies that may underestimate the more subtle forms of coronary heart disease.

Definitional idiosyncrasies among the studies mean that diagnostic terms used in one study do not necessarily mean the same thing when used in another. Moreover, a few studies included second and subsequent attacks of coronary heart disease among their values for total incidence rather than limiting themselves exclusively to first occurrences of the disease. While none of these studies adequately represents the national experience, their methodological dissimilarities suggest that pooling their results may be neither practical nor rewarding.

For our purposes, the ideal incidence study should satisfy four criteria:

1. The subjects included in the study should either constitute or closely approximate a probability sample of the national population.
2. The diagnostic subcategories should be structured to include all forms of coronary heart disease and to reflect standard diagnostic criteria.
3. Contributions to incidence should be limited to first manifestations of each diagnostic form of the disease.
4. A long-term prospective study rather than a short-term surveillance study is recommended in order to document adequately the more subtle, as well as the more overt, forms of the disease.[2]

Although the ideal incidence study does not yet exist, the Framingham Heart Study (not included in the group just critiqued) does incorporate its main features. In our opinion, the Framingham study has accumulated incidence data for first occurrences of coronary heart disease in a typical population that reflect all cases of the disease more accurately than any other study. Information from this study forms the basis for our estimates of the national incidence of coronary heart disease.

The Framingham Heart Study

The Framingham Heart Study is a long-term epidemiological investigation of atherosclerotic cardiovascular disease. The study, from its inception in 1948 and for a period of 20 years thereafter, conducted biennial examinations of a representative sample of Framingham, Massachussetts residents initially free of cardiovascular disease. Results are reported by Shurtleff (1974) and others.[3] One of the study's primary objectives was to document the first occurrences of cardiovascular disease, its component diseases (including coronary heart disease), and the various diagnostic subcategories of the component diseases in the Framingham population.

A survey of the literature and discussions with experts familiar with the study's methodology suggest several factors that support the use of Framingham data in formulating national incidence estimates. First, the town of Framingham, Massachusetts includes people in all walks of life. Furthermore, the town's population was, and is, quite stable and thus has been suitable for the 20 years of follow-up studies necessary to test the original hypotheses held by the study's designers. Second, the use of standardized biennial clinical examinations has permitted the collection of a wide variety of information about the characteristics of the people in the study both before and after their development of cardiovascular disease, as well as a standardized clinical evaluation of changes in their cardiovascular status. Third, the study is one of the few that has developed comprehensive incidence rates for both men and women. Fourth, the incidence data cover a wider range of ages (a 45-year span) than do most other sources. And fifth, the Framingham Heart Study has a national reputation for technical excellence and reliability.

Disease Etiology

In addition to the analysis of incidence, the Framingham Heart Study also has investigated the etiology of cardiovascular disease. The results of this investigation are reported by Kannel (1976). We summarize them here.

The Framingham data suggest that a number of variables, often referred to as *atherogenic variables*, operating through a variety of biological mechanisms contribute to the increased risk of coronary heart disease. Included in the group are hypertension (high blood pressure), high serum lipid levels in the blood, impaired glucose tolerence, cigarette smoking, and obesity. The Framingham experience, however, indicates the difficulty involved in specifying for any one of the these variables the point at which a normal level or value ends and an abnormal level begins. At virtually any level of each variable, the risk may vary widely depending on coexisting factors. The risk of coronary heart disease in an individual is most accurately assessed through simultaneous analysis of all atherogenic variables.

Kannel also reminds us that coronary heart disease, like other forms of atherosclerotic cardiovascular disease, is primarily a result of the aging process and, as such, is preventable only to the extent that one can retard this process. All known risk factors taken together, although related to age, do not account for more than a small portion of the age-related trend in coronary heart disease. For this reason, age is an important determining variable, especially in individuals who would otherwise be classified as at low risk for coronary heart disease.[4]

Diagnostic Categories of Coronary Heart Disease

To estimate the national incidence of coronary heart disease, we have subdivided the total disease cases into four mutually exclusive diagnostic categories: myocardial infarction (MI), sudden death, coronary insufficiency (CI), and angina pectoris uncomplicated (APU). The first three categories, which encompass the more severe forms of coronary heart disease, comprise what are popularly referred to as "heart attacks." Although other classification schemes exist, the approach used here represents what we feel is the best and most natural synthesis of alternatives presented in the literature and suggested by experts interviewed during the course of our research. The definitions developed for the disease categories reflect this process. The definitions are analogous to those of the Framingham Heart Study and represent a consensus of professional opinion.

Myocardial Infarction. Of the three forms of heart attack (sudden death, myocardial infarction, or coronary insufficiency), myocardial infarction is by far the most frequent and hence the most familiar to the lay public. In simplest terms, a *myocardial infarction* is the damage or death of an area of the myocardium, the heart muscle, that occurs when one or more of the three coronary arteries that supply oxygenated blood to the heart are occluded (a situation frequently precipitated by the buildup of atheromatic fatty deposits on the arterial walls).[5] The major symptom, from the patient's perspective, is severe, prolonged chest pain. In clinical terms, a recent myocardial infarction is diagnosed when changes occur on electrocardiographic tracings indicating an inversion of T waves, the loss of R wave potentials, and/or the development of Q waves. Other important diagnostic tools include laboratory tests for detecting unusually high levels of serum enzymes, such as glutamic oxalacetic transaminase lactic dehydrogenase,[6] or of CPK isoenzymes.

Although most myocardial infarctions cause significant pain or produce other symptoms that cause them to be *recognized* by the patient, some do not. Myocardial infarctions in this class are *unrecognized* by the patient at the time of their occurrence. In incidence studies, such as the Framingham Heart Study, that rely on physician-initiated (as opposed to patient-initiated) contact between the population at risk for the disease and medical investigators, a significant number of the myocardial infarctions unrecognized at the time of their occurrence are eventually diagnosed. These have often occurred weeks or perhaps months before discovery in examination.

Because of their nature, unrecognized myocardial infarctions do not receive the medical attention nor generate the treatment-related costs characteristic of clinically recognized MIs. In the case of the Framingham study, for instance, approximately 23 percent of the myocardial infarctions that were diagnosed were initially unrecognized and thus would not have received treatment in a population with patient-initiated doctor visits.[7] As a consequence, an estimate of direct treatment costs for the nation that was based on unadjusted Framingham incidence data for myocardial infarction would seriously overestimate the true magnitude of those costs. To avoid such a miscalculation, appropriate downward adjustments have been made in the Framingham incidence rates before formulating national incidence estimates.

Myocardial infarctions frequently lead to death within 30 days of the attack. We have classified these deaths as fatal myocardial infarctions. Patients surviving beyond 30 days are defined as nonfatal MIs. This distinction becomes important in assigning initial and follow-on treatment costs, as well as in determining lost earnings resulting from forgone productivity. Although the proportion of MIs that are fatal varies significantly with age and sex, an overall average computed from the Framingham data indicates that approximately 17 percent of all first myocardial infarctions are fatal.

Sudden Death. A separate incidence category, *sudden death*, is established apart from fatal myocardial infarction to include all deaths that occur within 60 minutes of the heart attack. In most instances, sudden death is caused by a myocardial infarction involving arrhythmias (irregular heart beats) and ventricular fibrillation (severe arrhythmias that significantly limit heart-muscle action).[8] However, it is also defined as a death to which no cause other than coronary heart disease can be attributed and for which no prior history of coronary heart disease, with the possible exception of angina pectoris, is apparent. As the Framingham Heart Study states, a sudden death has occurred

> ...if a subject, apparently well, was observed to have died within a few minutes (operationally documented as under one hour) from onset of symptoms and if the cause of death could not reasonably be attributed on the basis of the full clinical information and the information concerning death to some potentially lethal disease other than coronary heart disease.[9]

Coronary Insufficiency. The third form of heart attack, *coronary insufficiency*, includes cases of coronary heart disease where the symptoms appear to be more severe than those of angina pectoris but less so than those of myocardial infarction. Coronary insufficiency often manifests itself as variable or progressively worsening forms of angina and therefore is frequently alluded to in the medical literature as *unstable angina pectoris*. Coronary insufficiency is diagnosed when a patient experiences prolonged, ischemic chest pain of more than 15 minutes duration that may be accompanied by transient electrocardiographic changes but is not accompanied by serum enzyme changes that are indicative of heart-muscle death.[10] In general, coronary insufficiency is a state in which the coronary circulation is insufficient to meet the full metabolic demands of the heart muscle at rest, yet sufficient to prevent myocardial infarction. Coronary insufficiency is a frequent precursor to myocardial infarction, and its victims, for the most part, receive medical treatment that at least initially resembles that given myocardial infarction patients.

Angina Pectoris Uncomplicated (APU). *Angina pectoris* is the least severe and often the first manifestation of coronary heart disease in an individual. Classically, it is characterized by a brief recurrent chest pain of up to 15 minutes' duration brought on by moderate to severe exertion that is relieved by discontinuance of that activity.[11] The essential determinant of anginal pain is its occurrence with exertion, excitement, or emotional upset— circumstances that increase the pulse rate and the demand of the heart muscle for an increased blood supply. The discomfort of angina diminishes with rest, the administration of nitroglycerin, or other changes enabling a lowering of the pulse rate. The resting electrocardiogram (ECG) of an angina patient is usually normal, although recording the electrocardiogram during exercise often shows abnormalities that confirm the diagnosis of angina.

It is not unusual for chest pains to accompany myocardial infarction or coronary insufficiency or to develop subsequent to either of these conditions. However, *angina pectoris uncomplicated* (APU), our fourth incidence category, is defined to include only those cases of angina pectoris where the patient has not previously experienced other forms of coronary heart disease and did not develop other forms soon after the angina disorder.[12] The restriction of angina pectoris incidence to APU patients is consistent with our objectives to include in the annual incidence totals only those people presenting first instances of coronary heart disease.

Framingham Compared with Other Studies

Although incidence data from the short-term surveillance studies mentioned earlier may not be indicative of nationwide patterns of coronary heart disease, they do, nevertheless, provide useful points of comparison for corresponding data from the Framingham Heart Study. Data from four of these studies were selected for comparison: (1) a 3-year study of coronary heart disease incidence among members of the Health Insurance Plan (HIP) of Metropolitan New York reported by Shapiro et al. (1969), (2) a 1-year study of myocardial infarction and sudden death among residents of Nashville, Tennessee, published by Hagstrom et al. (1971), (3) a 1.5-year study of myocardial infarctions occurring among males in Middlesex County, Connecticut, published by Eisenberg et al. (1961), and (4) a 1-year survey of heart disease incidence in Framingham, Massachusetts, the Framingham Cardiovascular Disease Survey (CVDS), performed by Margolis et al. (1976).

Since short-term surveillance studies typically underestimate the "softer," more subtle end points of coronary heart disease, such as angina pectoris, the comparison of the four short-term studies with the Framingham Heart Study has been limited to two of the "harder" end points of the disease, sudden death and myocardial infarction. Incidence rates for these two disease types derived from data in the five studies are presented in table 3–1. Unfortunately, certain methodological and definitional differences among the short-term studies prevent a rigorous comparison of their results with those of the Framingham study. Despite this, there is still a remarkable order-of-magnitude similarity between the age- and sex-specific findings of Framingham and the findings of each of the other studies. Because of their peculiarities in defining sudden deaths, this similarity is perhaps best seen in the cases of the New York and Nashville studies by combining the sudden death and myocardial infarction categories and comparing the aggregate incidence rates with corresponding rates derived from Framingham. In a similar vein, the MI category of the Middlesex County study already includes sudden deaths and, for this reason, also should be compared with the aggregate sudden death plus MI results of Framingham.

All the short-term studies demonstrate general trends in the epidemiology of heart attacks that are duplicated in the Framingham Heart Study results.

Table 3-1

Annual Incidence Rates per 10,000 Population for Sudden Death and Myocardial Infarction (MI) as Reported in Selected Studies

Author: Locale: Dates of Study:	Shurtleff, 1974 Framingham, Mass. (Framingham Heart Study) 1948–1968		Margolis, 1976 Framingham, Mass. (Framingham CVDS) 1970–1971		Shapiro, 1969 Metropolitan New York (HIP) 1961–1964		Hagstrom, 1971 Nashville, Tenn. 1967–1968		Eisenberg, 1961 Middlesex County, Conn. 1957–1958	
	Sudden Death	*MI*	*Sudden Death*[a]	*MI*[a]	*Sudden Death*[b]	*MI*[b]	*Sudden Death*	*MI*	*Sudden Death*[c]	*MI*[c]
Males										
35–44	3.0	19.0	5.0	18.0	3.1	11.1	5.6	17.0	—	19.0
45–54	10.0	43.0	3.0	34.0	16.1	39.3	14.8	47.6	—	63.0
55–64	27.0	93.0	11.0	63.0	34.6	59.3	48.3	85.6	—	140.0
65–74	13.0	116.0	11.0	140.0	—	—	54.3	108.7	—	—
All ages	11.0	49.0	6.0	43.0	16.7	35.1	23.1	51.8	—	64.0
Females										
35–44	0.0	2.0	0.0	5.0	0.0	0.7	2.6	2.0	—	—
45–54	2.0	8.0	0.0	20.0	2.8	4.0	4.6	11.2	—	—
55–64	4.0	18.0	10.0	5.0	9.0	17.8	15.4	25.5	—	—
65–74	14.0	34.0	13.0	39.0	—	—	19.7	56.5	—	—
All ages	3.0	11.0	4.0	14.0	3.5	6.5	8.4	17.7	—	—
Comments:	First attacks only; unrecognized MIs included.		First attacks only; some unrecognized MIs included.		First attacks only; study based on definite and possible MIs; *sudden death within 48 hours;* some unrecognized MIs included; only ages 35–64 surveyed.		First and subsequent attacks included; *sudden death defined as death within 24 hours.*		First attacks among white males only; study based on definite and probable MIs; *MI category includes sudden deaths;* only ages 35–64 surveyed.	

[a] Abstracted from James R. Margolis, Richard F. Gillum, Manning Feinleib, Robert C. Brasch, and Richard R. Fabsitz, Community surveillance for coronary heart disease: The Framingham cardiovascular survey. Comparisons with the Framingham heart study and previous short-term studies, *American Journal of Cardiology* 37(1): 63, 1976 (Table 1). Reprinted with permission.

[b] Abstracted from Sam Shapiro, Eve Weinblatt, Charles W. Frank, and Robert V. Sager, Incidence of coronary heart disease in a population insured for medical care (HIP). Part II, *American Journal of Public Health* 59(6): 9, 1969 (Table 1). Reprinted with permission.

[c] Abstracted from Henry Eisenberg, William R. Feltner, Gerald H. Payne, and Charles A. Haddad, The epidemiology of coronary heart disease in Middlesex County, Connecticut, *Journal of Chronic Diseases* 14(2): 230, 1961 (Table II). Reprinted with permission of Pergamon Press, Ltd.

Each study shows that the incidence rates for sudden death and myocardial infarction increase significantly with age and, with few exceptions, are markedly higher for males than females. In addition, the incidence of sudden death, which represents rapidly fatal heart attacks, is consistently less than the incidence of myocardial infarction, which represents attacks that are predominately nonfatal in the short run. These similarities between Framingham and the other studies corroborate the representative nature of the Framingham results and further justify their use in developing national incidence estimates.

One possible drawback in using the Framingham data stems from the underrepresentation of minorities in the town, where only 1 percent of the residential population is black.[13] Epidemiological indications of possible racial differences in incidence rates derive from such local studies as the Nashville study mentioned earlier and a 7-year follow-up study published by Cassel et al. (1971) on the incidence of coronary heart disease in Evans County, Georgia. These differences, however, are far from consistent for the two sexes or across different diagnostic categories. The Nashville findings, for instance, indicate that white men had a higher incidence of myocardial infarction than black men, but there was no difference in the incidence of sudden death between black and white men. However, while there was no apparent difference in the incidence of myocardial infarction between white and black women, black women appeared to have a slightly higher incidence of sudden death. The Evans County study indicated only minor differences in the incidence of coronary heart disease between black and white women, but did find that the incidence of the disease was lower for black than white men in every occupational category except rural sharecropper. This finding suggests that physical activity rather than genetic racial factors are primarily responsible for the observed differences in incidence—since only as share-croppers did whites engage in as demanding physical labor as did blacks.

In sum, the evidence for systematic racial differences in incidence rates seems fragmentary at best and does not justify deriving race-specific incidence-rate estimates. Also supporting this conclusion is the analysis by Gordon and Garst of National Health Survey data on the prevalence of coronary heart disease.[14] They reported little apparent racial differences on a national level in the age- and sex-specific prevalence rates for adults. These data indicate, moreover, that the Framingham sample, despite its under-representation of blacks, is an adequate basis for estimating national incidence rates.

Declining Incidence

As in the case of stroke (see chapter 4), the decline in annual deaths resulting from coronary heart disease in the United States has progressed from being regarded as a possible statistical quirk to being generally accepted as incontrovertible. Unlike stroke, however, there are no extensive data enabling a direct measurement of the role of falling incidence in the mortality decline. Stern (1979) indeed comments that at present there is little if any information on what is occurring concerning the incidence of new coronary heart disease events. Between 1968 and 1976, the age-adjusted decline in coronary heart disease mortality amounted to 20.7 percent. Transitions between the sixth, seventh, and eighth revisions of the International Classification of Diseases, Adopted Code make it impossible to obtain precise numerical estimates of comparable CHD mortality in earlier years. Nevertheless, the general trends seem to have been rising age-adjusted mortality between 1949 and 1957, followed by a more gradual and diminishing rate of increase between 1957 and 1968 (judgment based on data in Stern, 1979).

A number of explanations have been put forward for the drop in coronary heart disease mortality and include (1) the absence of a major influenza epidemic in the United States since 1968, (2) dietary trends (the proportion of cholesterol in the average American diet having declined by 11 percent since the late 1950s), (3) reduced smoking, (4) increased exercise, (5) improved control of hypertension, (6) the increased use of coronary-care units, (7) improved emergency medical services, and (8) coronary artery bypass graft surgery (Stern, 1979). The first five factors would constitute primary prevention of CHD and might well be responsible for declines in incidence as well as in mortality. The known relationships between many of these factors and incidence support the supposition that incidence has indeed declined. The sixth through eighth factors would constitute secondary prevention measures and would lower mortality without affecting incidence.

The analytic dilemma we faced was how to estimate incidence decline in recent years without firm data. We decided to take a middle road and assume that age-adjusted incidence rates in 1975 were 10 percent lower than those observed in the Framingham study between 1948 and 1968. A person believing that secondary prevention is primarily responsible for the decline in mortality would argue that we are making too large an adjustment to the Framingham data; another, emphasizing the role of primary prevention and perhaps drawing parallels from the observed trends in stroke incidence, would argue that our adjustment is too small.

Calculation of National Incidence Estimates

Using Framingham data—adjusted for the 10 percent decrease just mentioned—incidence rates disaggregated by age and sex have been computed for each of the four subcategories of coronary heart disease. Estimates were first made for males and females in five age groups: 35 to 44,

45 to 54, 55 to 64, 65 to 74, and 75 and above. Because of the small size of the Framingham population at risk over 75, incidence rates for this age group were assumed equal to the corresponding rates for people aged 65 to 74.[15]

Heart disease among those under 35 is relatively rare and not addressed by the Framingham study. To extend the Framingham data to the age groups under 35, two sets of mortality/survival data were used: (1) national mortality statistics (from NCHS, 1978) on the number of people in different age groups who died from CHD in 1975, and (2) our best estimates of the survival rates following CHD incidence for those in the under-35 age groups. As a best gauge for survival following incidence for people in the under-35 groups, we assumed that year-by-year mortality patterns would be similar to those observed in the Framingham sample for the next youngest age groups providing adequate data for accurate estimates of survival. For men, these survival rates were observed for initial MIs between 35 and 54; for women, between 35 and 64.

The survival-rate figures enabled us to estimate the proportion of persons with initial CHD incident below the age of 15 who would die in each of the next two age intervals (that is, 15 to 24 years and 25 to 34 years). The process was repeated for incident CHD in each of the next two intervals. These calculations together with the national data on the number of deaths from CHD in 1975 led to the estimates that CHD annual mortality rates for people 0 to 14 years of age were 0.14 percent of those for people between 35 and 44, that mortality for people between 15 and 24 was 0.79 percent of that for people between 35 and 44, and that mortality for people between 25 and 34 was 12.4 percent of that observed between 35 and 44. We further assumed that incidence patterns paralleled mortality patterns across these age groups (that is, that the annual incidence rate of CHD under 15 was 0.14 percent of that between 35 and 44, and so on).

A final adjustment was necessary owing to the absence of sudden deaths for women under 45 in the Framingham sample. This seemed to result from the inability of the limited sample to reflect accurately the frequency of rare events. To estimate female sudden deaths in these age groups, we presumed that the ratio of sudden deaths to myocardial infarctions within each younger age group was the same as the ratio in the age group 45 to 54.

We sought to use the most recent available data in estimating incidence rates. For myocardial infarction, sudden death, and angina pectoris uncomplicated, the rates reflect the Framingham 16-year follow-up data. For coronary insufficiency, 14-year follow-up data were available for the 35 to 44 age group and 18-year follow-up data for each of the other age groups. Incidence rates based on this information and on the calculations described are presented for the Framingham population free of coronary heart disease in the first four columns of table 3–2. To convert these rates to analogous incidence rates for the U.S. general population, the Framingham rates were

Table 3-2

Annual Incidence Rates of Coronary Heart Disease for Framingham Population Free of Coronary Heart Disease and for U.S. Population

	Annual Incidence Rate per 10,000 for Framingham Population Free of CHD				Estimated Annual Incidence Rate per 10,000 for U.S. General Population[c]			
	Sudden Death[a]	MI (Recognized)[a]	CI[b]	APU[a]	Sudden Death	MI (Recognized)	CI	APU
Males								
0–14	0.004	0.02	0.01	0.01	0.004	0.02	0.01	0.01
15–24	0.02	0.10	0.06	0.06	0.02	0.10	0.06	0.06
25–34	0.34	1.6	1.0	0.89	0.34	1.6	1.0	0.89
35–44	2.7	13.1	8.1	7.2	2.7	13.1	8.1	7.2
45–54	9.0	29.8	9.9	24.3	8.8	29.1	9.6	23.1
55–64	24.3	64.4	9.9	67.5	23.9	63.2	9.7	64.3
65–74	11.7	80.4	17.1	50.4	11.2	76.4	16.3	45.5
75+	11.7	80.4	17.1	50.4	11.3	77.1	16.4	45.5
Females								
0–14	0.001	0.002	0.001	0.005	0.001	0.002	0.001	0.005
15–24	0.003	0.01	0.007	0.03	0.003	0.01	0.007	0.03
25–34	0.05	0.17	0.11	0.45	0.05	0.17	0.11	0.45
35–44	0.44	1.3	0.90	3.6	0.44	1.3	0.90	3.6
45–54	1.8	5.6	2.7	13.5	1.8	5.5	2.7	13.2
55–64	3.6	12.5	11.7	52.2	3.6	12.4	11.6	51.0
65–74	12.6	23.6	9.9	58.5	12.1	22.7	9.5	54.1
75+	12.6	23.6	9.9	58.5	12.2	22.9	9.5	54.1

[a]Computed from data in the Framingham Heart Study, Section 26, as cited in Margolis et al. (1976, Table 1, p. 63). Original incidence rates for myocardial infarction (MI) have been multiplied by 0.77 to eliminate the estimated 23 percent of MIs that are unrecognized. See text for description of methods used to adjust for declining incidence and to calculate incidence rates for the younger age groups.

[b]Computed from data in the Framingham Heart Study, Section 6, Table 6–5, and Section 30, Table 4–1.

[c]Incidence rates for the U.S. general population have been estimated from analogous rates for the Framingham population free of coronary heart disease by multiplying the Framingham rates by the proportion of the national population free of coronary heart disease (in the case of MI, CI, and sudden-death rates, from national CHD prevalence data presented in Wilder (1974) and Gordon and Garst (1965). Proportionality factors for each age and sex cohort have been developed by multiplying by the proportion of the national population free of heart attack). These factors range in value from a low of 0.904 for men 65 years of age and older to a high of about 1.000 for men and women under the age of 45.

Table 3–3
Annual Incidence of Coronary Heart Disease, by Age, Sex, and Diagnostic Type, United States, 1975

	1975 U.S. Population[a] (Thousands)	Sudden Death		MI (Recognized)	
		Incidence Rate per 10,000[b]	Total Incidence	Incidence Rate per 10,000[b]	Total Incidence
Males					
0–14	27,365	0.004	10	0.02	50
15–24	20,356	0.02	43	0.10	211
25–34	15,356	0.34	515	1.6	2,506
35–44	11,153	2.7	3,011	13.1	14,655
45–54	11,492	8.8	10,135	29.1	33,404
55–64	9,344	23.9	22,288	63.2	59,042
65–74	6,027	11.2	6,726	76.4	46,052
75+	3,145	11.3	3,538	77.1	24,257
Total	104,238	4.4	46,266	17.3	180,177
Females					
0–14	26,284	0.001	2	0.002	5
15–24	19,913	0.003	7	0.01	21
25–34	15,581	0.05	86	0.17	261
35–44	11,671	0.44	517	1.3	1,576
45–54	12,280	1.8	2,210	5.5	6,742
55–64	10,434	3.6	3,757	12.4	12,960
65–74	7,847	12.1	9,534	22.7	17,797
75+	5,383	12.2	6,588	22.9	12,303
Total	109,393	2.1	22,701	4.7	51,665
Total population	213,631	3.2	68,967	10.9	231,842

[a]From *Current Population Reports*, Series P-25, Number 614.

[b]Calculated from data in Framingham Heart Study, Sections 6, 26, and 30, by methods described in text.

multiplied, in the case of APU, by estimates of the proportion of the national population free of all forms of coronary heart disease and, in the case of myocardial infarction, coronary insufficiency, and sudden death, by the proportion of the national population free of heart attack.[16] Rates for the general population are displayed in the last four columns of table 3–2. These rates were then applied, as shown in table 3–3, to the 1975 U.S. population to produce an estimated number of first cases of coronary heart disease in each age, sex, and diagnostic group. The estimated total number of cases in 1975 is 659,926, of which 231,842 are myocardial infarctions, 68,967 are sudden deaths, 75,151 are occurrences of coronary insufficiency, and 283,966 are occurrences of angina pectoris uncomplicated.

CI		APU		Total CHD	
Incidence Rate per 10,000[b]	Total Incidence	Incidence Rate per 10,000[b]	Total Incidence	Incidence Rate per 10,000[b]	Total Incidence
0.01	31	0.01	28	0.044	119
0.06	130	0.06	116	0.24	500
1.0	1,545	0.89	1,373	3.87	5,959
8.1	9,034	7.2	8,030	31.1	34,730
9.6	11,066	23.1	26,579	70.6	81,184
9.7	9,083	64.3	60,051	161.0	150,464
16.3	9,818	45.5	27,447	149.4	90,043
16.4	5,152	45.5	14,322	150.3	47,269
4.4	45,859	13.2	137,946	39.4	410,248
0.001	3	0.005	13	0.009	23
0.007	14	0.03	57	0.050	99
0.11	174	0.45	697	0.78	1,218
0.90	1,050	3.6	4,202	6.29	7,345
2.7	3,316	13.2	16,246	23.2	28,514
11.6	12,115	51.0	53,250	78.7	82,082
9.5	7,486	54.1	42,444	98.5	77,261
9.5	5,134	54.1	29,111	98.7	53,136
2.7	29,292	13.3	146,020	22.8	249,678
3.5	75,151	13.3	283,966	30.9	659,926

Summary of Incidence Results

The annual incidence results displayed in table 3–3 reflect several trends indicative of the epidemiology of coronary heart disease. Four of the more important trends are

1. Regardless of diagnostic type, coronary heart disease is significantly more common in men than in women. The likelihood of sudden death, myocardial infarction, or coronary insufficiency is 1.8 to 4 times greater for males than for females. Men also seem to be at slightly greater risk for angina pectoris uncomplicated.

2. The chief manifestation of coronary heart disease in men is myocardial infarction, which accounts for 44 percent of presenting com-

plaints. Next in frequency are angina pectoris uncomplicated (34 percent) and sudden death (11 percent). In women, the presentation pattern is different. The major manifestation is angina pectoris uncomplicated, which accounts for 58 percent of presenting complaints, followed at a distance by myocardial infarction (21 percent). In fact, the incidence of APU in women is so large that women account for the majority (51.5 percent) of total APU incidence.

3. For both sexes and most diagnostic types, incidence increases sharply with age up to 65 and, in some instances, to 75. The majority of all incidence cases (59 percent) occur in people under the age of 65—with striking differences between the sexes. Nearly two-thirds (66 percent) of the incident events among males occur before the age of 65, while less than one-half of those for females occur in these younger ages. The overall age distribution characterizes coronary heart disease as a condition initially affecting people of middle and middle-to-old age, in contrast to other chronic diseases, such as cancer or stroke, which predominantly affect older people.

4. An analysis of all heart attacks incident in 1975 reveals their high immediate mortality. Over 10 percent of all first coronary events are sudden deaths. One-month mortality from first coronary events (sudden deaths plus MIs fatal within 1 month) is roughly 15 percent. These proportions are nearly doubled when APU is excluded.

Mortality and Life Expectancy

Available Data

On average, patients with coronary heart disease have higher mortality rates and lower life expectancies than individuals of similar age and sex in the general population. Specific mortality rates and survival patterns vary depending on the severity of the disease and the situation. Some individuals—sudden death victims—die before receiving any medical attention; others—patients suffering fatal myocardial infarctions—die in the hospital; and still others die months or years later. Data from the Framingham Heart Study indicate that about 30 percent of patients suffering a first heart attack die as a direct result of the attack. Approximately half the survivors have recurrences within 8 years. Second attacks are fatal in approximately 50 percent of the cases. For the group as a whole, however, mortality appears to be highest during the immediate post-heart-attack period—the first 24 hours—and then gradually tapers off.[17] In comparison with stroke victims, death tends to follow the initial heart attack much more rapidly than it does the cerebrovascular accident.

Mortality for first heart attack survivors substantially exceeds that of demographically matched populations for a considerable period after the attack (our own calculations from raw data indicate that this time is at least 6 years for males and females 65 years of age and older, 8 years for females under 65, and 13 years for males under 65). Although the excess mortality of heart attack survivors is not due to coronary heart disease exclusively, the principal cause of their future deaths is linked to their higher risk for subsequent fatal attacks. For this reason, there is little practical need to differentiate between the mortality associated with initial heart attacks and that associated with other complicating conditions (for example, subsequent strokes or congestive heart failures). Even if there were, such a procedure lies beyond current epidemiological capability. Our approach here will be simply to associate all mortality in excess of that for matched populations with the initial heart attack.

For our purposes, the most representative and most useful survival statistics come from population-based studies. These avoid the problems of selectivity biases associated with hospital-based studies or studies that select patients exclusively from participants in group medical plans. The population study used in estimating incidence—the Framingham Heart Study—also has followed its disease population over time and has reported survival by age, sex, and type of coronary heart disease. Our survival rates are derived from the results of this study. As we will show, these rates are remarkably consistent with similar results derived from data in other (not all population-based) studies of coronary heart disease patients.

Determinants of Mortality in Heart Attack Patients

Various studies—Framingham Heart Study, Weinblatt (1968), Pell and D'Alonzo (1964), and Fulton (1969)—all indicate that mortality following a heart attack worsens as age increases. In general, older heart attack patients compare less favorably with matched persons in the general population than do younger patients. Furthermore, an analysis of selected data from the Framingham study indicates that if one considers annual mortality rates, this trend is more pronounced for males than for females.

The type and severity of the heart attack affect survival. For example, the most severe form of the heart attack—sudden death—results in virtually instantaneous fatalities. However, the majority of patients suffering a first myocardial infarction do not suffer immediate death. Those patients, nevertheless, have life expectancies markedly shorter than those for the general population. Moreover, most epidemiologists of coronary heart disease believe that patients experiencing a first coronary insufficiency have the same general survival prognosis as patients suffering a first myocardial infarction and surviving at least the first 30 days (nonfatal MIs). The primary reason for this similarity lies in the relatively equivalent likelihood of each class of patient suffering future, fatal MIs. As indicated earlier, mortality following a second or subsequent heart attack is greater than that following a first attack.

Mortality in the Framingham Heart Study

The population-based study from Framingham reports survival data by age, sex, and type of coronary heart disease, enabling us to disaggregate the heart disease survival population along these dimensions. Data from the Framingham study on survival of heart disease victims as of the 20-year follow-up are available for victims of two forms of disease: myocardial infarction (exclusive of sudden death) and angina pectoris uncomplicated. The data are presented for men and women aged 35 to 74 by 5-year age groups and those aged 75 and over. Information on the numbers in groups having coronary heart disease and still alive at the beginning of each postattack interval, the numbers dying of any cause during the interval, and numbers withdrawing for lack of further follow-up time at 20 years (there were assumed to be no other losses owing to follow-up) were presented for each of the preceding age, sex, and diagnostic groups. For myocardial infarctions, all intervals but the first were single years. The first interval was broken into two subintervals, one encompassing the first 30 days following the attack and the other the period from 30 days to 1 year after the attack. For patients with angina pectoris uncomplicated, all intervals were single years.

Grouping Myocardial Infarction Patients by Age and Sex

As table 3–4 shows, the number of individuals in the population at risk suffering first myocardial infarctions is relatively small for certain 5-year age groups. This is especially true of women under the age of 50 and of both men and women over 75. While these sample sizes were adequate for reasonably accurate calculation of age- and sex-specific incidence rates, they are insufficient for precise determination of annual survival probabilities. To increase the group sizes—and thereby obtain more reliable age- and sex-specific survival rates—the data have been aggregated into broader age groups. For men, the enlarged age groups are 35 to 54 years, 55 to 64 years, and 65 years and older. These groups contain 75, 101, and 60 patients, respectively. For women, the age groups are 35 to 64 years and 65 years and older. They contain 45 and 36 patients, respectively.

Table 3–4

Distribution of First Myocardial Infarctions, by Age and Sex, Framingham Heart Study

Age at Diagnosis	Number Experiencing a First MI			
	Males		Females	
35–39	3		0	
40–44	13	} 75	2	
45–49	33		3	} 45
50–54	26		10	
55–59	50		12	
60–64	51	} 101	18	
65–69	33		17	
70–74	19	} 60	16	} 36
75+	8		3	
	236		81	

Source: Framingham Heart Study, Section 32, Tables II-8 and II-13.

Calculation of Survival Rates for
Myocardial Infarction Patients

Survival data on myocardial infarction patients from the Framingham study are presented by age and sex in the left section of tables 3–5 and 3–6. The age-at-diagnosis breakdowns used in the tables reflect the aggregation process discussed earlier.

Cumulative probabilities of survival for patients in each age and sex group have been computed in the standard manner. Both the methodology and the resulting probabilities are described in the right section of tables 3–5 and 3–6. As these tables show, patients surviving a first MI have a high mortality rate during the first year following their attacks and a still higher mortality rate during the first 30 days (reflecting the significant incidence of postattack, inhospital deaths). In addition, half the males aged 35 to 64 surviving initial attacks die within roughly 12 years. Half the female survivors under 65 die within 8 years. Of individuals aged 65 or older at the initial event, half will die within 5 or 6 years. The diminishing survivor groups shrink sample sizes and have led us to limit our calculations of survival rates to 13 years for males under 64, 8 years for females under 65, and 6 years for people 65 or older.

To calculate indirect and some direct costs, survival probabilities to age 99 are needed. Survival beyond the last interval in tables 3–5 and 3–6 is accordingly assumed to follow the conditional probabilities of survival for the U.S. general population. Thus, for males with myocardial infarction at age

40, the survival rates presented in table 3–6 are assumed to apply until age 53. Life tables then indicate the probability of surviving from 53 to 54 to be 0.9881. The probability that a 40-year-old male would survive for 14 years after a myocardial infarction is thus estimated to be 0.9881 × 0.4688, or 0.4632. Unique life tables, from age at myocardial infarction incidence to 99, have been generated in this way for all age groups and both sexes. Each of these life tables also has been considered representative of the survival experience of coronary insufficiency patients of corresponding age and sex. (Specifically, the portion of each of these life tables covering the period beyond the first 30 days after the attack is considered representative of the CI survival experience.) Survival of patients under 35 is assumed to mimic the patterns in tables 3–5 and 3–6 for the next older age groups for the periods indicated in the tables. Thereafter, survival is presumed to revert to that of

Table 3–5
Survival Data and Life Table for Females, Based on the Framingham Heart Study Data for Myocardial Infarction Patients

Age at Diagnosis	I^a	L^b	D^c	W^d	L^{*e}	Q^f	P^g	CP^h
35–64	0–30 days	45	6	0	45	0.133	0.867	0.867
	30 days–1 year	39	3	0	39	0.077	0.923	0.800
	1–2 years	36	2	1	35.5	0.056	0.944	0.755
	2–3 years	33	2	2	32	0.062	0.937	0.708
	3–4 years	29	2	2	28	0.071	0.929	0.657
	4–5 years	25	2	2	24	0.083	0.917	0.602
	5–6 years	21	1	1	20.5	0.049	0.951	0.573
	6–7 years	19	2	3	17.5	0.114	0.886	0.508
	7–8 years	14	2	1	13.5	0.148	0.852	0.432
65+	0–30 days	36	10	0	36	0.278	0.722	0.722
	30 days–1 year	26	0	0	26	0	1.000	0.722
	1–2 years	26	0	3	24.5	0	1.000	0.706^i
	2–3 years	23	1	0	23	0.043	0.956	0.691
	3–4 years	22	2	5	19.5	0.103	0.897	0.620
	4–5 years	15	0	3	13.5	0	1.000	0.590^i
	5–6 years	12	1	3	10.5	0.095	0.905	0.561

Source: Computed from data in the Framingham Heart Study, Section 32, Tables II-8 and II-13.

[a]Time interval past disease onset.
[b]Number alive at beginning of interval.
[c]Number dying during interval.
[d]Number withdrawn at end of interval.
[e]Adjusted number at risk = $L - W/2$.
[f]Probability of dying during interval = D/L^*.
[g]Probability of surviving interval = $1 - Q$.
[h]Cumulative probability of survival, $CP_n = P_1 \cdot P_2 \cdots P_n$.
[i]These CP estimates are derived by using linear interpolation.

the general population. Epidemiological proof that survival patterns of heart attack patients revert to those of the general population at specific times following incidence does not yet exist. However, the experts we questioned on this point felt that our assumptions represented a reasonable first approximation.

Table 3–6
Survival Data and Life Table for Males, Based on the Framingham Heart Study Data for Myocardial Infarction Patients

Age at Diagnosis	I[a]	L	D	W	L*	Q	P	CP
35–54	0–30 days	75	3	0	75	0.040	0.960	0.960
	30 days–1 year	72	3	0	72	0.042	0.958	0.920
	1–2 years	69	1	0	69	0.014	0.985	0.907
	2–3 years	68	1	4	66	0.015	0.985	0.893
	3–4 years	63	2	2	62	0.032	0.968	0.864
	4–5 years	59	4	2	58	0.069	0.931	0.804
	5–6 years	53	2	2	52	0.038	0.961	0.774
	6–7 years	49	4	4	47	0.085	0.915	0.708
	7–8 years	41	3	0	41	0.073	0.927	0.656
	8–9 years	38	1	12	32	0.031	0.969	0.635
	9–10 years	25	2	4	23	0.087	0.913	0.580
	10–11 years	19	1	2	18	0.056	0.944	0.548
	11–12 years	16	1	2	15	0.067	0.933	0.511
	12–13 years	13	1	2	12	0.083	0.917	0.469
55–64	0–30 days	101	12	0	101	0.119	0.881	0.881
	30 days–1 year	89	3	0	89	0.034	0.966	0.851
	1–2 years	86	3	0	86	0.035	0.965	0.822
	2–3 years	83	5	0	83	0.060	0.940	0.772
	3–4 years	78	4	2	77	0.052	0.948	0.732
	4–5 years	72	6	5	70	0.086	0.914	0.669
	5–6 years	61	3	2	60	0.050	0.950	0.635
	6–7 years	56	3	5	53.5	0.056	0.944	0.600
	7–8 years	48	1	4	46	0.022	0.978	0.586
	8–9 years	43	2	1	42.5	0.047	0.953	0.559
	9–10 years	40	2	6	37	0.054	0.946	0.529
	10–11 years	32	3	4	30	0.100	0.900	0.476
	11–12 years	25	1	2	24	0.042	0.958	0.456
	12–13 years	22	2	3	20.5	0.098	0.902	0.411
65+	0–30 days	60	16	0	60	0.267	0.733	0.733
	30 days–1 year	44	3	1	43.5	0.069	0.931	0.683
	1–2 years	40	3	3	38.5	0.078	0.922	0.629
	2–3 years	34	3	6	31	0.097	0.903	0.568
	3–4 years	25	4	3	23.5	0.170	0.830	0.471
	4–5 years	18	0	2	17	0	1.000	0.454[b]
	5–6 years	16	1	5	13.5	0.074	0.926	0.436

Source: Computed from data in the Framingham Heart Study, Section 32, Tables II-8 and II-13.
[a]Symbols I, L, D, W, $L*$, Q, P, and CP are as defined in table 3–5.
[b]This CP estimate is derived by using linear interpolation.

Framingham Compared with
Other Mortality/Survival Studies

Little's study (1967) of male Canadian heart attack victims found that approximately 25 percent experienced sudden death, 20 percent died inhospital (and thus corresponded broadly with our category of fatal myocardial infarctions), and 15 percent of the hospital survivors died within 1 year of the attack. By aggregating mortality data on men experiencing either sudden deaths or myocardial infarctions in the Framingham sample, the two studies may be directly compared. The cumulative probabilities of survival for 1 hour, 30 days, and 1 year following the attack are presented below for both studies:

Time after Attack	Little (1967)	Framingham Heart Study
1 hour	0.750	0.739
30 days	0.563	0.621
1 year	0.478	0.598

Over the short run, the survival experiences of patients in the two studies appear similar. Little's data did not permit a comparison of survival rates beyond the first year after the attack.

Selected data gathered recently by McNeer (1975) on a group of 522 male patients hospitalized with acute myocardial infarctions provide another comparison with the Framingham results. McNeer's sample was drawn from individuals treated at the Duke Medical Center Coronary Care Unit. He determined that, of the patients treated in the coronary-care unit who survived 4 days, 87 percent would survive 6 months. Although the Framingham data permitted the direct calculation of short-term survival probabilities for only 1 hour, 30 days, and 1 year past attack, interpolation procedures yielded estimates of the probabilities of surviving intermediate periods. We calculated that the average Framingham patient had a 0.722 chance of surviving 4 days and a 0.611 chance of surviving 6 months. Consequently, the conditional probability of a male patient in the Framingham sample surviving 6 months, given that he survives 4 days, is estimated to be $0.611 \div 0.722$, or 0.846. This estimate is consistent with McNeer's result of 0.870 and further argues for the general representativeness of the Framingham mortality/survival experience.

Weinblatt's (1968) frequently cited study of heart attack survival reported the experiences of 881 male patients insured by the Health Insurance Plan (HIP) of New York. This study provides survival data disaggregated by the age of the patient at the time of the attack. Selected survival rates based on these data are compared in table 3–7 with similar

Table 3–7
Survival Probabilities from the Weinblatt and Framingham Heart Studies, by Age, for Male Heart Attack Patients

Time After Initial Attack	Males Aged 45–54		Males Aged 55–64		Males All Ages[b]	
	Weinblatt	FHS	Weinblatt	FHS	Weinblatt	FHS
1 hour	—	0.761	—	0.686	—	0.739
1 day	0.722	—	0.650	—	0.692	—
1 month	0.692	0.732	0.579	0.585	0.640	0.621
1 year	0.666[a] ·	0.704	0.553[a]	0.568	0.615[a]	0.598
2 years	0.639[a]	0.690	0.526[a]	0.551	0.588[a]	0.575
3 years	0.611[a]	0.676	0.498[a]	0.525	0.561[a]	0.547
4 years	0.583[a]	0.646	0.470[a]	0.500	0.534[a]	0.511
4.5 years	0.569	0.630[a]	0.456	0.478[a]	0.521	0.494[a]
5 years	—	0.614	—	0.455	—	0.477

Source: Computed from data in the Framingham Heart Study, Section 32, Tables II-8 and II-17; and Weinblatt (1968).

[a]Estimated by linear interpolation.

[b]Includes patients younger than 45 years and older than 64 years.

rates developed from the Framingham data. The table shows a reasonable similarity of survival experiences across the two studies with closest correspondence between the studies for male heart attack patients aged 55 to 64 (the 10-year age group with the highest incidence).

Pell and D'Alonzo (1964), using a sample of 1331 male myocardial infarction patients who were employees of E.I. duPont de Nemours and Company, found that the 5-year survival rate for patients who lived at least 30 days was 0.740. The 95 percent confidence interval surrounding this estimate was 0.700 to 0.780. This interval brackets a corresponding 5-year survival rate of 0.768 derived from the Framingham data. An analysis of intermediate-term survival rates, conditional on the male myocardial infarction patient surviving at least 30 days, shows essential consistency across the Weinblatt, Pell and D'Alonzo, and Framingham studies. A comparison of survival rates among the three studies is presented in table 3–8.

These limited comparisons of the Framingham mortality data with other studies have revealed no fundamental inconsistencies. All studies reviewed that presented short-term survival data substantiated the high initial mortality rates found among heart attack patients in the Framingham study. Those studies which considered survival experiences past 1 year also were in basic agreement with Framingham. Age-specific mortality data were presented in the Weinblatt (1968) study, showing generally close agreement. Another study providing not only age- but sex-specific short-term survival data was conducted in Edinburgh, England in 1967 (Fulton, 1969). Although a

Table 3–8
Comparison of Survival Rates among Three Studies

Time after Initial Attack	MI Survival Rate Conditional on Surviving 30 Days		
	Weinblatt[a]	*Pell and D'Alonzo*	*Framingham*[a]
1 year	0.961	0.905	0.963
2 years	0.919	0.868	0.926
3 years	0.877	0.818	0.881
4 years	0.834	0.778	0.823
4.5 years	0.814	0.759	0.796
5 years	0.802	0.740	0.768

[a]Estimated from data in table 3–7.

detailed comparison of the two studies was not feasible, a broad consistency was found between the Edinburgh and Framingham results.

Survival of Angina Pectoris Uncomplicated (APU) Patients

By definition, no short-term deaths are caused by angina pectoris alone. APU patients do, however, experience a lower life expectancy relative to age- and sex-matched individuals in the general population. As for transient ischemic attacks in cerebrovascular disease, we have ascribed these reductions to the subsequent more serious conditions suffered by these patients. (APU patients do experience a higher likelihood of developing more severe forms of coronary heart disease than their age- and sex-matched peers in the general population.) This process enables us to avoid double counting of the lowered life expectancy by counting, for instance, the lowered life expectancy resulting from APU first, and then that from subsequent fatal MIs or strokes.

With this perspective in mind, we have developed two types of life tables based on the Framingham data for APU patients. The first, presented in table 3–9, is a standard life table that presents cumulative probabilities of survival for a period of 10 years past incidence. The second, presented in table 3–10, is a unique life table since the end point D described in the table involves either death, the occurrence of a heart attack, or the occurrence of both events together. For our purposes, the latter life table is more significant because it enables us to avoid the problem of double counting when estimating the long-run direct costs associated with coronary heart disease. If, in our study, an APU patient has a heart attack in the future, he is no longer considered part of the APU population, but rather is counted in the

Table 3–9
Life Tables Based on the Framingham Heart Study Data for Patients with Angina Pectoris Uncomplicated

		I[a]	L	D	W	L^*	Q	P	CP
Males, all ages	0–1 year	126	4	0	126	0.032	0.968	0.968
	1–2 years	122	4	11	117.5	0.051	0.949	0.919
	2–3 years	107	3	4	105	0.029	0.971	0.893
	3–4 years	100	3	4	98	0.031	0.969	0.865
	4–5 years	93	4	11	87.5	0.046	0.954	0.826
	5–6 years	78	4	4	76	0.053	0.947	0.782
	6–7 years	70	5	7	66.5	0.075	0.925	0.723
	7–8 years	58	4	4	56	0.071	0.929	0.672
	8–9 years	50	3	5	47.5	0.063	0.937	0.629
	9–10 years	42	4	5	39.5	0.101	0.899	0.566
Females, all ages	0–1 year	141	3	0	141	0.021	0.979	0.979
	1–2 years	138	4	15	130.5	0.031	0.969	0.949
	2–3 years	119	2	10	114	0.017	0.982	0.932
	3–4 years	107	3	5	104.5	0.029	0.971	0.905
	4–5 years	99	2	7	95.5	0.021	0.979	0.886
	5–6 years	90	1	4	88	0.011	0.989	0.876
	6–7 years	85	1	8	81	0.012	0.988	0.865
	7–8 years	76	4	7	72.5	0.055	0.945	0.818
	8–9 years	65	0	7	61.5	0	1.000	0.810[b]
	9–10 years	58	1	7	54.5	0.018	0.982	0.803

Source: Computed from data in the Framingham Heart Study, Section 32, Table II-1.
[a]Symbols I, L, D, W, L^*, Q, P, and CP are as defined in table 3–5.
[b]This CP estimate is derived by using linear interpolation.

incidence population of heart attacks in that future year. We assume that he would stop generating the annual costs associated with angina pectoris and would start generating costs characteristic of heart attack patients. The use of a life table for APU patients with multiple end-point events (that is, death or heart attack) ensures that the stream of APU-specific costs is truncated at the appropriate time.

In tables 3–9 and 3–10, the cumulative probabilities for patients of each sex are not disaggregated by age at diagnosis. As a result, we expect that the probability values in the tables will prove to be slight overestimates for the older and slight underestimates for the younger APU patients. This inaccuracy should not be serious, since in disaggregating by age, 10-year survival experience is found to be more or less the same for younger and older patients. Furthermore, after the first 10 years, age-specific information is incorporated by assuming that patients who survive this period will experience the same conditional annual survival rates as their age- and sex-matched peers in the general population.[18]

Table 3–10
Life Tables Based on the Framingham Heart Study Data for Patients with Angina Pectoris Uncomplicated, Where the End Point Involves Death or Heart Attack

	I [a]	L [b]	D [c]	W [a]	$L*$ [d]	Q [e]	P [f]	CP [g]
Males, all ages 0–1 year	126	6	2	125	0.048	0.952	0.952
1–2 years	118	7	9	113.5	0.062	0.938	0.893
2–3 years	102	8	4	100	0.080	0.920	0.822
3–4 years	90	4	4	88	0.045	0.954	0.784
4–5 years	82	6	9	77.5	0.077	0.923	0.724
5–6 years	67	4	4	65	0.061	0.938	0.679
6–7 years	59	6	7	55.5	0.108	0.892	0.606
7–8 years	46	6	4	44	0.136	0.864	0.523
8–9 years	36	0	4	34	0	1.000	0.497 [h]
9–10 years	32	3	3	30.5	0.098	0.902	0.472
Females, all ages 0–1 year	141	6	0	141	0.043	0.957	0.957
1–2 years	135	5	15	127.5	0.039	0.961	0.920
2–3 years	115	5	9	110.5	0.045	0.955	0.878
3–4 years	101	4	4	99	0.040	0.960	0.843
4–5 years	93	2	7	89.5	0.022	0.978	0.824
5–6 years	84	3	4	82	0.037	0.963	0.794
6–7 years	77	1	8	73	0.014	0.986	0.783
7–8 years	68	4	6	65	0.061	0.939	0.735
8–9 years	58	1	6	55	0.018	0.982	0.721
9–10 years	51	2	7	47.5	0.042	0.958	0.691

Source: Computed from unpublished data on APU patients surveyed in the Framingham Heart Study.

[a] Symbols I and W are as defined in table 3–5.
[b] Number of patients alive and free of heart attack at the beginning of the interval.
[c] Number of patients who either died or experienced a heart attack (MI or CI) during the interval.
[d] Adjusted number at risk $= L - W/2$.
[e] Probability of dying or experiencing a heart attack during interval $= D/L*$.
[f] Probability of surviving and not experiencing a herat attack during interval $= 1 - Q$.
[g] Cumulative probability of surviving and not experiencing a heart attack, $CP_n = P_1 \cdot P_2 \cdots P_n$.
[h] This CP estimate is derived by using linear interpolation.

Life Expectancies

The estimated life expectancies for persons with APU, for persons with first myocardial infarctions (exclusive of those leading to sudden death), for persons with coronary insufficiency, and for people in the general population are presented in table 3–11. The values in the table show substantially shortened life expectancies for both APU and heart attack patients.

A curious and at first glance counterintuitive result in the table is that female myocardial infarction and coronary insufficiency patients under 65

Table 3–11

Life Expectancy Following Angina Pectoris Uncomplicated, Coronary Insufficiency, and Myocardial Infarction *(Years)*

Age at Diagnosis	Angina Pectoris Uncomplicated	Myocardial Infarction[a]	Coronary Insufficiency[b]	General Population
Males				
0–14	37.6	31.3	32.6	62.2
15–24	31.4	26.4	27.5	50.7
25–34	26.2	22.4	23.3	41.6
35–44	21.4	18.6	19.4	32.5
45–54	17.1	15.5	16.1	23.9
55–64	13.8	10.4	11.8	16.4
65–74	10.4	4.8	6.6	10.5
75+	6.1	3.7	5.1	6.1
Females				
0–14	56.9	27.6	31.8	69.7
15–24	47.6	23.2	26.8	58.0
25–34	40.0	19.6	22.6	48.3
35–44	32.7	16.2	18.7	38.8
45–54	26.1	13.0	15.0	29.8
55–64	20.1	10.1	11.7	21.5
65–74	14.1	7.0	9.7	14.1
75+	8.2	5.1	7.1	8.2

Source: Calculations based on data in tables 3–5, 3–6, and 3–9 and survival probabilities of the general population.

[a]Incorporates survival experience of fatal and nonfatal MIs.

[b]As indicated in text, CI patients are estimated to have same survival patterns as MI patients who survive at least 30 days (that is, nonfatal MIs).

years of age have a shorter life expectancy than male patients of a corresponding age. This result seems counterintuitive since survival data for the general population indicate that females of each age have longer average life expectancies than males of the same age, and in the absence of any startling evidence to the contrary, we would expect the same relationship to hold among MI and CI patients. A possible explanation for this dichotomy may lie in the different methods used to aggregate age intervals for male and female MI patients prior to the calculation of survival probabilities and life expectancies. Recall that the raw Framingham data used to derive survival rates consisted of a larger sample of men and women (roughly a ratio of 3:1). This permitted us to establish three age groups for men—35 to 54, 55 to 64, and 65 and older—while having only two groups for women—under 65 and 65 and older. Since approximately two-thirds of the women in the group under 65 were, in fact, between the ages of 55 and 64, it is reasonable to expect that the use of this aggregated sample would result in an overestimate of the true mortality rates and hence an underestimate of true survival rates and life expectancies for female patients under 55. (This holds for CI as well as MI patients because the survival experience of MI patients in the sample who survived at least 30 days was considered indicative of the corresponding experience of CI patients.) This observation does not, however, explain the relatively shorter life expectancies observed for women compared with men in the 55 to 64 age group. Whether this phenomenon is typical of the MI and CI patient populations at large or is merely characteristic of the particular patient sample observed remains to be determined.

Direct Costs of Heart Disease

The direct costs of coronary heart disease constitute expenditures for medical treatment at onset of the disease and for later treatment. To estimate the direct costs in 1975 associated with sudden death, recognized myocardial infarction, coronary insufficiency, and angina pectoris uncomplicated, it is first necessary to develop a generalized treatment model. The model, described in the following paragraphs, quantifies treatment requirements after a patient is diagnosed as having one of the four forms of the disease. The model is a necessary simplification of several medical procedures applied in treating heart disease patients.

The Coronary Heart Disease Treatment Model

The sequence of treatment for coronary heart disease varies from patient to patient. In order to develop total-cost numbers, we first estimate average treatment patterns for each of the major disease categories. Figure 1–3 presents a schematic overview of the treatment model. Note that a distinction is made between the rapidly fatal forms of coronary heart disease (sudden death, fatal myocardial infarction) and the remaining subcategories, which have a more favorable prognosis. This differentiation is important since the rapidly fatal group generates direct costs for only a month or less following the initial attack, while patients in the other subcategories usually generate treatment needs and costs for several years past incidence. Future costs for patients in the latter group are significant and generally consist of two parts— costs of annual follow-on care and costs of treating recurring heart attacks. The following paragraphs summarize the treatment model as it applies to each of the four diagnostic categories. A more complete analysis follows in the next subsection.

    The medical care required by a sudden-death victim is essentially limited to emergency services, including both emergency transportation and care in an emergency medical facility. A person experiencing a myocardial infarction, however, receives extensive medical attention. In approximately 50 percent of the cases, the MI patient uses emergency transportation and requires emergency medical treatment. All MI patients, whether or not they receive emergency services, receive inhospital care. Those who survive initial hospitalization will need annual follow-on care as outpatients, and if they have subsequent heart attacks, they will need further inhospital care. The medical resources necessary to treat coronary insufficiency (CI) are similar to those required for MI, except that CI patients can expect to undergo surgery more frequently and often need extensive annual follow-on care.

The typical patient with angina pectoris uncomplicated has fewer medical needs than the MI or CI patient, since the majority of APU patients require outpatient care only. A small proportion of APU patients, however, requires hospitalization, and a fraction of these undergoes surgery. While APU patients are at high risk of developing more severe forms of coronary heart disease, the costs of treating the advanced forms of the disease (MI, CI, or sudden death) should not be associated with the initial anginal disorder, but rather with the later, more severe disease.

Estimating Direct-Cost Components

To calculate treatment costs, we must specify and estimate costs for the individual components of the model just described. For a coronary heart disease patient in the first year of disease these treatment components could include emergency services (transportation and emergency room care) and initial hospitalization plus follow-on care (physician visits, laboratory tests, x-ray, drugs). For MI and CI patients, additional care may be necessitated by a recurrent attack. In later years, treatment will include annual follow-on care and care for possible recurrences.

We have, in our analysis, not measured the costs of (1) prevention programs, such as special diets, exercise programs, and education programs; (2) special nursing care, (3) attendant and nursing home care, (4) vocational rehabilitation, and (5) training for medical professionals. These charges will be reflected in our analysis only to the extent that they are included in hospital per-diem charges. These exclusions could be questioned by noting the significance of nursing home costs, particularly those for cancer and stroke patients. However, it has been noted by epidemiologists (for example, Kannel) that coronary heart disease is "more lethal than disabling."[19] Similarly, Weinblatt et al. have noted that a substantial majority of MI survivors return to work within 1 year after the initial attack.[20] This suggests that CHD patients do not have significant charges for nursing home care or for vocational rehabilitation. Attendant care, when necessary, is provided at

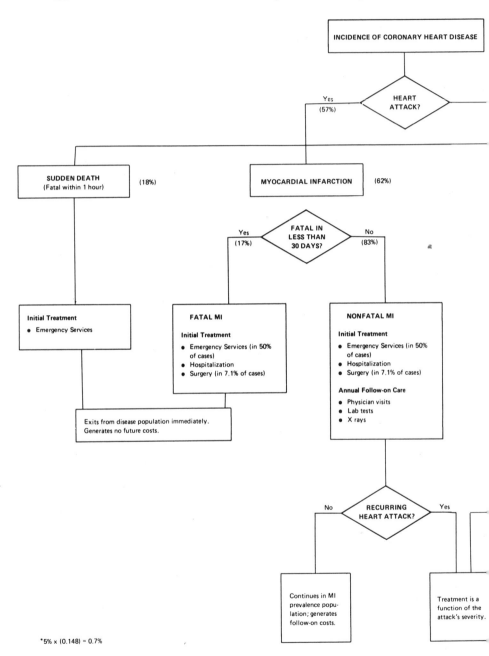

Figure 3–1. Generalized Treatment Model for Coronary Heart Disease.

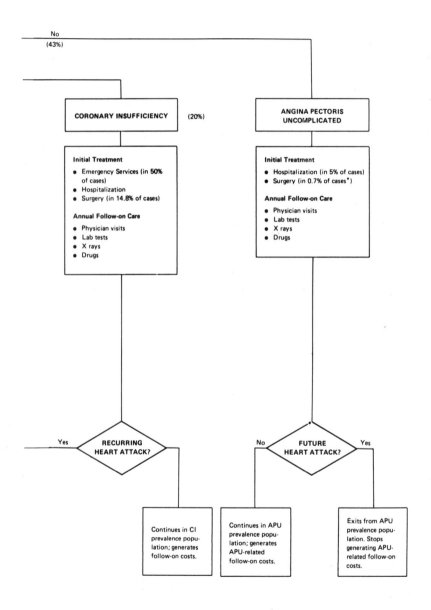

home and is limited. Even for older patients, four-fifths of whom return to the labor force, it is difficult to determine whether the remaining one-fifth use nursing homes or attendant care. For those who do, such use may be necessitated by other health problems. In sum, the best available evidence suggests that the categories of costs excluded from our analysis are negligible in magnitude.

Emergency Services. Among coronary heart disease patients, emergency transportation is used by victims of sudden death, coronary insufficiency, and myocardial infarction. A review of the literature suggests that patients with APU tend to be diagnosed during nonemergency visits to cardiologists, internists, or general practitioners. In virtually no case is emergency transportation used. Our interviews with emergency room physicians indicate that those few APU patients receiving emergency medical attention almost never require ambulance transportation.[21]

Ambulance use is similar for patients with either coronary insufficiency or myocardial infarction. Victims of first heart attacks are frequently unaware of incipient coronary heart disease and therefore do not recognize their symptoms for what they are. In these cases, the victims drive or are driven by family or friends for care. Ambulances are not used. While data indicating the national proportion of ambulance utilization for MIs or CIs are limited, we estimate the figure to be 50 percent. This estimate represents a synthesis of opinions obtained from interviews with emergency room physicians and cardiologists.[22] These physicians also emphasized the differences of situation among those suffering subsequent MIs and CIs. These people, having a history of heart attacks, recognize the threat confronting them and tend, almost universally, to engage ambulances or mobile coronary care units (MCCUs) for assistance.

In the case of sudden death, we have assumed that all victims will be transported to an emergency room in an ambulance or MCCU.[23] Although death, in some cases, is instantaneous and medical care is therefore unnecessary, the patient is usually taken to an emergency room where death can be confirmed by a physician.

Much has been written concerning the value and effectiveness of the MCCU. Nevertheless, its use in the United States in 1975 was relatively limited compared with that of the regular ambulance.[24] Hence, in our estimate of emergency transportation costs, we assume that every patient uses a standard ambulance. The average ambulance charge is estimated to be $60 in 1975. This figure includes the standard base rate of $40, an average urban-rural mileage charge of $15 (15 miles at $1 per mile), and an oxygen charge of $5. Cretin estimates that the average charge for an MCCU is $100.[25] Since less than 2 percent of patients transported use an MCCU, the underestimation of total emergency transportation costs through our assumption seems small.

With the exception of immediate lifesaving efforts, such as resuscitation, defibrillation (reestablishment of normal heart rhythms using electric shock), or the application of oxygen, little emergency medical care is administered outside of a hospital room. We have assumed, accordingly, that every heart disease patient who requires emergency transportation also receives care in a hospital emergency facility. The extent of that care will vary from patient to patient. The sudden-death victim who is dead on arrival at the hospital will receive minimal treatment compared with that given the patient with nonfatal but life-threatening MI. The CI patient may have electrocardiogram or laboratory results that do not indicate myocardial infarction. He may nevertheless be considered in a preinfarction condition and treated similarly to the definite MI patient.

Cost items in the average emergency room include physician fees and ancillary charges, including inhospital drugs, laboratory and x-ray fees, and a flat emergency room floor charge. Two estimates will be applied: an average charge for the sudden-death victim, dead on arrival, and an average charge for all other patients, including both those who die in the emergency room and those who survive to be transferred to an intensive or coronary care unit.

The emergency room cost for sudden deaths is assumed to be the same as that estimated for motor vehicle fatalities who are dead on arrival (DOA) at the emergency room. This is estimated to be $36 (see chapter 6). The average 1975 emergency room charge for MI and CI patients (the non-DOAs) was $190 and included an average floor charge of $48, ancillary services of $112, and physician fees of $30.[26] This figure was derived from an average cost for these victims in Massachusetts in 1977, adjusted to 1975 national levels. The floor charge and physician fees tended to be standard, not varying by degree of complication of illness. The ancillary charges, however, varied according to the type of treatment involved and ranged from a low charge generated by care for certain CI patients to a higher cost for those patients in shock, suffering cardiac arrest (stoppage of heart pumping action), or needing defibrillation.

Hospitalization. Patients suffering recognized myocardial infarctions and coronary insufficiency and a portion of those with angina pectoris uncomplicated are hospitalized. As with emergency care, actual treatment varies with the severity of the disease.

Patients who have MIs or CIs are hospitalized initially in a conventional intensive care unit (ICU) or specialized coronary care unit (CCU) and are then transferred to a nonintensive or convalescent area. Some CI patients, along with a smaller proportion of MI patients, require surgery. APU patients, when they require hospitalization, generally do not need the level of care provided in an intensive or coronary care unit.

Hospitalization costs for patients not undergoing surgery are estimated by multiplying the average per-diem charge for treatment in a coronary care unit by the number of days spent in a CCU, and by multiplying the average per-diem charge for convalescent bed care by the number of days of such care, summing the results, and adding the total to the average charges for physician visits in the CCU and convalescent care areas. If a patient requires surgery, additional charges must be included to cover the costs of surgeons' services and operating room facilities and personnel.

Acton (1973) estimated that the per-diem charge in a CCU is between 2 to 3 times that of a regular ward accommodation. According to the American Hospital Association, the average per-diem charge for inpatient care was approximately $136 in 1975.[27] This figure includes ancillary services: basic medical-surgical supplies, room and board, and routine nursing care. Acton's findings coupled with the estimate of hospital per-diem charges of $136 suggest that the average charge per day in a CCU lies somewhere between $272 and $408. Cretin has estimated that the per-diem charge in a CCU in 1975 was $325.[28] Since this latter figure is consistent with the values derived from Acton's work, we have used this amount as an average per-diem estimate applicable to all patients treated in a CCU or ICU.

The length-of-stay data used in the analysis have been gathered by the 1975 Professional Activities Survey (PAS).[29] The PAS data, taken from a representative sample of U.S. hospitals, provides information on average length of stay for patients with myocardial infarctions and angina pectoris. The length-of-stay data for coronary insufficiency patients were derived from estimates in the literature and our discussions with medical experts.

Physician fees are an important factor in any estimate of hospitalization costs. Since the treatment of heart disease requires the services of such specialists as internists, cardiologists, and cardiac surgeons, we would ideally wish to determine the fees charged by each. *Medical Economics* has published median fees charged in 1975 for initial and follow-up hospital visits made by internists, from which we have derived average charges of $38.46 and $13.28, respectively.[30] Unfortunately, no such estimates of cardiologists' fees are available. Cardiologist fees are accordingly assumed to be those of internists—an assumption that will bias our estimates downward. Costs occasioned by the use of a cardiac surgeon's services are included in our estimate of the costs of surgery. Estimates of surgical charges will be developed more fully in our discussions of MI, CI, and APU hospitalization costs.

Fatal Myocardial Infarction. Patients with fatal myocardial infarctions, by definition, survive at least 1 hour past their attacks but die within 30 days.

Virtually all succumb prior to hospital discharge. The vast majority of these deaths occur after the patient has left the emergency room and has been placed in an intensive or coronary care unit. Unlike sudden deaths, patients with fatal MIs generate inhospital costs. These costs may include charges for care received in the CCU, for time spent in the regular ward, and for physicians' and surgeons' services.

It is difficult to estimate CCU mortality for patients with fatal myocardial infarctions dying after the first day. Acton's data suggest that 56.6 percent of all fatal MIs die within 1 day.[31] If we assume that the times of death for the remaining 43.5 percent of fatal MIs are distributed uniformly between 1 and 30 days, then the fatal MI surviving 1 day will succumb, on average, 15.5 days after the attack.

Fatal MIs who die within 24 hours require an average of 1 day of CCU care ($325), with one initial ($38.46) and one follow-up physician visit ($13.28). In 1975 this meant an average total cost of $377 per patient. For the second group of fatal MIs—those who survive past 24 hours and die an average of 15.5 days after their attacks—Cretin estimates that the first 4.5 days of their hospital stay will be spent in the CCU, leaving an average of 11 days of less intensive care.[32] Assuming an average of two physician visits per day of CCU care and 1.5 visits per day of less intensive care, this implies a hospitalization cost of $3322 per patient: $1463 for 4.5 CCU days at $325 per day, $1496 for 11 days of normal hospitalization at $136 per day, $38 for one initial physician visit, and $325 for 24.5 follow-up visits at $13.28 per visit. By computing a weighted average of these two figures (that is, 56.6 percent of $377 plus 43.5 percent of $3322), we obtain an average hospitalization cost for all fatal MIs amounting to $1652. This figure does not include possible surgical charges—estimated later.

Nonfatal Myocardial Infarction. The nonfatal myocardial infarction patient, like the fatal MI who lives past 1 day, will spend an average of 4.5 days in a coronary care unit (CCU), incurring the same costs derived in the preceding discussion. The patient is then transferred to a standard, ward-type bed where he receives primarily convalescent care. PAS data help indicate the length of stay in the regular ward. These data are based on live discharges and provide a breakdown by age. The average length of stay ranges from 10.5 days for the 35- to 44-year-old patients to 11.6 days for patients over 65. The average number of physician visits ranges from 15.75 to 17.40 for the same age groups.[33] A weighted average of the costs of less intensive care yields a figure of $1770 per patient. When we include the 4.5 days in the CCU, we arrive at an average inhospital charge of $3382 for the nonfatal MI patient who does not require surgery.

Surgical procedures are not performed frequently on MI patients. In fact, we estimate from PAS data that they are required in only 7.1 percent of all cases.[34] When surgery is performed, however, it is normally the coronary artery bypass graft. According to Mundth and Austen (1975), the average total hospitalization charge per case for this type of surgery is about $10,000. This figure is inclusive of basic hospital charges, surgical charges, and physician fees. To include the cost of surgery in our estimates of average hospitalization costs, we have added to each nonsurgical patient's costs a surgical component equal to 7.1 percent of the difference between $10,000 and the patient's nonsurgical hospital costs. For nonfatal MIs, this amounts to an additional $473 = 0.071 × ($10,000 − $3382), and for fatal MIs, an additional $596 = 0.071 × ($10,000 − $1652). With the surgical component included, the average total hospitalization costs for a nonfatal MI becomes $3855 (that is, $473 + $3382), and for a fatal MI, $2248 (that is, $596 + $1652).

Coronary Insufficiency. Patients suffering from coronary insufficiency are hospitalized in virtually all cases. Of these, 14.8 percent undergo surgery.[35]

Inhospital treatment for the CI patient may include narcotic analgesics provided in the emergency room, propranolol, and/or long-acting nitrates administered in the CCU to assuage pain, bed rest, sedatives, ECG monitoring, and the use of digitalis or anticoagulants to treat medical complications such as congestive heart failure.[36] Coronary insufficiency produces acute anginal symptoms, is frequently incapacitating, and may fail to respond to nonsurgical medical management. In such cases, cardiac catheterization is often performed to determine the extent of ischemic damage, and this is followed by coronary bypass surgery.

Like the typical MI patient, the average CI patient spends approximately 4.5 days in a CCU or ICU, requiring nine physician visits. Discussions with several cardiologists suggest, however, that the average length of stay for CI patients following discharge from the CCU to less intensive care is shorter than the corresponding length of stay for MI patients. Their consensus indicated an average stay of about 5.5 days, with 1.5 physicians visits per day, while our earlier estimate for MI patients was 11 days, with the same rate of physician visits.[37] Taken together, these data indicate an average hospitalization cost per case of $2476 for CI patients not requiring surgery. Because 14.8 percent of the patients receive bypass surgery, an additional $1114 [that is, 0.148 × ($10,000 − $2476)] must be added to reflect average surgical expenses above and beyond basic hospital charges and physician fees. This yields an estimate of average total initial hospitalization costs per case of $3590 (that is, $1114 + $2476).

Angina Pectoris Uncomplicated. Most patients with angina pectoris are treated exclusively as outpatients. Selected drugs (usually nitroglycerin) taken as needed or as prophylaxis normally will suffice to control the angina pain. If the pain is sufficiently disabling, however, inhospital treatment is recommended. To obtain the proportion of the APU incidence population requiring hospitalization, we assumed that it would be the same as the proportion of the APU prevalence population also requiring hospitalization. This is estimated at 5 percent.[38] Of those hospitalized, we assume that the fraction requiring coronary bypass surgery is the same as for coronary insufficiency patients—14.8 percent.

According to PAS data, the average length of stay for hospitalized angina patients ranges from 5 days for people aged 35 to 44 to 6.5 days for those over 65. The average number of inhospital physician visits per patient ranges from 10 to 13 over these same age groups.[39] For patients not requiring surgery, virtually all medical care is provided in a less intensive convalescent setting. Based on the length-of-stay and physician-visit data, we calculate the average cost of this care to be approximately $970. To account for the estimated 14.8 percent of patients requiring bypass, an additional $1336 [that is, $0.148 \times (\$10,000 - \$970)$] must be included to cover average surgical expenses in excess of basic nonsurgical hospital charges. Totaling these two figures, the estimate of average total initial hospitalization costs per case becomes $2306 for the 5 percent of angina patients who are hospitalized.

Annual Follow-on Care. With the exception of intensive, specialized care for heart attack recurrences, the medical care administered to coronary heart disease patients following initial hospitalization is normally provided on an outpatient basis. Routine follow-on care for these patients includes drug treatment, laboratory tests, and physician visits.

We estimate that nonfatal MI, CI, and APU patients alike require an average of five physician visits per year, at a total cost of about $70—one initial visit at $20.60 and four follow-up visits at $12.30 each.[40] During these visits, physicians administer electrocardiograms and chest x-rays along with routine laboratory tests. The frequency with which they are ordered depends on the physician and the individual patient's condition. For each case, however, we estimate that an average of two such procedures are performed annually.[41] At 1977 Massachusetts rates adjusted to 1975 national levels, the costs of these tests and procedures average approximately $40 per year.

Drugs prescribed vary according to the coronary heart disease diagnostic category and to its severity. In the case of myocardial infarction, for example, the anginal chest pain that precedes attacks might disappear at its cessation. This development would relieve the individual, if only temporarily, of the need for medication. We do not therefore attribute annual drug costs to these patients. Coronary insufficiency, however, may be complicated by congestive heart failure or hypertension. In such cases, patients will require medication. At 1975 prices, the average cost of prescription drugs used in outpatient treatment of coronary insufficiency is estimated at $88 per patient.[42] A similar costing procedure indicates that for APU patients, the annual cost of drugs is $21.[43]

To calculate the average annual cost per patient for follow-on care, we sum the costs of drugs, laboratory tests and other procedures, and physician visits. These amount to $110 per nonfatal myocardial infarction, to $198 for coronary insufficiency, and to $131 for angina pectoris uncomplicated.

Treatment of Heart Attack Recurrences. The expected cost for treatment of second and subsequent heart attacks is a function of both the recurrence likelihood and the per-case treatment costs.

A review of the literature and discussions with epidemiologists suggest that the likelihood of a heart attack recurrence is high compared with the risk of a first attack for an unafflicted individual. This observation is confirmed by unpublished data on heart attack recurrences in the Framingham population.[44] When these Framingham data are disaggregated by age and sex, it also appears that the risk of a recurrence to patients surviving at least 30 days past the initial attack (essentially all nonfatal MI and CI patients) remains fairly constant during each year of survival. The data show that this trend exists for at least 14 years past the first heart attack and may extend further. Furthermore, the risk of recurrences varies considerably by sex and is significantly greater for patients over 65 at the time of first attack. Per-patient estimates of the annual recurrence risk have been calculated from the Framingham experience and are presented by age and sex below:

Age at First Attack	Males	Age at First Attack	Females
< 55	0.0728		
55–64	0.0867	< 65	0.1412
65+	0.1145	65+	0.2308

As for first heart attacks, the recurrent attack may take the form of a death within 1 hour (sudden death), fatal MI, nonfatal MI, or CI. Cretin found that heart attack recurrences were 47 percent more likely than first heart attacks to result in fatalities.[45] From our previous results on incidence and mortality, it is possible to calculate the proportion of first heart attacks of each diagnostic type. By adjusting these proportions to reflect the enhanced likelihood of death following a recurrence, we also can estimate the distribution of recurrent heart attacks by type. The results for both first and recurrent attacks are presented on an age- and sex-specific basis in table 3–12.

We assume that the cost of treating a recurrent heart attack is the same as the cost of treating a first attack of the same type. This cost is limited to

Table 3-12
Proportional Distribution of First and Recurrent Heart Attacks by Diagnostic Type

Age at First Attack	First Attack				Recurrent Attack			
	Sudden Death	MI		CI	Death < 1 hour	MI		CI
		Fatal	Nonfatal			Fatal	Nonfatal	
Males								
< 55	0.1606	0.0237	0.5690	0.2467	0.2361	0.0348	0.5086	0.2205
55–64	0.2455	0.0778	0.5767	0.1000	0.3609	0.1144	0.4472	0.0775
65+	0.1075	0.1962	0.5393	0.1570	0.1579	0.2884	0.4289	0.1248
Females								
< 65	0.1342	0.0657	0.4269	0.3732	0.1972	0.0966	0.3768	0.3294
65+	0.2745	0.1416	0.3682	0.2157	0.4035	0.2081	0.2449	0.1435

Source: Derived from data in tables 3–3, 3–5, and 3–6 and Cretin (1977, p. 149).

charges for emergency services and initial hospitalization. Given our assumption, one may estimate the treatment cost for a typical recurrence by taking a weighted average of the treatment costs for the four possible types of heart attack. Based on earlier results (summarized in table 3–14), these costs range from $96 for a death within 1 hour to $4105 for a nonfatal MI, with intermediate values of $2498 and $3840 for a fatal MI and CI, respectively.[46] Calculating the average cost of a recurrent heart attack requires multiplying the chance of each type of recurrence (found in table 3–12) by the cost per type of recurrence and summing. The procedure for calculating the average cost of treating a recurrence for a male heart attack victim, aged 40 at the time of first attack, is shown as:

Average cost
of treating $= \$3044 = (0.2361 \times \$96) + (0.0348 \times \$2498)$
a recurrence $+ (0.5086 \times \$4105) + (0.2205 \times \$3840)$

Similar results are summarized below for patients of different sex and age at first heart attack:

Males	Average Cost	Females	Average Cost
< 55	$3044	< 65	$3072
55–64	2454	65+	2115
65+	2978		

Our analysis requires estimates of the average annual recurrence costs for each year of survival following incidence. This is calculated by multiplying the likelihood of recurrence by the average treatement costs. The resulting values for average annual recurrence costs per patient are given in table 3–13. Since recurrence costs are generated only by first-attack survivors, the estimates in the table apply exclusively to nonfatal MI and CI patients.

Summary of Direct-Cost Components. Table 3–14 summarizes the values of the direct-cost components developed in the previous subsections. The values represent average costs for each of the coronary heart disease categories.

As the table indicates, the magnitudes of the initial treatment costs and the annual follow-on costs accruing to patients in different diagnostic subcategories differ substantially. The direct costs assigned to a sudden death, for example, are insignificant when compared with the costs of other patients. The costs of a typical patient in the other rapidly fatal category—fatal MI—are also relatively small, but not insignificant, averaging $2373. The direct costs for patients in each of the fatal categories cease soon after

Table 3–13
Average Annual Recurrence Costs per Patient, by Age
at First Heart Attack
(Dollars)

Age at First Attack	Average Annual Recurrence Costs[a]
Males	
< 55	222
55–64	213
65+	341
Females	
< 65	434
65+	488

Note: All costs are in 1975 dollars.
[a]Costs apply only to nonfatal MI and CI patients.

the initial attack. In contrast, those heart attack patients who survive initial hospitalization have average initial treatment costs of $3890 for nonfatal MIs and $3715 for CIs. They also generate average annual costs for follow-on care of between $110 and $198 and average recurrence costs of $318.

The hospitalization costs displayed for APU patients ($2306 per case) are different from those displayed for MI and CI patients, since the figures in the table apply only to the 5 percent of the APU incidence population that is hospitalized. To obtain an overall average for all APU patients, the costs must be multiplied by 0.05, yielding an estimated $115 per case. Each APU patient, regardless of hospitalization status, is assumed to generate the average annual follow-on costs shown—$131 per case.

Estimating Average Costs per Patient

The present values of average direct costs per patient for individuals in each incidence (age, sex, and diagnostic) category are calculated by discounting to the year of incidence the average direct costs incurred during each year of survival.

As an example of these cost calculations, we now work through the case of a male myocardial infarction victim who is 40 years old at the time of first heart attack. The calculation is performed in two parts, first for a fatal MI and then for a nonfatal MI. Each cost estimate is then weighted by the patient's likelihood of being fatal and nonfatal, respectively, and the results are summed to give an overall average for an MI patient of that age and sex.

For a fatal MI, direct costs are limited to those generated during the first year. We calculate that present-valued costs for this patient are

Table 3–14
Average Direct Costs per Patient: A Summary of Component Costs of Coronary Heart Disease by Diagnostic Type (Dollars)

Direct-Cost Category	Sudden Death	MI Fatal	MI Nonfatal	CI	APU Hospital	APU Nonhospital
Emergency services[a]						
Emergency transportation	60	30	30	30	—	—
Emergency medical care	36	95	95	95	—	—
Subtotal	96	125	125	125	—	—
Initial hospitalization						
Basic hospital charges	—	1459	3002	2243	786	—
Physician fees	—	193	380	223	184	—
Additional surgical charge[b]	—	596	473	1114	1336	—
Subtotal	—	2248	3855	3590	2306	—
Total initial hospitalization and emergency services costs	96	2373	3980	3715	2306	—
Annual follow-on costs[c]	—	—	110	198	131	131
Annual recurrence costs[d]	—	—	318	318	—	—

Note: All costs are in 1975 dollars.

[a]Estimates of emergency services costs for MIs and CIs reflect 50-percent utilization of such services by first heart attack patients.

[b]Surgical charges represent average surgical expenses *in excess* of basic hospital charges and physician fees.

[c]Follow-on costs apply during each year, including the first, that patient survives.

[d]Recurrence costs apply during each year, including the first, that patient survives. Estimates in table represent averages over all age and sex groups, while estimates used in actual analysis are age- and sex-specific.

$$PVC_{\text{fatal MI}} = (\$125 + \$2248) = \$2373$$

For a nonfatal MI, direct costs are generated during the first and subsequent years past the initial attack. At a discount rate of 6 percent, we have

$$PVC_{\text{nonfatal MI}} = FYC + AFOC \times \sum_{n=41}^{99} \frac{P_{40,s}^i(n)}{(1 + .06)^{n-40}}$$

where FYC = first-year costs
$AFOC$ = annual follow-on plus annual recurrence costs
$P_{40,s}^i(n)$ = the probability of a 40-year-old male victim of a nonfatal MI surviving to age n[47]

Since

$$FYC = (\$125 + \$3855 + \$110 + \$222) = \$4312$$

$$AFOC = (\$110 + \$222) = \$332$$

and

$$\sum_{n=41}^{99} \frac{P_{40,s}^i(n)}{(1.06)^{n-40}} = 8.981$$

it follows that

$$PVC_{\text{nonfatal MI}} = \$4312 + \$332 \times 8.981 = \$7294$$

Table 3–6 indicated that 4 percent of all 40-year-old male MI patients are fatal MIs. This means that a weighted average of the fatal and nonfatal costs is

$$PVC_{\text{MI}} = (0.04)PVC_{\text{fatal MI}} + (0.96)PVC_{\text{nonfatal MI}}$$
$$= (0.04 \times \$2373) + (0.96 \times \$7294) = \$7097$$

Costs of insurance administration are 4.5 percent of this, or $319. Hence, at the time of initial heart attack, the present value of the lifelong direct costs for a 40-year-old male MI is approximately $7416 (that is, $7097 + 319).

Similar estimates have been calculated for all patient subgroups with MI, CI, and APU. The results are shown in table 3–15. Several trends are evident in the values in the table. First, within each diagnostic type and age grouping, the costs for males are less than the corresponding costs for females. For MI and CI patients, this difference primarily results from the smaller likelihood of a heart attack recurrence for males than for females of the same age. For APU patients, the discrepancy is caused by the shorter period of time that male patients, on the average, remain alive and free of a heart attack than female patients. Second, although all cost estimates decrease with age, this phenomenon is more pronounced for APU patients than for MI or CI patients. This result is explained by recalling that angina patients generate proportionally more of their costs in the form of annual charges for follow-on care than do heart attack victims. The greater magnitude of direct costs for a CI patient than for an age- and sex-matched MI patient results from the fraction of MIs that are fatal in the short run and thus do not generate either large costs of initial hospitalization or any follow-on costs.

Summary of Total Direct Costs

By multiplying the cost estimates in table 3–15 by the numbers of patients in each incidence category we obtain estimates of total direct costs generated by patients in each category. Table 3–16 displays these estimates. We see that male coronary heart disease patients generate disproportionately more direct costs than female patients: 66 percent of the direct costs are for males, who constitute only 62 percent of the incidence population. Two factors explain this result. First, males experience proportionately more heart attacks than females—MIs accounting for 44 percent of all male CHD, but for only 21 percent of all female CHD. Second, males suffer a higher proportion of their heart disease at a younger age than females. Sixty-seven percent of the male CHD incidence population was under 65, versus only 48 percent of the female incidence population. Since per-patient costs decrease with age, the younger age of male patients partly offsets the greater per-person direct cost of female patients at all ages. We also see that CHD patients under the age of 65 account for 59 percent of all direct costs. This finding reemphasizes the character of the disease as affecting those of middle age and middle to old age.

Table 3–17 presents a breakdown of present-valued direct costs by diagnostic type and cost category. There we see that nearly half the total direct costs of $2491 million are incurred for hospitalization (over half, when one reflects that $55 million of insurance administration costs derive from hospitalizations). Over three-quarters of all hospitalization costs are for MI patients. Physician service charges account for the second largest portion of direct costs, $791 million. Laboratory fees amount to $182 million, while

Table 3–15
Present Value of Direct Costs, per Patient with Myocardial Infarction, Coronary Insufficiency, and Angina Pectoris Uncomplicated, by Age
(Dollars)

Age	MI	CI	APU
Males			
0–14	7728	8685	1538
15–24	7659	8593	1510
25–34	7556	8459	1465
35–44	7416	8273	1401
45–54	7247	8051	1321
55–64	6319	7300	1233
65–74	5551	6906	1150
75+	5330	6543	1074
All males	6270	7547	1229
Females			
0–14	8549	10030	1929
15–24	8473	9928	1896
25–34	8359	9776	1847
35–44	8189	9549	1774
45–54	7949	9230	1674
55–64	7636	8811	1543
65–74	6803	8843	1399
75+	6360	8136	1271
All females	7107	8781	1473
Total population	6457	8028	1353

Note: All costs are in 1975 dollars, discounted at 6 percent.

drugs, insurance administration, and emergency services each account for roughly $100 million. Physician service charges are two-thirds of hospitalization costs for CI patients and constitute over half of APU direct costs. Laboratory fees amount to over one-quarter of APU direct costs.

Indirect Costs of Heart Disease

Work Incapacity Resulting from Heart Attack

To calculate earnings forgone as a result of a heart attack, we compare earnings expectations at the age of first heart attack with those realized after the heart attack. The study by Weinblatt et al. (1966) examined the functional status of heart attack survivors. Using a population of male myocardial infarction patients, the proportion of patients who survived and who returned to work at different intervals after the initial attack was computed.

Table 3–16
Present Value of Total Direct Costs of Coronary Heart Disease,
by Age and Diagnostic Type; United States, 1975
(Thousands of Dollars)

Age	Sudden Death	MI	CI	APU	Total CHD
Males					
0–14	1	387	269	43	700
15–24	4	1,616	1,117	175	2,913
25–34	52	18,936	13,069	2,012	34,069
35–44	302	108,684	74,745	11,254	194,985
45–54	1,017	242,090	89,089	35,111	367,307
55–64	2,236	373,088	66,305	74,021	515,649
65–74	675	255,659	67,807	31,548	355,689
75+	355	129,273	33,706	15,389	178,723
All males	4,641	1,129,733	346,107	169,553	1,650,034
Females					
0–14	0	43	30	25	98
15–24	1	178	139	108	426
25–34	9	2,182	1,701	1,287	5,178
35–44	52	12,905	10,026	7,455	30,438
45–54	222	53,597	30,608	27,199	111,626
55–64	377	98,954	106,745	82,184	288,259
65–74	956	121,075	66,201	59,388	247,621
75+	661	78,243	41,774	36,981	157,659
All females	2,277	367,176	257,224	214,627	841,305
Total population	6,919	1,496,909	603,331	384,180	2,491,339

Note: All costs are in 1975 dollars, discounted at 6 percent.

For our purposes, an important aspect of the Weinblatt sample was its focus on persons who were employed prior to their heart attacks and who would have remained at their regular jobs if they had not experienced attacks.[48] Weinblatt's research indicated that the proportion of male MI patients who return to work is influenced by one's age at the time of initial attack. For male survivors under 45, virtually all return to work by the ninth month after the attack. For survivors aged 45 to 54, 94.2 percent return to work by 1 year after the heart attack, and for those over 55, 81.8 percent return to work by the thirteenth month after the attack.[49] We assume that these proportions also apply to female survivors.

It is not possible, with present data, to estimate possible losses resulting from the reduced "on-the-job" capabilities of heart attack victims who return to work. It will therefore be assumed that patients who return to work or homemaking tasks function at full preattack capacity. This assumption appears reasonable since heart attack survivors, unlike victims of other

Table 3–17
Present Value of Total Direct Costs of Coronary Heart Disease,
by Diagnostic Type and Direct-Cost Category
(Millions of Dollars)

Direct-Cost Category	Sudden Death	MI	CI	APU	Total CHD
Emergency services	7	61	24	0	91
Hospitalization	0	913	291	11	1215
Physician services[a]	0	402	189	201	791
Laboratory fees	0	57	23	102	182
Drugs	0	0	50	54	104
Insurance administration	0	64	26	17	107
Total	7	1497	603	384	2491

Note: All costs are in 1975 dollars, discounted at 6 percent.

[a]Physician services costs include both inhospital and outpatient charges, as well as surgical charges.

chronic illness, such as stroke or spinal cord injury, do not suffer the types of physical disabilities that would limit vocational performance.[50]

Calculating the Value of Work Performed by
Heart Attack Survivors

To estimate the expected earnings of heart attack patients following their attacks, the incidence of heart attacks may be divided into two groups—the rapidly fatal types of heart disease (sudden death and fatal MIs) and the nonfatal types (nonfatal MIs and CIs). Only the latter group has subsequent earnings. Inasmuch as CI and nonfatal MI patients have similar survival patterns, we also assume that they have similar expected earnings streams following their initial disease episodes.

Using Weinblatt's data and survival data from this analysis, we have developed age- and sex-specified estimates of (1) the fraction of potential first-year productivity actually generated by heart attack survivors ($\alpha_{l,s}$) and (2) the proportion of previously employed nonfatal MIs surviving and returning to work (or to homemaking tasks) 1 year after their first attacks ($\beta_{l,s}$). These values are displayed in tables 3–18 and 3–19. The values in table 3–19 (for $\beta_{l,s}$) represent the multiplication of the values of two intermediate parameters. The first is the proportion of nonfatal MI patients of that age and sex who survive at least 1 year past first attack, and the second is the fraction of those first-year survivors who were working before their attacks and who return to work 1 year later. The second parameter is our best estimate of the

Table 3–18
Proportion of Potential Productivity Actually Generated by Nonfatal
Myocardial Infarction Patients during the Year Following First Attack

Age at First Attack	Male	Female
< 44	0.6061	0.5952
45–54	0.5997	0.5888
55–64	0.4642	0.4722
65+	0.4540	0.4722

Source: Derived from data on MIs in Weinblatt et al. (1966) and data abstracted from tables 3–5 and 3–6. Results are assumed to apply also to CI patients.

proportion of normal vocational capability maintained by heart attack survivors compared with that of a matched heart-disease-free population.

Incorporating the values for $\alpha_{l,s}$ and $\beta_{l,s}$, we can model the expected postmorbid earnings of a heart attack survivor as

$$PVPM = [\alpha_{l,s} \cdot Y_s(l) \cdot E_s(l)]$$

$$+ \left\{ \beta_{l,s} \cdot \left[\sum_{n=l+1}^{85} P_{l+1,s}^i(n) \cdot Y_s(n) \cdot E_s(n) \cdot \left(\frac{1+\gamma}{1+r} \right)^{n-l} \right] \right\}$$

where all other parameters are as defined in chapter 2. The first term on the right side of the equation represents average first-year earnings, and the second term represents the present value of average earnings generated in subsequent years by nonfatal MI and CI patients. The second term reflects our expression of future earnings for heart attack survivors as a proportion of the earnings for comparable heart-disease-free individuals, but with the

Table 3–19
Proportion of Previously Employed Nonfatal Myocardial Infarction
Patients Surviving and Returning to Work or Homemaking Tasks
1 Year after First Attack

Age at First Attack	Male	Female
< 44	0.9583	0.9231
45–54	0.9027	0.8696
55–64	0.7779	0.7551
65+	0.7495	0.7431

Source: Derived from data on MIs in Weinblatt et al. (1966) and data abstracted from Tables 3–5 and 3–6. Results are assumed to apply also to CI patients.

added qualification that these earnings will accrue over a significantly reduced lifespan.

Based on our model, the expected first-year earnings of a 40-year-old male nonfatal MI patient are $9646, and the present-valued earnings in later years are $127,482. These sum to $137,128. As indicated earlier, this result also applies to a male CI patient of like age and thereby represents a first-order estimate of the average postmorbid earnings for a CI patient in the male 35-to-44 age group.

Victims of fatal MIs do not generate postmorbid earnings. As a result, the expected earnings of an average myocardial infarction patient are calculated by multiplying the earnings of a nonfatal MI by the proportion of MIs that are nonfatal. For 40-year-old male patients, 4 percent of first myocardial infarctions are fatal and 96 percent are nonfatal. The present-valued average earnings of a 40-year-old male MI patient thus are

$$0.96 \times \$137,128 = \$131,643$$

This serves as our best estimate of the average postmorbid earnings for male MI patients aged 35 to 44 years.

Forgone Earnings per Heart Disease Patient

Average forgone earnings for heart attack patients of different age, sex, and diagnostic type have been estimated by subtracting their average postmorbid earnings from the expected earnings of demographically matched unafflicted individuals. The results are presented in table 3–20.[51] Because sudden-death cases, like fatal MIs, do not generate postmorbid earnings, their losses are equivalent to the earnings expectations of matched unafflicted persons. For coronary insufficiency, the least severe type of heart attack, forgone earnings per patient range from 30 to 60 percent of the earnings of comparable heart-attack-free individuals. For patients with myocardial infarctions, the situation is even bleaker—with the range increasing to 32 to 65 percent of the earnings of disease-free individuals. The table also shows the relationship between sex and age and forgone earnings. Males, with higher earnings, have larger average forgone earnings for instances of heart disease occurring before the age of 65. After that age, female forgone earnings are larger. Aside from the two youngest age groups, average forgone earnings per incident case fall dramatically with the age of the patient.

Forgone earnings resulting from APU accrue entirely from productive time lost during treatment and recovery and not from reductions in life expectancy owing to excess mortality. Considerably less time, therefore, is lost to useful activity for APU patients than for heart attack victims. The

Table 3–20
Forgone Earnings per Heart Disease Patient, by Age
and Diagnostic Type
(Dollars)

Age	Sudden Death	MI	CI	APU
Males				
0–14	130,863	72,873	70,457	0
15–24	225,992	103,249	98,135	17
25–34	247,881	100,469	94,327	47
35–44	205,687	74,045	68,559	55
45–54	135,972	43,948	40,114	53
55–64	52,199	24,647	20,926	38
65–74	5,754	3,723	2,984	8
75+	533	320	242	0
Females				
0–14	92,241	60,251	55,343	0
15–24	156,059	93,003	83,330	15
25–34	153,131	87,953	77,954	32
35–44	126,642	70,397	61,769	32
45–54	87,150	47,554	41,479	32
55–64	39,950	23,077	20,489	21
65–74	11,682	7,326	5,649	9
75+	2,556	1,496	1,088	2

Note: All earnings figures are in 1975 dollars, discounted at 6 percent.

literature is silent on the actual number of days lost from work by the average APU patient. Based on discussions with physicians concerning the behavioral aspects of angina pectoris, we felt that it was appropriate to assume no lost days for those patients who do not require hospitalization. For APU patients hospitalized but not undergoing sugery, we estimate 2 weeks of vocational disability, and for those patients who undergo surgery, 3 months of vocational disability. Averaging over all APU patients, hospitalized or not, this means that slightly more than 1 day of vocational disability accrues per patient. This translates into average forgone earnings per capita of approximately $24.

Total Forgone Earnings Resulting from
Coronary Heart Disease

Total estimates of forgone earnings broken down by age, sex, and type of heart disease are calculated by multiplying the average figures—shown in table 3–20—by the incidence numbers. The results are shown in table 3–21. Individuals suffering myocardial infarctions account for the largest

Table 3–21
Present Value of Total Forgone Earnings of Coronary Heart Disease
Patients, by Age and Diagnostic Type, United States, 1975
(Millions of Dollars)

Age	Sudden Death	MI	CI	APU	Total CHD
Males					
0–14	1.3	3.6	2.2	0	7.1
15–24	9.7	21.8	12.8	0	44.3
25–34	127.7	251.8	145.7	0.1	525.2
35–44	619.3	1,085.1	619.4	0.4	2,324.2
45–54	1,378.1	1,468.1	443.9	1.4	3,291.5
55–64	1,163.4	1,455.2	190.1	2.3	2,811.0
65–74	38.7	171.5	29.3	0.2	239.7
75+	1.9	7.7	1.2	0	10.9
All males	3,340.1	4,464.8	1,444.6	4.4	9,253.9
Females					
0–14	0.2	0.3	0.2	0	0.7
15–24	1.1	2.0	1.2	0	4.2
25–34	13.2	23.0	13.6	0	49.7
35–44	65.5	110.9	64.9	0.1	241.5
45–54	192.6	320.6	137.5	0.5	651.2
55–64	150.1	299.1	248.2	1.1	698.5
65–74	111.4	130.4	42.3	0.4	284.6
75+	16.8	18.4	5.6	0.1	40.9
All females	550.9	904.7	513.5	2.2	1,971.3
Total population	3,891.0	5,369.5	1,958.1	6.6	11,225.2

Note: All earnings figures are in 1975 dollars, discounted at 6 percent.

component of total forgone earnings, 48 percent. While sudden deaths represent only one-tenth of the CHD incidence population, they generate 35 percent of total forgone earnings. (In addition, sudden-death victims average $56,418 in forgone earnings per patient. This is more than twice the corresponding per-capita figures for MI and CI patients.) Forgone earnings associated with APU constitute only 0.06 percent of the $11.2 billion disease total.

Men account for 82 percent of the total forgone earnings of coronary heart disease, despite representing only 62 percent of total incidence. This dominance of forgone earnings by men results from three factors. First, forgone earnings per patient are greater for men than for women of the same age—for people under the age of 65. Second, CHD tends to strike younger men than women. Finally, men experience a larger portion of their incidence in the form of more severe and lethal types of CHD.

CHD patients aged 65 and over account for only 5 percent of total forgone earnings, while constituting 41 percent of total incidence. This disproportionality results from the decreased earnings expectations of older people relative to their younger counterparts.

Summary and Sensitivity Analysis

Direct, Indirect, and Total Costs

Direct, indirect, and total economic costs of coronary heart disease broken down by age and sex are displayed in table 3–22. We see there the contrast between the patterns of the two main cost categories. Before the age of 54, indirect costs—for all age and sex groups—are many times larger than the direct costs. For those older than 65, direct costs outweigh the indirect. Persons under 65 account for 59 percent of all incidence, for 62 percent of all direct costs, 95 percent of indirect costs, and 89 percent of total CHD costs. Of the total costs of $13.717 billion, approximately 82 percent are indirect.

Table 3–22
Present Value of Direct, Indirect, and Total Costs of Coronary Heart Disease, by Age, United States, 1975
(Millions of Dollars)

Age	Direct Costs	Indirect Costs	Total Costs
Males			
0–14	0.7	7.1	7.8
15–24	2.9	44.3	47.2
25–34	34.1	525.2	559.3
35–44	195.0	2,324.2	2,519.2
45–54	367.3	3,291.5	3,658.8
55–64	515.6	2,811.0	3,326.6
65–74	355.7	239.7	595.4
75+	178.7	10.9	189.6
Total males	1,650.0	9,253.9	10,903.9
Females			
0–14	0.1	0.7	.8
15–24	0.4	4.2	4.6
25–34	5.2	49.7	54.9
35–44	30.4	241.5	271.9
45–54	111.6	651.2	762.8
55–64	288.3	698.5	986.8
65–74	247.6	284.6	532.2
75+	157.7	40.9	198.6
Total females	841.3	1,971.3	2,812.6
Total population	2,491.3	11,225.2	13,716.5

Note: All costs are in 1975 dollars, discounted at 6 percent.

The economic cost of heart disease in males exceeds that in females—partly because of greater incidence among males. Men account for 62 percent of total incidence, 66 percent of direct costs, 82 percent of indirect costs, and 80 percent of total costs. The three male age groups between 35 and 64 account for 69 percent of all CHD costs. The older two of these groups each have larger total costs than do all females. Peak costs for men occur at a younger age than for women: 45 to 54 years of age for men versus 55 to 64 years of age for women. Among men, 93 percent of all costs are due to incidence under 65; among women, 74 percent.

Table 3–23 disaggregates direct, indirect, and total costs of heart disease by the four major diagnostic types. Roughly half the total costs derive from myocardial infarctions. Sudden deaths occasion by far the largest costs per case, followed by CIs and MIs. Average economic costs of APU cases are a fraction of those for other forms of heart disease.

Sensitivity Analysis

Despite our attempts to use the most satisfactory data available and the most reasonable assumptions, we recognize that certain inaccuracies are possible in our economic analysis of coronary heart disease. For more effective use of our economic analysis in a policymaking context, we examine the more likely components of imprecision by means of sensitivity analysis covering six major possible sources of error: incidence, recurrence, mortality, direct costs, discounting, and indirect costs.

Incidence. All cost estimates for coronary heart disease are obtained by multiplying incidence by per-case costs. Any error in estimating incidence will therefore translate into an error of the same proportion in the cost figures. We are fortunate to have such an extensive and systematic sample as the Framingham study as the basis for our incidence estimates. Nevertheless, the

Table 3–23
Total Costs of Coronary Heart Disease by Diagnostic Type, Distinguishing Direct and Indirect Components

Diagnostic Type	Millions of Dollars			Average Costs per Person
	Direct Costs	Indirect Costs	All Costs	
Sudden Death	7	3,891	3,898	56,520
MI	1,497	5,369	6,866	29,615
CI	603	1,958	2,561	34,078
APU	384	7	391	1,377
Total CHD	2,491	11,225	13,716	20,784

Note: All costs are in 1975 dollars, discounted at 6 percent.

chance for error arises in the possible nonrepresentativeness of the Framingham data and in changing incidence trends over time. The Framingham data might be unrepresentative either because of geographic variation in coronary heart disease incidence or because of racial differences in incidence. As discussed earlier, the possibility of severe inaccuracy because of these errors does not seem great. Our method of adjusting for the decline in incidence would, for instance, be grossly imprecise only if the relationship between incidence and mortality changed drastically over the few years before 1975.

Relatively large proportional error is possible in estimating incidence among the younger age groups. Regarding such incidence, the Framingham study is mute—forcing us to extrapolate from older age groups using mortality data. Since the relationship between incidence and mortality may differ considerably between 20-year-olds and 40-year-olds, incidence estimates for the younger ages could be in error by as much as 20 percent. However, the same factor that bears responsibility for the error—the rarity of heart disease before the age of 35—also limits its impact. Suppose, for instance, that as a worst case, we did misestimate incidence in males between 25 and 34 by 20 percent. This error would translate into errors of only 0.3 percent among total direct costs and of only 0.9 percent among total indirect costs.

Recurrence. Data on recurrent heart attacks were scanty—forcing us to rely on unpublished figures from the Framingham study. An error in our estimates of recurrences is possible, but probably not of major impact for the overall cost estimates. Assume, for example, that by using the Framingham data we made an error of 20 percent in underestimating recurrence rates for males suffering nonfatal MIs and CIs between the ages of 35 and 44. This imprecision would have led to a corresponding underestimation of average annual recurrence costs for this incidence group, indicating that those costs should be $266 per year instead of the $222 per year quoted in our analysis. Under this set of circumstances, our estimate of total indirect costs would be low by approximately $11.6 million. This would represent an underestimation of direct costs of 6 percent for CHD patients in that age and sex group but of only 0.5 percent for all patients. Even in the extreme situation where recurrence rates for all nonfatal MIs and CIs were in error by 20 percent (in either direction), this would produce an error of just 4 percent in total direct costs and of 0.7 percent in total (direct plus indirect) costs.

Mortality. The declining mortality rates for CHD in the last two decades show that survival patterns for CHD patients may vary over time. The introduction of such new technologies as coronary artery bypass surgery may well affect mortality rates. Such changes in survival patterns (unaccounted for in our mortality analysis) would create errors in both direct and indirect costs. Potential errors in survival rates would bias the direct-cost estimates for MI, CI, and APU patients and the indirect-cost estimates for MI and CI patients. Table 3–24 illustrates the effect on costs of errors in the estimation of survival probabilities. If, for instance, we have underestimated all survival probabilities by 10 percent, the table shows that our estimate of direct costs would be low by approximately $108 million (that is, 2599 minus 2491), or 4 percent (since CHD patients would survive longer than we anticipated). At the same time, however, our figure for indirect costs would represent an overestimate of $1012 million (that is, 11,225 minus 10,213), or 9 percent, giving us a *net overestimate* of total costs of $904 million (that is, 13,716 minus 12,812), or 7 percent. Conversely, in the case of a 10 percent overestimate of the survival probabilities, our total-cost figure would represent a *net underestimate* of 7 percent.

Direct Costs. Since we have pieced together data on direct-cost components for heart disease from a variety of sources, our direct-cost estimates are vulnerable to error. The most critical components of the direct-cost data—hospitalization expenses and physician service charges—constitute over four-fifths of total direct costs (see table 3–17). An error of 10 percent in

Table 3–24
Sensitivity of Direct, Indirect, and Total Costs of Coronary Heart Disease to Changes in Survival Probabilities, by Diagnostic Type
(Millions of Dollars)

Diagnostic Type	Cost Category	Percentage Variation of Survival Probabilities from Original Values		
		−10 Percent	−0 percent	+10 Percent
Sudden death	Direct	7	7	7
	Indirect	3,891	3,891	3,891
	Total	3,898	3,898	3,898
MI	Direct	1,445	1,497	1,549
	Indirect	6,074	5,369	4,665
	Total	7,519	6,866	6,214
CI	Direct	577	603	630
	Indirect	2,266	1,958	1,650
	Total	2,843	2,561	2,280
APU	Direct	353	384	413
	Indirect	7	7	7
	Total	360	391	420
Total CHD	Direct	2,382	2,491	2,599
	Indirect	12,238	11,225	10,213
	Total	14,620	13,716	12,812

Note: All costs are in 1975 dollars, discounted at 6 percent.

estimating hospitalization costs would induce an error of approximately 5 percent in the direct-cost total. Comparable inaccuracy in estimating physician fees would result in a total-direct-cost error of about 3 percent. However, if all other direct-cost components (that is, emergency services, laboratory fees, drugs, and insurance administration expenses) were in error by as much as 10 percent, the total direct costs would consequently err by only 2 percent.

Discounting. The discount rate selected for this and the three other disease analyses has had significant influences on the present valuation of all future costs. This is demonstrated in table 3–25, where the effects of the choice of the discount rate on direct costs disaggregated by age and sex are displayed. Had all direct costs been discounted at 2 instead of at 6 percent, the present-valued total would have risen by 19 percent, to $2.955 billion. At a discount rate of 10 percent, present-valued direct costs would have fallen by 10

Table 3–25
Sensitivity to the Discount Rate of Total Direct Costs of Coronary Heart Disease, by Age
(Millions of Dollars)

	Discount Rate		
Age	*2 Percent*	*6 Percent*	*10 Percent*
Males			
0–14	1	1	1
15–24	4	3	2
25–34	45	34	29
35–44	247	195	170
45–54	445	367	326
55–64	596	516	468
65–74	390	356	333
75+	191	179	170
Total males	1,919	1,650	1,500
Females			
0–14	0	0	0
15–24	1	0	0
25–34	8	5	4
35–44	43	30	25
45–54	148	112	94
55–64	363	288	247
65–74	294	248	219
75+	178	158	144
Total females	1,036	841	733
Total population	2,955	2,491	2,233

Note: All costs are in 1975 dollars.

percent, to $2.233 billion. As one would expect, the proportional effects of the discount-rate choice are greater for younger victims, since their costs are, on average, spread over a greater time. At each age, the discount-rate choice has proportionately more effect on direct costs for women than for men.

The corresponding data for indirect costs are shown in table 3–26. These costs are spread over as long a period as direct costs but are not so heavily concentrated in the first year. As a result, discounting at different rates more strongly influences the estimates of indirect costs. The proportionate impact of the discount-rate choice again declines with rising age. The choice of a 2 percent discount rate would have increased indirect costs by 35 percent; discounting at 10 percent would have lowered them by 20 percent.

Indirect Costs. Our estimate of total indirect costs depends on our assumptions about (1) the discount rate, taken to be 6 percent; (2) the annual rate of productivity growth in the economy, estimated at 1 percent; and (3)

Table 3–26
Sensitivity to the Discount Rate of Total Indirect Costs of Coronary Heart Disease, by Age
(Millions of Dollars)

	Discount Rate		
Age	*2 Percent*	*6 Percent*	*10 Percent*
Males			
0–14	22	7	3
15–24	96	44	25
25–34	939	525	336
35–44	3,590	2,324	1,641
45–54	4,313	3,292	2,635
55–64	3,226	2,811	2,501
65–74	271	240	216
75+	12	11	10
Total males	12,469	9,254	7,366
Females			
0–14	2	1	0
15–24	9	4	3
25–34	87	50	33
35–44	374	242	172
45–54	893	651	507
55–64	879	698	579
65–74	336	285	246
75+	44	41	38
Total females	2,625	1,971	1,578
Total population	15,094	11,225	8,944

Note: All costs are in 1975 dollars.

the mode of valuing household labor, the market-value approach. Table 3–27 shows the sensitivity of indirect costs to changes in these analytical assumptions. We see there that alternative choices regarding these assumptions could lead to estimates of total indirect costs varying from as high as $20.5 billion to as low as $8.5 billion—a possible range of $12 billion. By adopting the market-value approach to evaluating household labor, our base-case estimate of $11.2 billion is in the lower part of this range. Had we followed the opportunity-cost method of valuation (and maintained the discount rate and productivity growth rate at their assumed levels), total indirect costs would have increased by approximately $2.6 billion, or 23 percent. In this scenario, women would have accounted for 23 percent of all indirect costs versus 18 percent under the market-value approach.

Other factors that significantly affect indirect costs include the estimates of the relative work rates of heart attack survivors (table 3–18 and 3–19), as well as the national figures providing employment and wage rates for the disease-free population. The chief possible source of imprecision here derives from our reliance on Weinblatt's (1966) data on work rates for heart attack survivors. These data might be atypical or outdated. If they are inaccurate, only the forgone earnings of MI and CI patients will be affected. To illustrate, we consider a hypothetical error of 10 percent in estimating relative work rates for the first, second, and subsequent years past the first heart attack. In this case, the expected postmorbid earnings of MI and CI patients also would be in error by 10 percent. This would alter the postmorbid earnings by approximately $1.120 billion and the forgone earnings by the same amount. This would represent an adjustment of 15

Table 3–27
Sensitivity of Total Indirect Costs of Coronary Heart Disease to the Discount Rate, Productivity Growth Factor, and Mode of Valuing Household Labor
(Billions of Dollars)

		Discount Rate	Rate of Productivity Growth		
			0 Percent	*1 Percent*	*2 Percent*
Market-value approach	Discount rate	2%	13.9	15.1	16.5
		6%	10.5	11.2	12.0
		10%	8.5	8.9	9.5
Opportunity-cost approach	Discount rate	2%	17.2	18.7	20.5
		6%	12.9	13.8	14.8
		10%	10.4	11.0	11.6

Note: All costs are in 1975 dollars.

percent in the indirect costs of the MI and CI patient groups and of 10 percent in the indirect costs of all CHD incident cases.

Conclusions from the Sensitivity Analysis

We have not considered all possible sources of imprecision and error in our calculations, but we have examined the most critical. Based on our sensitivity analysis, we infer that the most important sources of imprecision are the incidence data, the data on survival rates, the data on survivor work rates, and the analytical assumptions. All these potential sources of error have a substantial effect on indirect costs, an important result since indirect costs constitute 82 percent of total economic costs in our base-case analysis.

To refine the analysis reported here, highest priority should be placed on the four components just mentioned. While several minor issues affect CHD incidence estimates, the main source of imprecision appears to be the possible idiosyncratic trends in incidence over the past few years. Technological innovations in the treatment of heart disease and the recent reported decline in annual mortality owing to coronary heart disease suggest that continued reliance on the survival-rate data from Framingham may be inappropriate. Survivor work rates for CHD patients need to be updated. The vast shifts in the absolute value of indirect costs when we vary the analytical assumptions are disconcerting. While there is merit in trying to resolve the uncertainty in the key variables affected (that is, the discount rate, the productivity-growth factor, and the mode of valuing household labor), the large shifts in value caused by changing the assumptions do not diminish the utility of our estimates. As long as consistent assumptions are maintained across different illnesses, the ratios of the costs of one illness to those of another will vary less than the shifts in absolute totals suggest. The *comparative* economic costs of these illnesses, indicating relative economic magnitudes, hence are less sensitive to the variation in the analytical assumptions than the absolute costs.

Data in other parts of the analysis (for example, on recurrence and direct-cost components) are subject to error but have modest impact on disease-cost totals. Despite the imperfect data base, the eventual effects of total costs of errors in the direct-cost components are much less than similar errors in other variables. This occurs primarily because total direct costs are a small proportion of total economic costs for CHD.

In sum, our estimate of annual total costs of coronary heart disease at $13.7 billion must be interpreted in light of the possible errors brought out in the sensitivity analysis. Despite these possible sources of imprecision, we conclude with confidence that the incidence-based costs of coronary heart disease will substantially exceed those of stroke (see chapter 4), will be exceeded by those of cancer (see chapter 5), and will roughly parallel those of motor vehicle injuries (see chapter 6).

Notes

1. J.T. Doyle, A.S. Heslin, H.E. Hilleboe, P.F. Formel, and R.F. Korns, A prospective study of degenerative cardiovascular disease in Albany. Report of three years experience. I: Ischemic heart disease, *American Journal of Public Health* 47(April 1975):25–32; R.M. Hagstrom, C.F. Federspiel, and Y.C. Ho, Incidence of myocardial infarction and sudden death from coronary heart disease in Nashville, Tennessee, *Circulation* 44(November 1971):884–890; H. Eisenberg, W.R. Feltner, G.H. Payne, and C.A. Haddad, The epidemiology of coronary heart disease in Middlesex County, Connecticut *Journal of Chronic Diseases* 14(2):221–235; 1961; L. Kuller, M. Cooper, J. Perper, and R. Fisher, Myocardial infarction and sudden death in an urban community, *Bulletin of the New York Academy of Medicine* 49(6):532–543, 1973; W.J. Zuckel, R.H. Lewis, P.E. Enterline, R.C. Painter, L.S. Ralston, R.M. Fawcett, A.P. Meredith, and B. Peerson, A short-term community study of the epidemiology of coronary heart disease, *American Journal of Public Health* 49(12):1630–1639, 1959; S. Shapiro, E. Weinblatt, C.W. Frank, and R.V. Sager, Incidence of coronary heart disease in a population insured for medical care (HIP). Part II, *American Journal of Public Health* 59(6):1–101, 1969; J. Cassel, S. Heyden, A.G. Bartel, B.H. Kaplan, H.A. Tyroler, J.C. Cornoni, and L.G. Hames, Incidence of coronary heart disease by ethnic group, social class, and sex, *Archives of Internal Medicine* 128(6):901–906, 1971; and, J.R. Margolis, R.F. Gillum, M. Feinleib, R.C. Brasch, and R.R. Fabsitz, Community surveillance for coronary heart disease: The Framingham cardiovascular disease survey. Comparisons with the Framingham heart study and previous short-term studies, *American Journal of Cardiology* 37(1):61–67, 1976.

2. This requirement can be relaxed if immediate base-line incidence estimates are required or if the current study is to serve as a verification or updating of a prior more comprehensive study.

3. U.S. Department of Health, Education and Welfare, Public Health Service and National Institutes of Health, *The Framingham Study—An Epidemiological Investiation of Cardiovascular Disease*, Sections 1 through 32.

4. W.B. Kannel, Some lessons in cardiovascular epidemiology from Framingham *American Journal of Cardiology* 37(February 1976):271.

5. S. Cretin, Modeling the impact of treatment strategies on death from myocardial infarction, in T.R. Willemain and R.C. Larson (eds.),

Emergency Medical Systems Analysis (Lexington, Mass.: Lexington Books, D.C. Heath and Co., 1977), p. 147.

6. D. Shurtleff, *Some Characteristics Related to the Incidence of Cardiovascular Disease and Death: Framingham Study, 18-Year Follow-Up. The Framingham Study: An Epidemiological Investigation of Cardiovascular Disease,* Section 30 (1974), p. 18.

7. J.R. Margolis, W.B. Kannel, M. Feinleib, T.R. Dawber, and P.M. McNamara, Clinical features of unrecognized myocardial infarction—Silent and symptomatic, *American Journal of Cardiology* 32(1973):1–7. .

8. T.N. Yames, Sudden death related to myocardial infarction, *Circulation* 45(1972):27.

9. Shurtleff, *Some Characteristics Related to the Incidence of Cardiovascular Disease and Death,* p. 21.

10. Ibid., p. 20.

11. Ibid., pp. 17–18.

12. In the Framingham Heart Study, the operational definition of *angina pectoris uncomplicated* is angina pectoris that developed in an individual between two successive biennial examinations but where the individual remained free of any other manifestation of coronary disease during that period.

13. Derived from unpublished data of the 1970 U.S. Census.

14. T. Gordon and C.C. Garst, Coronary heart disease in adults, *Vital and Health Statistics Series* 11(10):5 and 13, 1965.

15. Assumptions based on limited unpublished data on the incidence of CHD in people over 75 received from Dr. Paul Sorlie of the Framingham Heart Study, January 1978.

16. For each age and sex cohort, estimates of the proportion of the national population free of all forms of coronary heart disease and free of heart attack were developed from national CHD prevalence data presented in Gordon and Garst, Coronary heart disease in adults, and C.S. Wilder, Prevalence of chronic circulatory conditions: United States, 1972 *Vital and Health Statistics Series* 10(94), 1974.

17. Cretin, Modeling and impact of treatment strategies on death from myocardial infarction, p. 149.

18. Data on the probability of an APU patient experiencing a heart attack later than 10 years past diagnosis are limited in the Framingham study and no comparable data are found in other studies. Consequently, in extending the cumulative probabilities of table 3–10 into the future, we have not incorporated the possibility of heart attacks occurring after the tenth year.

19. Kannel, Some lessons in cardiovascular epidemiology from Framingham, p. 276.

20. E. Weinblatt, S. Shapiro, C.W. Frank, and R.V. Sager, Return to

work and work status following first myocardial infarction, *American Journal of Public Health* 65(2):169–185, 1966. In this study, the author reported that after 1 year, all patients younger than 45 return to work, while 94.2 percent of all patients age 45 to 54 and 81.8 percent of all patients 55 to 64 return to work. This suggests that MI survivors do not experience severe disability. Interviews with Dr. Peter Urchak, August 25, 1977, and Dr. Peter Cohn, June 29, 1977, also strongly implied that MI patients do not have long periods of disability.

21. Based in part on an interview with Dr. Peter Cohn, Peter Brent Brigham Hospital, June 29, 1977.

22. Based in part on interviews with Dr. Paul Levine, October 6, 1977, and Dr. Michael Pozen, July 7, 1977.

23. D. Bendor and W. Fowkes, Sudden and unexpected death due to arteriosclerotic heart disease—Implications for mobile coronary care units, *Circulation* [Suppl. 3] 40(4):III-43, 1969.

24. S. Cretin, *A Model of the Risk of Death from Myocardial Infarction*, Technical Report No. 09-74 (Cambridge, Mass.: Massachusetts Institute of Technology, Operations Research Center, 1974), p. 16; H.A. Dewar, J.P.K. McCollum, and M. Floyd, A year's experience with a mobile coronary resuscitation unit, *British Journal of Medicine* 4(677):226–229, 1969; and S. Carveth, D. Olson, and J. Bechtel, Emergency medical care system *Archives of Surgery* 108(April 1974):528–530.

25. S. Cretin, Cost/benefit analysis of treatment and prevention of myocardial infarction, *Health Services Research* (Summer 1977):1978.

26. Synthesized from data found in the literature and figures obtained in an interview with Michael Hooley, Unit Manager, Emergency Room, Massachusetts General Hospital, July 21, 1977.

27. Abstracted from data found in American Hospital Association, *Hospital Statistics*, 1976.

28. Cretin, Cost/benefit analysis, p. 177.

29. Commission on Professional and Hospital Activities, *Length of Stay in PAS Hospitals by Diagnosis, United States, 1975* (Ann Arbor, 1976), pp. 90–91.

30. A. Owens, At last: Hard figures on how fast fees have been climbing, *Medical Economics* (October 13, 1975):106.

31. J.P. Acton, *Evaluating Public Programs to Save Lives: The Case of Heart Attacks*, Rand Corporation Report No. R-950-RC (Santa Monica, Calif.: Rand Corporation, January 1973).

32. Cretin, Cost/benefit analysis, p. 177.

33. *Length of Stay in PAS Hospitals*, pp. 90–91.

34. Ibid.

35. Ibid.

36. Based in part on information obtained in an interview with Dr. Peter Urchak, August 25, 1977.

37. Based in part on information obtained in an interview with Dr. Paul Levine, October 6, 1977.

38. The prevalence data were abstracted from information found in T. Dawber, F. Moore, and G. Mann, Coronary heart disease in the Framingham study, *American Journal of Public Health* 47(Suppl.):4–24, 1957; and also found in *Length of Stay in PAS Hospitals*, p. 91.

39. *Length of Stay in PAS Hospitals*, p. 91.

40. This estimate of 5 visits annually represents the average based on a variable pattern. For the nonhospitalized angina pectoris patient, we found that the number of visits annually ranged from 2 to 8.7 a year. For the hospitalized angina pectoris patient, the typical pattern involved a physician visit within 3 weeks of discharge and then 4 additional visits during the year. For the MI patient, physician visits varied according to the particular patient and physician and ranged from an initial visit 6 weeks past discharge and 2 subsequent visits during the year to a maximum of an annual visit 2 weeks past discharge and follow-up visits once every 3 weeks. Average physician fees per outpatient visit are derived from data in Owens, At last: Hard figures on how fees have been climbing, p. 102.

41. This estimate represents the average of a range running from one complete set of x-ray laboratory tests per year (the pattern followed by a general practitioner whose patients had to use outside laboratory facilities) to one complete set each visit (a pattern followed when the primary physician was a cardiologist with an office equipped for such services).

42. Based in part on information obtained in interviews with four cardiologists: Dr. Michael Pozen, July 7, 1977; Dr. Peter Urchak, August 25, 1977; Dr. Peter Cohn, June 29, 1977; and Dr. Paul Levine, October 6, 1977.

43. Ibid.

44. Based on unpublished data from the Framingham Heart Study giving the number of instances of second heart attacks following recognized MI 1 month, 1 year, and each subsequent year following the initial attack.

45. Cretin, Modeling the impact of treatment strategies, p. 149.

46. The cost of estimates for MI and CI include full utilization of emergency services. Consequently, $125 was added to the MI and CI initial treatment costs shown in table 3–14.

47. These probabilities are conditional on surviving 30 days.

48. The Weinblatt sample consisted of members of the Health Insurance Plan (HIP) of New York. Sixty-five percent of the members were insured through group contracts with governmental agencies, while trade union welfare funds insured about 20 percent of the sample.

49. Weinblatt, et al., Return to work and work status following first myocardial infarction, p. 173.

50. Kannel, Some lessons in cardiovascular epidemiology, p.276.

51. The productivity loss incurred by survivors of recurrences who are inactive during their recovery periods are not captured by our model. Sensitivity analysis, however, shows this exclusion to be minor: at most, 2 percent of forgone earnings, and in all likelihood, considerably less.

4 Stroke

The Stroke Syndrome

Cerebrovascular stroke in the United States consitutes a major cause of death and disability. The common term refers both to the long-term perspective of disease in the blood vessels of the brain (whose technical term is *cerebro-vascular disease* or *CVD*) and to the sudden episodes of severe mental affliction (*cerebrovascular accidents* or *CVA*s) that often dramatically signal presence of the disease. While technical distinction is made between heat stroke (an acute, dangerous reaction to heat exposure), paralytic stroke (sudden onset of paralysis owing to injury), and apoplectic stroke (sudden loss of consciousness owing to circulatory dysfunction), the use of the word *stroke* by itself refers only to the last of these three syndromes. We shall follow this terminological convenience.

Stroke results from two major causes: (1) arterial blockage resulting from emboli (undissolved matter in the blood) or from thrombi (blood clots), and (2) hemorrhage into the brain or into the subarachnoid space (the space between the innermost two of the three membranes surrounding the brain). Embolic and thrombotic strokes involve ischemia (interruption in the supply of blood to tissue) and infarction (resultant tissue death). These strokes may result from buildup of plaque in the major arteries of the neck and brain, from arteriosclerosis (hardening of the arteries) from thrombi related to arterial plaque or other causes, and from emboli. Emboli are associated with rupture of arterial plaques and with rheumatic heart disease, among other sources. Mild ischemia may be caused by temporary hypotension (low blood pressure), by vascular spasm, by compression or kinking of vessels, or by brain compression owing to tumor or hematoma (a swelling containing blood). Ischemia causing impairment for less than 24 hours is considered a *transient ischemic attack* (TIA). Episodes lasting more than a day followed by complete recovery are termed *reversible ischemic neurological deficits* (RINDs) but are so rare that we have excluded them from our analysis. Hemorrhagic strokes are most commonly related to hypertension, to vessel malformation, to ruptured aneurysms (abnormal bulges in blood vessels), and to altered states of blood coagulability. In addition to these direct causes, note also should be taken of factors that are epidemiologically related to strokes and contribute to inducing them. These include hypertensive vascular disease, diabetes mellitus, hypothyroidism, obesity, cigarette smoking,

133

hyperuricemia (excessive uric acid in the blood), and hyperlipidemia (excessive fat in the blood).

Since specific cerebral dysfunction—tissue death in part of the brain—may be either ischemic or hemorrhagic, immediate causal distinction is not always possible. A broad range of symptoms is associated with both stroke types and includes coma, convulsion, confusion, headache, hemiplegia (paralysis of one-half the body, generally that contralateral to the affected side of brain), vertigo, numbness, diploplia (double vision), and aphasia (speech difficulty). Clinical manifestations are useful in identifying the affected brain area or the occluded (blocked) artery.

Epidemiology

Stroke is predominantly an affliction of the aged, having an incidence of less than 1 per year per 10,000 persons under 35 and rising to a level of over 100 per year per 10,000 persons over 75 (see Incidence section of this chapter). Aggregate incidence for the United States in 1975 amounted to 1.8 per 10,000. Mortality rates have shown a similar relationship to age, rising from a rate of 3.2 deaths per year per 10,000 persons aged 45 to 54, to 9.2 for ages 55 to 64, to 30.3 for ages 65 to 74, and to 142.4 for persons over 75. A total of 194,038 deaths, or 9.11 per 10,000 of the whole U.S. population, were attributed to cerebrovascular disease in 1975 (NCHS, 1977). Age-adjusted mortality rates for nonwhites exceed those of whites.[1] Regional variation of stroke mortality within the United States has been identified. In particular, evidence points to significantly higher mortality among whites in the Southeast.[2] Whether this in an artifact of diagnostic terminology, however, remains problematic.[3] Variation in mortality across nations also has been noted. Adjusting for age, Japan has a death rate from stroke of more than twice that of the United States. Other nations with especially high rates are Finland, Scotland, Uruguay, and Italy, while Belgium, Mexico, and the Philippines have remarkably low rates.[4]

Among the types of CVD, an aggregation of several study results found that 69 percent were thrombotic or embolic infarctions, 12 percent were intracranial hemorrhages, 8 percent subarachnoid hemorrhages, and 11 percent unknown or other.[5] Hemorrhages have a sharply higher mortality rate than infarctions—30.6 percent of all first stroke victims with hemorrhage survive 1 year versus 56.1 percent of first stroke victims with infarction—and hence account for disproportionately more deaths.[6]

Therapy and Management

A number of measures can aid recovery from a cerebrovascular accident. These include anticoagulant therapy, antihypertensive agents, vasodilators (drugs that expand the blood vessels), and inhalation therapy. Critical in distinguishing between hemorrhagic and occlusive (embolic or throbotic) strokes and in localizing points of blockage is cerebral angiography (x-ray examination of the blood vessels in the head). Computerized tomography (CAT scans) are increasingly utilized in differential stroke diagnosis. Surgery may be performed to remove atherosclerotic plaque or to clip intracranial aneurysms. Rehabilitation programs are important in achieving maximum recovery of brain function.

Improvements in population-based management of stroke may be attained along sociomedical dimensions. Heightened awareness of risk factors for stroke and behavior modifications for high-risk individuals may reduce incidence and severity. Eliminating delay in inaugurating rehabilitation is thought to bring about more complete recovery.[7]

Transient Ischemic Attacks (TIAs)

Temporary loss of neurological (brain) function occurs in transient ischemic attacks (TIAs). These are defined to be "episodes of temporary focal dysfunction of vascular origin" lasting no more than 24 hours.[8] (Other definitions set variant time limits for the TIA. Twenty-four hours is the most common limit.) They are distinguished from "completed," "permanent," or "persistent" strokes. Commonly ascribed causes for TIAs include, among others, microemboli, sludging, local ischemia, or hypertension.[9] Most TIAs last a matter of minutes: a median 14 minutes for TIAs of the carotid artery system (the two major arteries in the front of the neck and their branches) and a median 8 minutes for TIAs of the vertebral-basilar system (the two major arteries in the back of the neck leading to the back of the brain and their branches). Nine-tenths of all TIAs in the carotid system (CAS TIAs) terminate within 6 hours; nine-tenths of vertebral-basilar TIAs (VBS TIAs), within 2 hours.[10]

Conclusive localization of the TIA (distinguishing between origin in the carotid or vertebral-basilar system) is not always possible. Attacks are accordingly classified as definite or suspected instances of each type.[11] Dizziness, ataxia (spasticity), and diploplia are common in VBS TIAs, while dysphasia (speech impairment), one-side weakness, and sensory complaints predominate in CAS TIAs.[12] Among all TIAs (including recurrences and TIAs subsequent to stroke), CAS TIAs are more likely to be followed by cerebral infarction than are VBS TIAs. VBS TIAs are more likely to be followed by repeat TIAs.[13] Endarterectomy (surgical reaming and cleaning out of occuluded arteries) is felt to be more efficacious for carotid TIAs.

Epidemiology of TIAs

Through the age of 64, males are nearly twice as likely as females to have TIAs. Thereafter, female incidence roughly parallels that of males. Male predominance is greater among CAS TIAs.[14]

The incidence of TIAs among blacks is thought to be slightly higher than that among whites. Rates of TIA incidence observed in populations with few blacks (Rochester, Minnesota) have been found similar to rates in an area with a substantial black population (Evans County, Georgia).[15] Since the latter figures are based on individual recall, they may represent a substantial underestimate. For lack of definitive data, we make the conservative assumption that rates within the two racial groups are the same.

Consequences and Therapy

Transient ischemic attacks do not in themselves cause deaths but are associated with reduced life expectancy. This is seen in table 4–1, which compares the survival of persons with a history of stroke experiencing first TIAs with their actuarial expectancy. Only 28.9 percent of those with TIA survived 10 years beyond their first attack, in comparison with an expected 10-year survival rate of 52.2 percent. Figuring prominently among eventual causes of death for TIA victims are cerebrovascular and cardiovascular events. Twenty-nine percent of the deaths in this population were ascribed to cerebrovascular causes; 13 percent to cerebral infarction; 9 percent to intracranial hemorrhage; and 7 percent to strokes of unknown type. Heart

Table 4–1
Survival of Persons after First Transient Ischemic Attack (TIA)
in Comparison with Actuarial Expectancy

Years after Diagnosis	Survival Rate	Adjusted Normal Survival Rate
0	1.000	—
1/12	0.960	—
3/12	0.919	—
6/12	0.899	—
1	0.857	0.946
2	0.802	0.894
3	0.727	0.843
4	0.666	0.793
5	0.620	0.745
6	0.553	0.698
7	0.492	0.652
8	0.454	0.607
9	0.345	0.564
10	0.289	0.522

Source: Abstracted from J.P. Whisnant, A population study of stroke and TIA: Rochester Minnesota, In *Stroke*, edited by Gillingham, Mawdsley, and Williams (Edinburgh: Churchill Livingstone, 1976), p. 35 (Table 15). Reprinted with permission.

Note: Based on sample of 88 males and 110 females, averaging 70 years of age in Rochester, Minnesota, 1966–1969.

disease was listed as the cause of death in 44 percent of the group, while other (26 percent) and unknown (1 percent) causes accounted for the remainder of the deaths.

Therapy for TIA patients aims to prevent completed strokes. Surgical intervention—endarterectomies—has been shown in certain cases to improve survival.[16] Anticoagulants and antiplatelet-aggregating therapies are frequently prescribed but to date have not demonstrated conclusive efficacy.[17] Antihypertensive regimens are indicated for hypertensives.[18]

Incidence

Data Deficiencies

Owing to idiosyncrasies in the manner by which strokes are managed and recorded, accurate data on incidence are difficult to secure. This is indicated in figure 4–1. In the best of all possible worlds for the epidemiologist, all cases of stroke are brought to medical attention, diagnosis is accurate, and complete records are kept and are accessible. This enables direct and simple calculation of incidence. In reality, however, not all cases of stroke appear in the medical system, medical records themselves are inconsistent and subject to error, and certification of death cause is yet less accurate.[19] That accurate certification of death does not ensure accurate reporting was shown by one study (Florey, 1967), which found that only 73 percent of strokes reported on death certificates were so included in published mortality data. The figure indicates, moreover, that documentation is least adequate for cases that never find their way into medical or death records. Thus, to capture all occurrences of stroke, including those which survive and do not receive medical attention, all members of a defined population must be surveyed. It would be useful, in addition, to investigate all deaths to determine whether new strokes not otherwise noted are implicated. If one were interested only in the direct medical costs of stroke, reliance on medical records would suffice. We are, however, concerned with indirect costs (largely forgone earnings owing to impairment or death) and nonmedical costs (for example, attendant care for possibly unreported strokes). This forces us to piece together a model of incidence, capturing strokes not represented or poorly documented in medical records and death certificates.

Population-Based Studies

While the ideal incidence study does not exist, several studies incorporating its main features have been reported. Since 1948, the well-known Framingham Heart Study has conducted biennial examinations of a sample

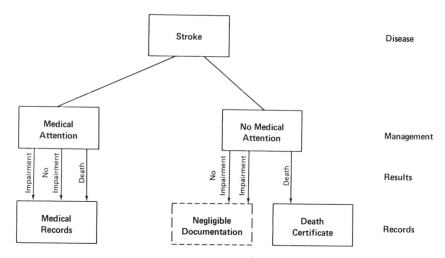

Figure 4–1. Schematic Representation of Recorded Information on Stroke

of Framingham, Massachusetts residents initially free of cardiovascular disease. The study constitutes one of the more methodologically thorough investigations of heart disease and stroke ever undertaken. Results are provided through an ongoing series of monographs, of which, for our purposes, the most important is by Shurtleff (1974). Since, however, the initial population ranged in age from 30 to 62, the data are accordingly restricted. In particular, there are very few cases in the older age groups, among whom the incidence of stroke is highest. Moreover, the population is partially selected, since those with preexisting cardiovascular disease at the beginning of the study were excluded.

Four studies have been performed that did not include thorough monitoring of a population, but which attempted to discover all cases of stroke in a defined group. These investigations reviewed death certificates and hospital records for residents of specified areas and either reviewed physicians' records or requested physicians to report all cases of stroke in residents of the region. Matsumoto et al. (1973) reported the results of such a study on the residents of Rochester, Minnesota over the period 1955 to 1969. Extensions to the mid-1970s of Matsumoto's work on the same population are reported by Furlan (1979), Garraway (1979a) and Garraway (1979b). Alter et al. (1970) conducted a similar study in 1965–1966 in the communities of Fargo, North Dakota and Moorhead, Minnesota. In both these studies, first strokes only were included in incidence figures. Two other studies, by Eisenberg et al. (1964) in Middlesex County, Connecticut and by Eckstrom et al. (1969) in three counties in central Missouri, include repeat as well as first strokes.

Numerous other studies of stroke incidence in populations have been performed—both in the United States and abroad. These studies used the same general method of reviewing medical records and death certificates to discover cases of stroke. An exception is the study of Heyman et al. (1971) in Evans County, Georgia, which included examination of the population. This work, in a departure from standard epidemiological practice, included both "definite" and "probable" strokes in its incidence computations. Age-specific incidence rates for both sexes combined from twelve studies are displayed in table 4–2.

General Findings on Incidence

From these studies, general conclusions about the epidemiology of stroke have emerged, as summarized by Stallones (1972). Incidence rates increase with age, are higher for males than for females, and are higher for blacks than for whites. A cooperative study of hospital records (Kuller, 1970) also indicated geographic variation within the United States, with the Southeast having the highest incidence rates. This variation had long been suspected because of differences in mortality rates between the Southeast and the rest of the country (Soltero, 1978).

Sex- and age-specific rates are available from the studies just mentioned. Most of the best studies, however, are from predominantly white populations and do not reflect racial differences. Oh (1971) has estimated that stroke incidence in blacks is at least 1.5 times that in whites, and this is borne out by the two available studies having incidence data on blacks and whites in the same population (Eckstrom, 1969; Heyman, 1971). When the number of strokes and the population at risk for whites and blacks from both studies are combined and the crude incidence rates are computed, the rate for black males is 1.44 times that for white males, and the rate for black females is 1.42 that for white females.

Geographic Difference

Regional variation is less easily catered to. Of the five most comparable U.S. studies (Eisenberg, 1964; Eckstrom, 1969; Alter, 1970; Matsumoto, 1973; and Shurtleff, 1974), none were conducted in the Southeast; four of five were carried out in New England or the North Central States. If incidence rates are truly higher in the Southeast, such regional data will lead to underestimating national rates. We believe, however, that this underestimation is not substantial. The same study (Kuller, 1970) of hospital morbidity that found higher rates in the Southeast also found the rates discovered in population studies to be intermediate in the range of rates derived from hospital studies.

Table 4–2
Age-Specific Incidence Rates per 10,000 per Year for All Types of Stroke (Excluding Transient Ischemic Attacks), as Reported in Population-Based Studies

Author: Locale:	Shurtleff, 1974 Framingham, Mass.	Eckstrom, 1969 Central Missouri	Eisenberg, 1964 Middlesex County, Conn.	Alter, 1970 Fargo, N.D. and Moorhead, Minn.	Matsumoto, 1973 Rochester, Minn.	Heyman, 1971 Evans County, Ga.
Dates of Study:	1950–1968	1965	1957–1958	1965–1966	1955–1969	1960–1969
Rates for Both Sexes at Age:						
<35	—	1.0	0.2	0.8	0.4	0.3
35–44	—	0	1.0	6.0	4.0	12.0
45–54	14.0	1.0	11.0	17.0	11.0	39.0
55–64	30.0	32.0	40.0	35.0	36.0	44.0
65–74	80.0	59.0	94.0	108.0	79.0	—
75–84	—	229.0	219.0	343.0 ⎫	⎫ 216.0	—
85+	—	479.0	507.0	516.0 ⎭	⎭	101.0
Comments:	Selected population originally free of cardiovascular disease; first strokes only.	White only; "major" strokes only (deficit persisting 72 hours after onset).	Population 98 percent white.	First strokes only; population 99.6 white	First strokes only.	Whites only; based on definite or probable stroke examination.

Author: Locale:	Whisnant, 1971 Rochester, Minn.	Carpenter, 1972 Western Penn.	Acheson, 1971 Oxford, Eng.	Zupping, 1976 Estonia	Aho, 1974 Finland	Stallones, 1972 Midpoint Estimates for U.S. from Published Studies
Dates of Study:	1945–1954	1968	1963	1970–1973	1972	
Rates for Both Sexes at Age:						
<35	0.2	1.0	0.4	1.0	3.0	2.0
35–44	3.0	2.0	2.0	1.0	2.0	10.0
45–54	16.0	16.0	33.0	6.0	12.0	10.0
55–64	37.0	66.0	33.0	16.0	36.0	35.0
65–74	108.0	139.0	71.0	44.0	49.0	90.0
75–84	249.0 }	395.0 }	219.0 }	133.0	159.0	200.0
85+		655.0		293.0	441.0	400.0
Comments:	First strokes only.	"Major" strokes only.	—	First stroke only.		All races; first strokes only.

By consistently relying on population rates instead of hospital rates, we limit the extent of any underestimation.

Type of Stroke

We have noted that completed strokes are not a single entity but a range of conditions arising from a variety of pathological mechanisms. Since treatment and prognosis vary by category, it is important to distinguish among the types. A common breakdown of stroke in epidemiological studies is into cerebral thrombosis, cerebral embolism, cerebral hemorrhage, and "ill-defined" or "other." It is, however, not always possible to distinguish the types readily in a clinical situation or from medical records—particularly if such tests as angiography, lumbar puncture, or CAT scan have not been performed. A more accurate picture of the relative frequencies of the types can be obtained from the results of an autopsy series, but this does not fully capture the relative frequency of occurrence since survival rates vary by the type of stroke. Further clouding the issue are the varying rules for classifying observed strokes into types. One study, for example, may classify a stroke as embolic in type only if there is a definite source of embolus. Another study may allow cases with suspected sources to be classified as embolic. We have therefore followed the broader classification of cerebral infarction, which includes embolic and thrombotic strokes, and hemorrhage, including cerebral and subarachnoid. This common distinction is followed by Eisenberg (1964) and USDHEW (1980), among others.

Most population studies that report stroke incidence by type also include an "ill-defined/other" category that includes cases in which there was not enough information to classify by type of stroke. Following the lead of several authors (Whisnant, 1976; Matsumoto, 1973; and Stallones, 1972) who have concluded that these cases overwhelmingly comprise cerebral infarctions, we assume that all in this category are infarctions.

The incidence of different types of stroke is thought to vary by age, with younger groups having a higher occurrence of subarachnoid hemorrhage (Stallones, 1972). The proportion of cerebral infarction/other and hemorrhagic strokes found in several of the older incidence studies is presented in table 4–3. These proportions have been weighted by the number of cases in the study and an average of 80 percent cerebral infarction/other and 20 percent hemorrhagic strokes obtained. These figures replicate the results obtained by Kurtzke (1976) with a slightly different group of studies and are close to the 25 percent hemorrhage, 75 percent cerebral infarction/other estimated by the Epidemiology Study Group (Stallones, 1972).

Our own estimates of the proportions of the two main types of stroke derive from separate calculations of the incidence of each. As will be seen,

Table 4–3
Proportion of Types of Stroke Reported in Incidence Studies

			Type of Stroke	
Study	Locale	Total Number of Cases	Cerebral Infarction and Other	Hemorrhage
Wolf, 1977	Framingham, Mass. (22-year follow-up)	267	0.83	0.17
Matsumoto, 1973	Rochester, Minn.	993	0.84	0.16
Eisenberg, 1964	Middlesex County, Conn.	191	0.64	0.36
Alter, 1970	Fargo, N.D.	408	0.77	0.23
Weighted average		1859	0.80	0.20

we estimate that 14 percent of all first strokes occurring in 1975 were hemorrhagic. These figures suggest that the decline in hemorrhagic incidence may exceed that for infarcts. The explanation may, however, derive simply from altered population ratios. Infarcts predominate most over hemorrhages in the older age groups. With population increases in the older groups, a consequence is a rise in the proportion of all strokes that are infarctive.

Secular Trends

A thornier problem is posed by the variability of incidence over time. Observing the Rochester, Minnesota area for over 25 years, Matsumoto (1973) found a steady decrease in annual incidence from 1955 on. Mortality also has been decreasing (*Statistical bulletin of the Metropolitan Life Insurance Company*, 1975). Notwithstanding these findings, epidemiologists of cerebrovasular disease were reluctant as recently as the mid-1970s to consider trends in incidence to be definitely confirmed. Mortality data might, after all, have reflected artifacts resulting from changes in classification methods as well as in survival-pattern trends. (Matsumoto [1973] documented a striking degree of imprecision in the recording of strokes on death certificates.) A practical consideration (as will be shortly seen) was that admission of incidence trends required delicate adjustment for dates of incidence—a considerable complication in an already complex methodology.

With the publication of a trio of articles in 1979 (Furlan, 1979; Garraway, 1979a and Garraway, 1979b) the decline in incidence became irrefutably documented. The trend encompasses both hemorrhagic and infarctive strokes. As a result, epidemiological attention has turned to measuring and explaining the reduced incidence. The extent to which it may be due to behavioral changes (better exercise, less stress), to better personal health habits (less smoking and lower blood cholesterol), to better medical preventive measures (better control of hypertension, endarterectomies), or other factors is currently conjectural.

Recent examination of mortality shows similar trends (Soltero, 1978). Data from the National Center for Health Statistics show drops of at least 25 percent for all 10-year age groups over 35 for whites of both sexes between 1960 and 1975. Parallel patterns were found among nonwhites. Because of the imprecision in measuring incidence, the role of declining incidence as a factor in reduced mortality remains unclear.

Alternative Approaches

The challenge posed to incidence-based cost calculations is to obtain best estimates of 1975 incidence. One possible methodology would be to aggregate data from a number of studies. This approach would offer the advantages of increasing the data pool and of straddling some geographic variation. The drawback is that tenuous adjustments would have to be made to reflect the dates when each study measured incidence.

We felt that a superior alternative would be to base our estimates exclusively on the most recent data—thus minimizing the imprecision inherent in the needed adjustments. These data derive from experience in Rochester, Minnesota. A major advantage over many previous studies of incidence is that separate estimation of hemorrhagic and infarctive strokes is enabled. We describe first the methods used in estimating hemorrhagic incidence.

Hemorrhagic Incidence

The five main steps in gauging the incidence of hemorrhages were (1) identifying a primary data base, (2) adjusting for the two main types of hemorrhage, (3) disaggregating to more age groups, (4) setting in 1975 terms, and (5) adjusting for race.

Step 1. Identifying a Primary Data Base. We felt that the best available data (which were derived from the period 1945–1976) were provided by Furlan (1979). These data are broken down by sex and by five age groupings: under 45, 45 to 54, 55 to 64, 65 to 74, and over 75.

Step 2. Adjusting for the Two Main Types of Hemorrhage. A shortcoming of the Furlan data is that they apply exclusively to intracerebral hemorrhage. To extend these data to comprise all hemorrhages, adjustments must be made to account for subarachnoid hemorrhages. These adjustments were based on data from Matsumoto (1973), who found 38 percent more subarachnoid hemorrhages than cerebral hemorrhages for persons aged 64 or less and 76 percent fewer subarachnoid hemorrhages than cerebral hemorrhages for those over 65. We presumed that the same ratios would apply to the Furlan data, which derived, after all, from the same basic population (the Matsumoto data for 1945 through 1976).

Step 3. Disaggregating to More Age Groups. To break the Furlan data down into narrower age groups, few specific incidence data were available—in large part because of the infrequency of all strokes under the age of 45. To enable a best first approximation of incidence in the four age groups under 45, we assumed a constant relationship between incidence and mortality within these ages. A similar assumption enabled the disaggregation of data on persons over 75 into two age groups. Any errors introduced by these assumptions do not affect the overall magnitude of estimated incidence, just its disaggregation to the different age groups.

Step 4. Setting in 1975 Terms. Using data from Furlan (1979) and NCHS (1979*b*), we adjusted the data arising from steps 1 to 3 to 1975 terms by multiplying by a factor of 0.570. We assumed conservatively that two-thirds of the decline in mortality in the 1970s was due to falling incidence. Had we assumed that incidence was falling at the same rate as mortality, the adjustment factor would have been 0.544. [This factor was obtained in the following way. First, we divided the age-adjusted incidence rate of Furlan for 1945 to 1976 into the comparable rate for 1969 through 1976, obtaining a factor of 0.603. From the midpoint of Furlan's latter interval (1969 to 1976) to the middle of 1975 is 2.5 years. The average annual rate of decline in age-adjusted mortality rates during the mid-1970s was 3.4 percent. Assuming that two-thirds of this rate of decline occurred for 2.5 years reduces the adjustment factor of 0.603 to 0.570.]

Step 5. Adjusting for Race. The estimates cited earlier (Eckstrom, 1969; Heyman, 1971, Oh, 1971), placing age-adjusted black incidence 50 percent above white incidence, were made when age-adjusted mortality rates for blacks exceeded those for whites by at least 50 percent (Soltero, 1978). By 1975, the ratio of black to white mortality for strokes had fallen to 1.38. We accordingly presumed that Furlan's (1979) incidence rates for an over-whelmingly white population would have to be multiplied by 1.4 for blacks. This supposition, combined with data on the proportions of nonwhites in the different age and sex groups, enabled calculation of incidence rates for the total population within each of these groups. These are displayed in table 4–4.

Table 4-4
Annual Incidence of Stroke, by Age and Type of Stroke,
United States, 1975

Age	Estimated Incidence Rate for Hemorrhages (per 100,000)	Estimated Number of Hemorrhages[a]	Estimated Incidence Rate for Infarcts (per 10,000)	Estimated Number of Infarcts[a]
Males				
0-14	0.57	155	0.73	199
15-24	0.94	191	1.53	311
25-34	2.79	429	3.47	533
35-44	9.18	1,024	11.64	1,298
45-54	30.52	3,507	52.25	6,005
55-64	60.89	5,690	218.28	20,396
65-74	78.45	4,728	638.18	38,463
75-84	72.88	1,846	1,331.11	33,717
85+	133.77	820	1,828.06	11,206
Total males	17.64	18,390	107.57	112,128
Females				
0-14	0.56	147	0.22	59
15-24	0.90	179	0.48	95
25-34	2.59	404	1.03	160
35-44	8.24	962	3.35	391
45-54	16.29	2,001	14.69	1,804
55-64	56.32	5,876	162.56	16,961
65-74	44.69	3,507	380.29	29,841
75-84	64.45	2,654	962.87	39,651
85+	107.91	1,365	1,287.83	16,291
Total females	15.63	17,095	96.22	105,253
Total population	16.61	35,485	101.76	217,381

[a]Based on resident population, all races, July 1, 1975, from *Current Population Reports*, Series P-25, Number 614, Table 1; and methodology described in text.

Infarctive Incidence

The four steps in estimating the 1975 incidence of infarctions included (1) identifying a primary data base, (2) disaggregating to more age groups, (3) setting in 1975 terms, and (4) adjusting for race.

Step 1. Identifying a Primary Data Base. Best recent data are those of Garroway (1979*b*). These pertain to all first infarctive strokes in Rochester, Minnesota between 1970 and 1974. In line with accepted practice, these strokes include embolic and thrombotic infarctions and strokes of unknown type.

Step 2. Disaggregating to More Age Groups. Garraway's data distinguished five age groups: under 55, 55 to 64, 65 to 74, 75 to 84, and over 85. We disaggregated the youngest age group in two steps. First, we used Matsumoto's (1973) data to break down the rates for groups aged under 35, 35 to 44, and 45 to 54. Second, mortality data were used to disaggregate the under 35 groups—following the same methodology as for hemorrhages.

Step 3. Setting in 1975 Terms. As with hemorrhages, we assumed that two-thirds of the decline in mortality between 1972 and 1975 could be ascribed to falling incidence. This led us to multiply Garraway's figures by a factor of 0.931.

Step 4. Adjusting for Race. This step was the same as for hemorrhages.

Incidence of All Completed Strokes

The results of these incidence calculations are shown in table 4–4, where the separate incidence rates estimated for hemorrhages and infarctions have been multiplied by the resident U.S. population in the various age and sex groups. Table 4–5 displays the combined incidence of hemorrhagic and infarctive strokes. We see from the two tables that the majority of both types of stroke occurs for those over 55: 75 percent of all first hemorrhages and 95 percent of all first infarcts. The rates of incidence for both stroke types rise with age (with two exceptions that may represent idiosyncrasies of the data sets used). Hemorrhages occur somewhat earlier than infarcts. The age group with the greatest number of first hemorrhages for both sexes is 55 to 64 years. Greatest numbers of first infarcts occur for males between the ages of 65 to 74, and for females, a decade later. Stroke incidence is slightly higher among males, who are estimated to have had 52 percent of all first hemorrhages and of all first infarcts in 1975.

Incidence of Transient Ischemic Attacks (TIAs)

Data on three aspects of TIA occurrences are required: (1) an estimate of first TIAs occurring in 1975 in patients without a history of stroke; (2) an estimate of TIA recurrence following a first TIA in 1975 but without completed stroke; and (3) an estimate of TIA occurrence after completed stroke or strokes, the first of which occurred in 1975. Of these, data on the first are by far the soundest. Only bits and pieces of data indicate TIA recurrence rates and patterns of TIA subsequent to stroke. For computing direct inpatient costs, these are not serious defects because data on

Table 4–5
Total Incidence of Stroke, by Age, United States, 1975

	1975 U.S. Population (Thousands)[a]	Total Stroke Incidence Rate Proportion (Per 10,000)	Total First Strokes	Proportion Hemorrhagic
Males				
0–14	27,365	1.29	354	0.44
15–24	20,356	2.47	502	0.38
25–34	15,356	6.26	962	0.45
35–44	11,153	20.82	2,322	0.44
45–54	11,492	82.77	9,322	0.37
55–64	9,344	279.17	26,086	0.22
65–74	6,027	716.63	43,191	0.11
75–84	2,533	1,403.99	35,563	0.05
85+	613	1,961.83	12,026	0.07
Total males	104,239	125.21	130,328	0.14
Females				
0–14	26,284	0.78	206	0.71
15–24	19,913	1.38	274	0.65
25–34	15,581	3.62	564	0.72
35–44	11,671	11.59	1,353	0.71
45–54	12,280	30.99	3,805	0.53
55–64	10,434	218.87	22,837	0.26
65–74	7,847	424.98	33,348	0.11
75–84	4,118	1,027.73	42,305	0.06
85+	1,265	1,395.73	17,656	0.08
Total females	109,393	111.84	122,348	0.14
Total population	213,632	118.37	252,676	0.14

Source: Aggregation of elements in table 4–4.
[a]From *Current Population Reports*, Series P-25, Number 614.

hospitalization for TIA are reasonably good. Even though data do not permit definitive distinction of first TIAs, recurrent TIAs, and TIAs susbsequent to stroke, inaccuracies in estimating the breakdown will only have the effect of ascribing hospital costs to the wrong year.

The best data on incidence of first TIAs derive from a study of Rochester, Minnesota patients having first TIAs between January 1, 1955 and December 31, 1969.[20] These incidence rates are shown in the second column of table 4–6. Although the population studied was overwhelmingly white, rates obtained for populations with large proportions of blacks are similar.[21] Accordingly, we assume the estimated rates apply nationally. Multiplying these rates by 1975 population figures provides an estimate of first TIA incidence in 1975 in the rightmost column of table 4–6. This indicates that

Table 4–6
Incidence of First Transient Ischemic Attacks (TIAs), United States, 1975

	1975 U.S. Population (thousands)	Estimated Incidence (per 10,000)	First TIAs in 1975
Males			
0–44	74,230	0.2	1,485
45–54	11,492	2.1	2,413
55–64	9,344	9.6	8,971
65–74	6,027	26.3	15,851
75+	3,146	26.7	8,397
Total males	104,239	3.6	37,117
Females			
0–44	73,449	0.04	294
45–54	12,280	1.2	1,474
55–64	10,434	5.0	5,218
65–74	7,847	19.2	15,066
75+	5,383	30.6	16,469
Total females	109,393	3.5	38,521
Total population	213,632	3.5	75,638

Source: Data abstracted from J.P. Whisnant, A population study of stroke and TIA: Rochester, Minnestoa, in *Stroke*, edited by Gillingham, Mawdsley, and Williams (Edinburgh: Churchill Livingstone, 1976), p. 33 (Table 11). Reprinted with permission.

approximately 3.5 individuals in 10,000 (1 in 2825), or a total of 75,638, suffered first TIAs in 1975. The average age of first TIA victims was 69.3 years: 66.6 among males and 71.8 among females.

Recurrence

Basic Recurrence Rates

Among survivors of a first stroke, a leading cause of death is stroke recurrence (Ford, 1966). First stroke survivors are at much higher risk for future stroke than the demographically matched stroke-free population. Since we are estimating the total, present-discounted costs of cerebrovascular disease for all persons with first stroke in 1975, an accurate estimate of the recurrence pattern is required. Our estimate is based on unpublished data from the Framingham Heart Study, which gives, by age and sex groups, the number of second strokes occurring in the stroke victim group for each year past the first stroke. Individuals exit from the group at risk for a second stroke when they die or have a second stroke. Using a life-table approach, it is possible to

Table 4–7
Average Annual Recurrence Rates

	Age at First Stroke		
	Less than 55	*55 to 64*	*More than 65*
Males	0.037	0.095	0.098
Females	0.043	0.049	0.072

Source: Unpublished data from the Framingham Heart Study (see text).

compute for age and sex groups the probability of having a second stroke in each year past the first stroke. These probabilities have remained generally constant over time. Marquardsen (1969), in a follow-up study of hospitalized stroke patients, found the annual recurrence rate to be independent of the length of time elapsed since stroke. Taking advantage of this evidence, we have averaged the annual probabilities through year 9 after stroke of having a second stroke to arrive at single annual recurrence rates for age and sex groups. These are displayed in table 4–7.

Interpretation of Findings and Other Results

Table 4–7 shows that the probability for a person who has had one stroke of having a second is considerably higher than the probability of a previously stroke-free person having a first stroke. We note, for example, from our incidence rates that the annual probability of a 60-year-old male having a first stroke is 0.0028; if he has had one stroke, his annual probability of having another is 0.095. This is a thirtyfold increase.

These estimates from Framingham data accord well with results from other studies. Matsumoto (1973) found that of those who survived 1 month, 10 percent had a recurrence within 1 year; 5 percent of the survivors of the second year had a recurrence in the third year. Marquardsen (1969) found an annual recurrence rate of 0.08 for males and 0.099 for females. Matsumoto (1973) found that of 694 patients surviving more than 1 month after a first stroke, 140 patients had one recurrence, 25 had two, 5 had three, and 3 had four. In order to take third and subsequent strokes into account, we have applied our recurrence rates to all stroke survivors, not only to those who have not yet had a second stroke.

Matsumoto (1973) found that recurrent strokes had, for the most part, the same distribution of type and stroke as did first strokes. Precise data on the breakdown of subsequent strokes by type are not available, however. Therefore, we have not distinguished between hemorrhagic and infarctive subsequent strokes. All types of first strokes were assumed to have the same rate of recurrence. Evidence that this may not be completely true is provided by Ford (1966), who found that embolic strokes recur more frequently than any other type. However, because all types of stroke were represented in Framingham sample, the overall rate—based on that sample— is not biased by this assumption.

Computed Numbers of Recurrences

The number of recurrent strokes occurring in each year past 1975 has been estimated in line with the preceding assumptions. For each age group (l), sex group s, and type t of first completed stroke, the probability of a recurrence in the mth year following stroke is given by

$$\left[\frac{P_{l,s}^{t}(l + m - 1) + P_{l,s}^{t}(l + m)}{2}\right] \cdot (R_{l,s})$$

where $P_{l,s}^{t}(l + m - 1)$ and $P_{l,s}^{t}(l + m)$ are the probabilities that a person of sex s and age l at first stroke of type t will survive to ages $l + m - 1$ and $l + m$, respectively, and $R_{l,s}$ is the age- and sex-specific recurrence rate taken from table 4–7. The first factor is the average chance of being alive at any time in the mth year following stroke—calculated by taking the mean of the probabilities of being alive at the beginning and the end of that year. Note that the recurrence rate $R_{l,s}$ is a function of the age at first completed stroke and not a function of age at the time of possible recurrence. Multiplying the preceding expression by the incidence broken down by age, sex, and type of stroke yields the expected number of recurrences for each of these groups for each year after stroke.

The annual expected numbers of recurrences are shown in table 4–8 for each year through June 30, 1990, broken down by sex and by type of first stroke. Within this period, a total of 85,795 recurrences are expected to occur for persons experiencing first strokes in 1975. A further 21,755 recurrences are expected in this group between July 1, 1990 and June 30, 2062. The total of 107,550 recurrences is roughly two-fifths of the number of first strokes in 1975.

The annual number of recurrences is, at 12,197, greatest for the first year following stroke and thereafter falls steadily. By the sixth year after stroke, the level of recurrences falls to less than one-half the first-year level. Whereas males suffered only 52 percent of first strokes in 1975, they are estimated to have 59 percent of the recurrences. This occurs because men over 55 have a greater rate of recurrences than do women of comparable ages—a factor that outweighs the greater mortality rates among men.

Table 4–8
Stroke Recurrence for Persons with First Strokes in 1975

	Males		Females		
	After Hemorrhage	After Infarct	After Hemorrhage	After Infarct	Total
First year (1975–1976)	570	6,808	373	4,446	12,197
Second year (1976–1977)	487	5,393	318	3,495	9,693
Third year (1977–1978)	452	4,650	296	3,021	8,419
Fourth year (1978–1979)	420	4,027	276	2,621	7,344
Fifth year (1979–1980)	393	3,502	258	2,283	6,436
Sixth year (1980–1981)	367	3,079	241	1,979	5,666
Seventh year (1981–1982)	350	2,862	234	1,877	5,323
Eighth year (1982–1983)	333	2,649	227	1,770	4,979
Ninth year (1983–1984)	316	2,441	219	1,659	4,635
Tenth year (1984–1985)	298	2,240	211	1,547	4,296
Eleventh year (1985–1986)	281	2,047	203	1,436	3,967
Twelfth year (1986–1987)	264	1,863	195	1,327	3,649
Thirteenth year (1987–1988)	247	1,690	187	1,222	3,346
Fourteenth year (1988–1989)	231	1,529	178	1,119	3,057
Fifteenth year (1989–1990)	216	1,381	170	1,021	2,788
All years (1975–2062)	7,395	56,110	5,880	38,165	107,550

Recurrence of Transient Ischemic Attacks (TIAs)

Estimating TIA recurrence patterns on the basis of existing epidemiological evidence is tenuous. The best data we found on both repeat TIAs and the sequencing of TIAs and completed strokes derives from a study by Baker.[22] These data were based on a population of male veterans followed for an average of 41 months beyond their hospitalized TIAs and are displayed in table 4–9. We note that twenty-six of the seventh-nine patients, or 33 percent, had had prior cerebral infarction. (TIAs are physiologically and epidemiologically more closely related to infarctive than to hemorrhagic strokes. This explains why Baker restricted the focus to the relationship

Table 4–9
Influence of Prior Cerebrovascular Disease on Occurrence
of New Cerebral Events in Hospitalized Transient Ischemic
Attack (TIA) Patients

CVD before Study Stroke	Number of Patients	CVD Following Hospitalized TIA	
		New TIA	New CI
No Prior CI	53	31	11
Prior CI	26	14	7

CVD = cerebrovascular disease
TIA = transient ischemic attack
CI = cerebral infarction
All cells show numbers of patients

Source: Abstracted from R.N. Baker, J.C. Ramseyer and W.S. Schwartz, Prognosis in patients with transient cerebral ischemic attacks, *Neurology* 18: 1160 (Table 9), 1968. Reprinted with permission.
Note: Sample group consisted of 79 patients hospitalized for transient ischemic attack.

between TIAs and infarctive strokes.) Since this group represented a sequence of TIAs present in the hospital situation and excluded only those with subjective symptoms (for example, giddiness, vertigo, syncope, and paresthesia), we estimate that 33 percent of all hospital admissions for TIA are subsequent to cerebral infarction.

Hospitalization of Initial Transient Ischemic Attacks
(TIAs) and Recurrences

For purposes of attributing costs, we are not so much interested in all TIAs, but concentrate instead on those leading to hospital admissions. In particular, we do not want to include those with many recurrences except in the proportion that they appear in hospitals. That multiple recurrences ought not to be too heavily weighted is indicated by findings that persons with many recurrences are at relatively low risk for subsequent stroke (Toole, 1977) and for hospitalization for any specific TIA. A handle on this is provided by Baker (1971), who relates that 16 percent of all patients hospitalized with TIA were in fact hospitalized for their first TIA. Unfortunately, he does not indicate how many of these already had had cerebral infarction. Evidence on the number of first TIAs occurring after completed strokes is provided by Marshall (1964), who among 600 consecutive cases of cerebrovascular disease found 29 such instances. The timing of these episodes is not, however, revealed.

Fitting this evidence together as best we can, we obtain the breakdown on

Table 4–10
Past Histories of Patients Hospitalized for
Transient Ischemic Attacks (TIAs)
(Percent)

	No Prior Cerebral Infarction	Prior Cerebral Infarction
No prior TIA	13	3
Prior TIA	54	30
Total	67	33

Source: Baker (1971), extended by assumptions discussed in text.

all patients hospitalized for TIAs shown in table 4–10. The row sums and column sums for the table are taken from Baker, leaving 1 degree of freedom. With the further assumption that 3 percent of all TIA patients are hospitalized with prior cerebral infarction but without prior TIA, the table is completely determined. We base this assumption on Marshall's evidence that 5 percent of his 600 cases fit this category—not all of which were hospitalized for such TIAs (or would have been in the United States). Sensitivity analysis (see later section) reveals that little inaccuracy is introduced by the assumption (since the row and columns sums are not affected by it).

Intervals between Initial Cerebrovascular Disease (CVD)
and Subsequent Transient Ischemic Attacks (TIAs)

Table 4–10 suggests that 54 percent of all TIA hospitalizations occur for second or later TIAs but before completed stroke. To determine how long after the first TIA these are likely to occur, we refer to a group of forty-six hospitalized TIA patients studied by Marshall (1964), of whom only one developed a major episode during follow-up. The lengths of time over which multiple TIAs were experienced were 1 year or less for nineteen patients (41 percent) 1 to 3 years for seventeen patients (3 percent), 3 to 5 years for three patients (7 percent), and 5 to 10 years for seven patients (15 percent). The mean time between first and last attack is 2 years. We assume that attacks leading to hospitalization will occur in the middle of this interval or 1 year after first TIA. Data on the timing of TIAs after completed stroke are even less reliable. For want of alternative evidence, we assume that the pattern of TIAs following first stroke resembles the pattern following first TIA prior to stroke. On this basis, we estimate the mean time lapse between first stroke and subsequent hospitalized TIA to be 1 year. Sensitivity analysis shows that the possible inaccuracy of this assumption has minimal impact on final results.

Mortality and Life Expectancy

General Wisdom

Varied patterns of survival are observed for stroke victims. Some die before receiving any medical attention; others die in the hospital; still others die years later. Mortality is highest for the immediate stroke period—the first 4 weeks—then drops off.[23] However, death tends not to follow the cerebro-vascular accident as rapidly as it does the myocardial infarction.

For a considerable period after the stroke, mortality for stroke survivors substantially exceeds that of demographically matched populations. While stroke victims are at higher risk for future strokes, the excess mortality is not exclusively due to CVD.[24] To sort out the mortality caused by initial strokes lies beyond current epidemiological capability. Instead, our approach is simply to associate all mortality in excess of that for matched populations with the initial stroke.

Determinants of Mortality

Ford (1966) reports general agreement that survival, both short- and long-term, worsens as age increases. Eisenberg (1964) shows that older stroke patients compare less favorably with matched persons in the general population than do younger patients. After age is taken into account (females tend to have strokes at older ages than males), sex has not been shown to be consistently related to differences in either early or late prognosis. Type of stroke affects immediate survival. Ford estimates that 1-month mortality following hemorrhage is twice that following thrombosis. However, the type of stroke has not been shown to be so consistently related to long-term survival. Eisenberg (1964) states that "those cerebral hemorrhage victims who lived one month appeared to have as good, if not better, five-year survival than the cerebral thrombosis victims."[25] This assertion is corroborated by the National Survey of Stroke (USDHEW, 1980), which found that 49.4 percent of 1-month hemorrhage survivors were alive 5 years after their stroke as compared with 42.5 percent of 1-month infarct survivors. The severity of the stroke and initial condition of the patient also affect survival. Patients who are in a coma shortly after their stroke are more likely to die in a short time than those stroke victims who are responsive. The more severe is the stroke (the greater residual impairment), the less favorable are the long-term prospects for survival. Mortality after a first stroke seems to be similar to that after a recurrent stroke. Previous stroke history seems thus not to affect survival prospects (Ford, Katz, 1966).

Difficulties Estimating Survival

Problems of data analysis in estimating survival following first completed strokes in 1977 resemble those encountered in estimating incidence. Data are scanty and insufficient for desired disaggregation by age, sex, and diagnostic type. Moreover, as Garraway (1979b) indicates, survival has been improving over the years—with gains ranging from a 2 percent improvement in 1–month postinfarction survival through a 16 percent improvement in 5–year survival. Such trends make the inference of current survival from older data tenuous and argue for reliance on most recent data. Since, however, more breakdowns of older data are available, we have examined them in order to better interpret more recent data.

Older Data

Figures on poststroke survival in Framingham (Shurtleff, 1974) and Middlesex (Eisenberg, 1964) were analyzed. We found (1) that survival rates following hemorrhagic strokes for most age and sex groups and for most lengths of survival were roughly 60 percent of comparable rates for infarctive strokes; (2) that survival seems best described in terms of three parameters indicating 1–month, 1–year, and 5–year survival [That is, an initial high rate of mortality prevails during the first month following stroke; a lower but still high rate prevails during the rest of the first year; and a still lower rate of mortality describes survival from the first through fifth years. It is problematic whether stroke survivors exhibit greater mortality than age- and sex-matched individuals after the fifth year following first stroke. While evidence suggests continuing greater mortality for stroke survivors, these data are somewhat outdated and do not reflect the substantial improvement in long-term survival for stroke victims described by Garraway (1979b)]; and (3) that significant sex-based differences in survival do not exist for stroke victims aged under 65 [for stroke victims aged over 65, there seemed reasonable evidence, despite small sample sizes, that male mortality exceeded female mortality substantially (that is, by more than the excess of male over female mortality in the general population of these ages)].

Calculating Survival

In accordance with these findings, survival following stroke was estimated in four steps: (1) identifying the primary data base, (2) disaggregating by type of stroke, (3) disaggregating into more age groups, and (4) disaggregating the older age groups by sex.

Step 1. Identifying the Primary Data Base. The most recent and extensive data derive from the recent Department of Health, Education and Welfare (DHEW) study based on 1365 initial strokes occurring between 1971 and 1976 (USDHEW, 1980). Of these, 199 were hemorrhagic and 1166 infarctive. The data were broken down into four age groups: under 65, 65 to 74, 75 to 84, and over 85.

Step 2. Disaggregating by Type of Stroke. Disaggregation of the age-based mortality rates into separate rates for hemorrhagic and infarctive strokes was based on the observed ratios of survival for the two types. The 1-month survival rate of hemorrhagic stroke patients was 54.3 percent of that for infarctive stroke patients. The corresponding ratios of survival rates at 1 and 5 years were 54.5 and 63.3 percent (USDHEW, 1980). Assuming that these rates would hold within the different age groups enabled disaggregating the age-specific survival rates into rates broken down by age and diagnostic type.

Step 3. Disaggregating into More Age Groups. Estimation of survival among stroke victims aged 0 to 14 was based on Schoenberg (1977 and 1978). The former article describes perinatal cerebral hemorrhages, noting no cases of survival beyond a few days. The latter article reports the survival experience of thirty-eight victims of infarctive strokes and of thirty-one victims of hemorrhagic strokes. The age range was from 0 to 14, but excluded perinatal strokes. To obtain survival rates for this age group, three adjustments were necessary for the data provided by Schoenberg (1978). First, the observed number of deaths was increased by 25 percent to account for the generally better survival of patients in the Mayo Clinic (Schoenberg's group) than in the general U.S. population. The figure of 25 percent is slightly less than the reported 28.5 percent difference in mortality rates for infarctive strokes as found in Garraway's (1979*b*) largely Mayo Clinic population and in the general U.S. population for the same years (USDHEW, 1980). Second, an adjustment was made to combine Schoenberg's figures with data on perinatal strokes—overwhelmingly hemorrhagic and overwhelmingly fatal within 1 month. This was done by presuming that eighty-nine of the ninety-four deaths before the age of 1 resulting from cerebral hemorrhage reported by NCHS (1979) in 1977 were due to perinatal events. The reduction by five deaths reflects the average annual rate of mortality from cerebral hemorrhage for ages 1 to 4. Similarly, five of the seven cerebral infarction deaths under age 1 were presumed to be due to perinatal events. All perinatal stroke deaths were presumed to arise from the pattern of mortality documented by Schoenberg (1978). Third, since Schoenberg's group had no deaths of hemorrhage survivors between 1 and 5 years after stroke, the 5-year survival rate for hemorrhage was adjusted to reflect the average mortality of the general population.

In the absence of data enabling the breakdown by age of survival for stroke victims aged 15 to 64, we assumed that all differences in survival across these ages paralleled the differences in the general population. For example, since 60-year-olds in the general population have a 5-year survival rate equal to but 93 percent of that for 40-year-olds, the same ratio was assumed to hold for stroke survivors.

Step 4. Disaggregating the Older Age Groups by Sex. The DHEW data are not broken down by sex. Analysis of the Framingham and Middlesex data indicates that distinction between male and female survival under the age of 65 is not critical (or statistically significant). For those over 65, survival among women exceeded that for men. Lacking adequate data on stroke survivors to make appropriate sex distinctions, we instead relied on general mortality data. For example, 5-year survival of 80-year-old men is 82 percent of that for 80-year-old women. We assumed the same ratio to hold for stroke survivors.

Interpreting Estimated Survival

The results of these calculations are shown in table 4–11. They are generally consistent with such other survival figures as those calculated for stroke survivors in the Framingham and Middlesex studies. The chief difference between the figures in table 4–11 and those of the New England studies occurs for hemorrhagic survival after the age of 75. The earlier studies found 5-year survival to be 2.3 percent—considerably lower than the corresponding figures in table 4–11. This discrepancy may result from the few (thirty) patients of these ages in the New England studies or from an as yet undocumented improvement in hemorrhagic mortality rates paralleling that for infarctive mortality (Garraway, 1979b). Other studies reporting stroke survival are by Howard (1963), Robinson (1968), and Acheson (1971). When chronology is taken into account, the figures reported by each of these is in accordance with table 4–11.

Table 4–11
Survival Following First Completed Stroke, United States, 1975

Age at Stroke		1 Month	1 Year	2 Years	3 Years	4 Years	5 Years
Hemorrhage							
Survival							
0–14		0.540	0.509	0.507	0.505	0.504	0.502
15–24		0.463	0.401	0.392	0.383	0.374	0.365
25–34		0.463	0.401	0.392	0.383	0.374	0.365
35–44		0.463	0.400	0.390	0.381	0.372	0.363
45–54		0.463	0.398	0.387	0.376	0.365	0.355
55–64		0.463	0.394	0.379	0.364	0.351	0.337
65–74	M	0.433	0.337	0.302	0.270	0.241	0.216
	F	0.433	0.344	0.314	0.287	0.263	0.240
75–84	M	0.381	0.249	0.210	0.176	0.149	0.125
	F	0.381	0.259	0.227	0.198	0.174	0.152
85+	M	0.295	0.153	0.111	0.080	0.058	0.042
	F	0.295	0.160	0.121	0.091	0.069	0.052
Infarct survival							
0–14		0.880	0.818	0.802	0.786	0.771	0.756
15–24		0.853	0.741	0.700	0.661	0.625	0.590
25–34		0.853	0.741	0.700	0.661	0.625	0.590
35–44		0.853	0.740	0.698	0.659	0.621	0.586
45–54		0.853	0.737	0.692	0.650	0.610	0.573
55–64		0.853	0.729	0.678	0.630	0.586	0.545
65–75	M	0.795	0.619	0.534	0.460	0.397	0.342
	F	0.795	0.633	0.558	0.491	0.433	0.381
75–84	M	0.699	0.459	0.373	0.304	0.247	0.201
	F	0.699	0.477	0.403	0.340	0.288	0.243
85+	M	0.542	0.280	0.195	0.136	0.095	0.066
	F	0.542	0.293	0.214	0.156	0.114	0.083

Source: USDHEW (1980), disaggregated by methods described in text.

As noted earlier, data were most sparse for the breakdown of survival rates between the ages of 15 and 64. It is therefore heartening to find the close agreement between the figures in table 4–11 and those for the mortality following cerebral infarction in young adults reported by Grindal (1978). Grindal's patients were aged between 15 and 40 and suffered inhospital mortality of 13.8 percent—a figure in line with the 1-month survival rate of 85.3 percent given in table 4–11 for these ages.

The figures in table 4–11 are based on the latest data available, which, with one exception, were restricted to 1970 or later. Only Schoenberg's (1978) data pertain to any earlier strokes—his covering the period from 1965 through 1974. Should there be a trend in mortality between first strokes suffered in the early 1970s and 1975, the figures shown in table 4–11 will not reflect it.

Extended Survival

Calculation of recurrences and of many direct costs (for example, nursing home costs) requires estimating the extended survival of stroke victims. To do this, we assume that survival patterns for the sixth and later years after stroke will be those of the general population.

Epidemiological proof that survival patterns of stroke patients revert to those of the general population at some time after stroke does not yet exist. Several studies, however, have found minimal differences between the mortality of long-term stroke survivors and that of the general population. Pincock (1957) concluded that the two survival patterns were indistinguishable. Katz (1966) observed that detectable differences in survival subsided 24 to 30 months after the stroke. Eisenberg (1964) found that there was a similarity of mortality rates for the general population and for the stroke groups 3 to 5 years after their cerebrovascular accident. Hutchinson (1975) found that after 5 to 7 years, the survival curve of stroke patients parallels that of the general population.

Life Expectancy after Stroke

The survival figures in table 4–11 enable calculation of life expectancies for stroke survivors. These are shown in table 4–12, where they also are contrasted with life expectancies for the general population. This contrast emphasizes the importance of strokes in younger persons. On the surface of table 4–11, it appears that strokes among the older population are more serious, inasmuch as they have greatest mortality in the immediate poststroke years. When, however, we measure the seriousness of strokes in terms of the expected loss of life years, we see that strokes in persons between 15 and 24 occasion the greatest loss of life expectancy: for males, 31.9 (that is, $50.7 - 18.8$) years for hemorrhages and 20.0 (that is $50.7 - 30.7$) years for infarcts; for females, 36.7 years for hemorrhages and 23.2 years for infarcts.

Transient Ischemic Attack (TIA) Mortality

Since, by definition, the TIA is temporary in nature, it follows that no deaths are directly due to it in the short run. We have noted in our introductory comments on TIAs the lower life expectancy of TIA victims vis-à-vis sex- and age-matched individuals free of TIAs. An analytical dilemma is posed: Do we treat the reduction in life expecancy as a consequence of the TIA or do we interpret the TIA merely as a signal that its victims belong to a class of

Table 4–12
Life Expectancy Following Hemorrhagic and Infarctive Strokes,
United States, 1975
(Life Expectancy in Years)

	Hemorrhage Victims	Infarct Victims	General Population
Males			
0–14	31.1	47.1	62.2
15–24	18.8	30.7	50.7
25–34	15.4	25.3	41.6
35–44	12.2	20.0	32.5
45–54	9.1	15.1	23.9
55–64	6.6	10.9	16.4
65–74	3.5	5.8	10.5
75–84	1.8	3.2	6.1
85+	0.8	1.4	4.0
Females			
0–14	35.0	52.8	69.7
15–24	21.3	34.8	58.0
25–35	17.9	29.2	48.3
35–44	14.4	23.6	38.8
45–54	11.1	18.2	29.8
55–64	8.0	13.2	21.5
65–74	4.4	7.2	14.1
75–84	2.3	3.9	8.2
85+	0.9	1.6	4.9

Source: Calculations based on table 4–11 and survival probabilities of the normal population (NCHS, 1980) following standard life-table techniques.

persons with shorter life expectancies? In the former case, significant forgone earnings extending over the long run would be ascribed to the TIA; in the latter, none.

We take the latter interpretation both because we believe it more true and because it leads to a more consistent and straightforward analysis. If we were to estimate the life reduction owing to TIA, it would be necessary first to distinguish TIA deaths from those resulting from stroke. Twenty-nine percent of TIA victims eventually die of stroke. Whisnant's figures (abstracted in table 4–1) do not provide sufficient detail to separate stroke deaths from other causes of premature death for TIA victims. Another 44 percent of deaths for TIA survivors are due to heart disease. Not unreasonably, epidemiologists have ascribed these life-year reductions not to TIAs, but to heart disease—as have we in chapter 3. For analytic accuracy and consistency (to avoid double counting), we ascribe deaths only to their direct causes and, hence, not to TIAs.

Direct Costs of Stroke

Overall Perspective

Perhaps the best data on direct costs of stroke will be found in the National Survey of Stroke. A few of the summary statistics of this study have been released (USDHEW, 1980). For purposes of calculating mortality, these were of sufficient detail to be used in our calculations. In the area of direct costs, the description of the methodology is appealing, but the details so far released have not been adequate for our purposes. (Total direct-care costs on a prevalence basis were found to be $3.259 billion—$1.376 billion for hospital care, $1.029 billion for nursing homes, $127 million for physician services, $699 million for other medical and social services, and $28 million for aids and appliances.) Detailed breakdowns will be released at a later date. To our regret, permission to use preliminary figures from this study in our own analysis was not forthcoming.

As a result, three main strategies were followed in estimating direct costs. First, costs of hospitalization were based largely on the experience of Blue Cross patients in Massachusetts, augmented by other data. Second, nursing home costs were estimated based on data from the National Nursing Home Survey (NCHS, 1979). Third, costs of rehabilitation services (inpatient, outpatient, and home), vocational rehabilitation, medical equipment and appliances, outpatient care, and miscellaneous paramedical expenses are based on a study by Emlet (1973).

Initial Hospitalization Charges for Stroke

Hospitalization costs for Blue Cross stroke patients in Massachusetts averaged $2976 per stay from July 1976 through June 1977 for all cerebrovascular admissions excluding TIAs. To adjust this to a national basis, we take into account that Massachusetts hospitalization costs exceeded national costs by 49.6 percent. Dividing $2976 by 1.496 yields an estimated national average hospital bill for stroke of $1989. To put this in 1975 terms, this figure must be further adjusted for 18 months' inflation (division by 1.191), yielding $1670.

Data on average length of stay in the Professional Activities Survey (PAS) hospitals for stroke patients, which was restricted to patients with single diagnoses and excluded those who died in the hospital, indicated an average stay of 11.97 days.[26] We estimate professional charges by average internist fees, which in 1975 were $38.46 for first visits and $13.28 for follow-up visits.[27] We assume one follow-up visit for each day beyond the first and arrive at a total of $184 (that is, $38.46 + 10.97 × 13.28) as the estimated professional fees for physician visits per stay.

Costs incurred for anesthesiology and interpretation of tests were figured from the 1974 California Relative Value Study calibrated by reference to the 1974 Medicaid fee schedule for Massachusetts.[28] This procedure essentially sets costs for the professional fees at reimbursement levels for Massachusetts Medicaid patients. Figures on the rates of special operations are provided by PAS (Commission on Professional and Hospital Activities, 1976) and Haerer (1971). PAS data indicate that operations were performed for 41.9 percent of single-diagnosis patients in stroke categories. Haerer's figures derive from the Mississippi Regional Medical Program Stroke Care Demonstration Unit and show that 1.5 percent of his patients had carotid endarterectomies, 1 percent had carotid explorations, 2 percent had craniotomies, and 0.5 percent had ventricular-auricular shunts.[29] Assuming that no patients had multiple operations (untrue, but the minuteness of the figures minimizes resulting errors), Haerer's figures apply to 5 percent of all stroke patients. To reconcile this with PAS data, we suppose that 36.9 percent (41.9 percent indicated by PAS to be operated on less the 5 percent linked by Haerer to specific procedures) had procedures for which the average professional fee was that for cerebral angiography. This procedure is likely to be the most common among these patients, and its charge is intermediate among fees for possible operations for stroke patients. Data on the relative frequencies of unilateral and bilateral angiography is taken from a detailed study of TIA patients (see subsequent paragraphs), with the same proportions assumed to hold for stroke patients undergoing the procedure. Weighting by appropriate frequencies and adding the costs of these procedures yields an average professional charge of $94 for stroke patients in 1974 in Massachusetts. These figures are adjusted to the 1975 average by division by 1.496 (Massachusetts rates divided by national rates) and multiplication by 1.123 (inflation in physician fees between 1974 and 1975). With these adjustments, the average professional fees for special tests are estimated to be $71 per hospitalization.

Totaling the institutional bill plus professional fees for inhospital visits and procedures brings the total expenses for a hospital stay to $1925. This indicates that the 252,866 first strokes occurring in 1975 incurred total costs of $487 million.

Hospitalizations for recurrence are assumed to have the same real costs set in terms of 1975 dollars. Discounting at 6 percent, we find the total hospitalization costs for all recurrences to be $123 million. The disaggregation of these costs by age and sex is provided in table 4–23 as part of the sensitivity analysis.

Nursing Home Costs

The National Nursing Home Survey indicates that 103,500 residents of nursing homes in the United States in 1977 had a primary diagnosis of stroke at their last examination. Staff personnel of that study reported (an unpublished data disaggregation) that, of these, 10,800 were under 65; 27,700 were between 65 and 74; 41,900 were between 75 and 84; and 23,100 were 85 or older.

These data suggest that older stroke survivors are more likely than younger stroke survivors to be placed in nursing homes. To quantify this tendency, we compared nursing home occupancy with nursing home eligibility—which we defined as the first 5 years of survivorship following first completed stroke. We realized that this coarse measure would not reflect eligibility based on recurrences, but considered this a minimal problem inasmuch as our goal was a general measurement of the effect of age on nursing home placement of stroke survivors. We found that 42 percent of recent initial stroke survivors (that is, those whose initial stroke occurred within the previous 5 years) aged over 85 were in nursing homes with a primary diagnosis of stroke. For stroke survivors between 75 and 84, the corresponding figure was 29 percent; for those between 65 and 74, it was 17 percent; and for those under 65, it was 7.1 percent.

To disaggregate the nursing home patients under 65 into finer age groups, similar relationships were presumed, based on consultation with stroke experts. We supposed that recent stroke patients—of both initial and subsequent strokes—between 45 and 54 were 0.6 as likely as those between 55 and 64 to be in nursing homes. Similarly, recent stroke patients between 0 and 34 were presumed 0.3 as likely as those between 55 and 64 to be in nursing homes; those between 35 and 44 were supposed 0.4 as likely as those between 55 and 64 to be in nursing homes. These suppositions enabled us to disaggregate those under 65 in nursing homes across the six component age groups. This method led to the estimates that of the 10,800 years spent by stroke patients under 65 in nursing homes in 1977, 27 were for those under 15, 43 were for those between 15 and 24, 84 for those between 25 and 34, 264 between 35 and 44, 1368 between 45 and 54, and 9014 between 55 and 64.

Many persons in nursing homes entered as the result of strokes occurring while they were in the previous age group. To disentangle age of nursing home residents from age at the critical stroke, we relied on the findings of Emlet (1973) that stroke patients under 55 in nursing homes have short stays, while those over 55 have stays of 1.581 years average duration. We accordingly assumed that those under 55 in nursing homes were predominantly there for strokes—initial or recurrences—occurring while in their current age group. For those over 55, we estimated that of 23,100 stroke patients over 85 in nursing homes, 2116 were there for strokes occurring before the age of 85. Similarly, 2906 of those between 75 and 84 and 1741 of those between 65 and 74 had their nursing-home-committal strokes in the next younger age groups.

Two further assumptions were then made. First, it was presumed that, adjusting for age, initial strokes were just as likely as recurrences to lead to nursing home care. This in line with the judgment of Ford and Katz (1966) that cerebrovascular history prior to the most recent stroke has little effect on subsequent experience. Second, we presumed that the decline in incidence rates was counterbalanced by the growth in the incident population. In fact, the annual decline in the incidence rates is roughly 2.3 percent, while the growth in the incident population is 2.1 percent (that is, if the incidence rates were unchanged, each succeeding year would have 2.1 percent more first strokes than the previous). These assumptions imply that the numbers of various age groups in nursing homes in 1977 equal the numbers of years people experiencing first strokes in 1975 would spend in nursing homes while in those age groups (unless a substantial shift in survival rates or nursing-home-committal rates is also occurring). (For example, we have estimated that 9014 patient-years were spent in nursing homes in 1977 by patients between 55 and 64. The assumptions of this paragraph imply that the group of persons suffering first strokes in 1975 will spend a total of 103,500 years in nursing homes with a primary diagnosis of stroke. Of these 103,500 patient-years, 9014 are assumed to be those of patients aged 55 to 64 while in nursing homes. Many of these 9014 patient-years are those of persons young in 1975 whose nursing home years between the ages of 55 and 64 therefore occur many years in the future.)

These data and assumptions lead to table 4–13, which shows that the estimated present value at 6 percent of nursing home charges resulting from strokes of persons whose incident strokes occurred in 1975 was roughly $821 million. Ten percent ($82.4 million) of these costs were incurred by persons whose first stroke was hemorrhagic. Fifty-one percent of the costs were for males, and 2.5 percent of the costs were for persons whose first stroke occurred before the age of 55.

Other Direct Costs

To estimate direct costs other than those of hospitalization and nursing homes, we rely on the report of Emlet (1973). His purpose was to estimate the costs and benefits of improved care for stroke patients. The study invoked a structured Delphi methodology to estimate 1972 stroke-care costs under assumptions of both current average and optimum care.

For present computational purposes, we focus on his estimates for

Table 4–13
Nursing Home Costs for Stroke Survivors, United States, 1975
(Thousands of Dollars)

Age at First Stroke	Hemorrhage	Infarction	Total
Males			
0–14	85	126	211
15–24	100	188	288
25–34	237	347	584
35–44	744	1,107	1,851
45–54	3,656	7,230	10,886
55–64	13,032	56,959	69,991
65–74	13,958	129,190	143,148
75–84	6,720	133,227	139,947
85+	3,431	48,648	52,079
Total males	41,963	377,022	418,985
Females			
0–14	86	40	126
15–24	100	63	163
25–34	241	116	357
35–44	761	375	1,136
45–54	2,265	2,434	4,699
55–64	11,689	38,815	50,504
65–74	10,125	96,850	106,975
75–84	9,532	153,068	162,600
85+	5,653	69,490	75,143
Total females	40,453	361,252	401,705
Total population	82,416	738,275	820,691

Source: National Nursing Home Survey (NCHS, 1979), disaggregated by methods described in text.
Note: Discounted at 6 percent; all costs are in 1975 dollars.

current average cost; a sense of possible future trends in costs may be obtained from the figures for optimum care. The panel convened for the estimation procedure included two neurologists, two physiatrists, one epidemiologist, one family practitioner, one hospital administrator, one nursing home administrator, one physical therapist, one social service worker, and one vocational counselor. For each of a number of parameters needed to gauge costs of stroke care, the panel members made individual estimates. Statistical summaries of these estimates were made and were used as a basis for panel discussions and for arriving at consensus estimates. The costs were estimated for the three-state region of Minnesota, North Dakota, and South Dakota.

Emlet's approach to the estimation problem began with identification of those patients with achievable benefits not achieved (ABNA). These are essentially those surviving initial hospitalization. The ABNA patients were then broken down into four groups of representative patients. These four groups comprised 78 percent of the total ABNA patients—excluding primarily patients with complicating conditions. Since we wish to focus on the costs of stroke as distinguished from those associated with simultaneous conditions, we are interested in the direct costs incurred by the four age groups set out by Emlet. For other survivors of initial hospitalization, we assume that their stroke-connected costs, as distinct from costs owing to their other conditions, are those of the average ABNA patients in the four groups.

Stroke survivors have been found to require on average 3.3 more physician visits annually than the general population.[30] We estimate the cost per visit in 1975 to be $11, on the basis of a report by Center for Health Services Research and Development of the American Medical Association (1978). This leads to estimated annual follow-on charges of $36. We assume that these will be incurred by all stroke survivors for their remaining lives.

Costs of rehabilitation services (inpatient, outpatient, and in the home), vocational rehabilitation, medical equipment and appliances, and miscellaneous paramedical expenses are also taken from Emlet. We adjusted Emlet's numbers to account for regional cost variations and for inflation between the time of his study (1972) and 1975. A final adjustment was necessary because Emlet's group noted the difficulties of discounting—for example, determining the appropriate rate—and took this as a pretext for not discounting. We consider this analytically incorrect and hence have further modified Emlet's figures by discounting those occurring more than 1 year after the initial stroke (as estimated by Emlet). The results of these

Table 4–14
Direct-Cost Components per Patient for Stroke Survivors Excluding Hospitalization Not Explicitly for Rehabilitation, Nursing Home Care, and Costs of Physician Visits

	Discounted at 6 percent
RS, inpatient[a]	937
RS, outpatient	555
RS, home	846
Vocational rehabilitation	82
Medical equipment and appliances	353
Miscellaneous paramedical expenses	1033
Total	3806

Source: Emlet study (1973), disaggregated by authors.

Note: All costs are in 1975 dollars.

[a]RS = Rehabilitation services.

computations are summarized in table 4–14. It should be noted that rehabilitation services occurring as part of the initial neurological hospitalization are reflected in its total charges (noted earlier) and hence are excluded from table 4–14. The minimal charges for vocational rehabilitation reflect the small percentage of stroke patients (less than 5 percent) estimated by Emlet to receive it. Miscellaneous paramedical expenses include the costs of home visits by nurses, home health aides, homemaker help, physical therapy, and transportation.

Cost items neglected in the analysis of Emlet include emergency services, home modifications, and drugs for outpatients (the estimates cover drugs in nursing homes and in extended-care facilities). Of these, the most significant are the medications. Anticoagulants may be used in treatment of infarctions, especially those of a progressive nature. Many physicians feel that these drugs ought not to be used in normal, nonprogressive infarctions. That the use of anticoagulants for infarctions is vastly less than that for TIAs is not disputed. Haerer, whose patients included 4.5 percent TIAs and 12.5 percent "miscellaneous others," found that only 6 percent were administered anticoagulants—both in the hospital and after discharge. Many of these were most likely TIA patients. While antihypertensive drugs are often administered after hemorrhagic strokes, Emlet evidently considered this to be treatment for the underlying condition and not for stroke per se. We follow Emlet's lead in excluding these cost categories in confidence that any bias so introduced is minute.

Summary of Direct-Cost Components

The various components of direct costs for completed strokes are displayed in table 4–15. As indicated there, the costs taken from Emlet are labeled *initial survival costs* and are assumed to occur primarily in conjunction with first strokes. Of the costs under this heading, Emlet assumes that all but one category will occur soon after the initial stroke. The exception is inpatient rehabilitation, which Emlet recognizes may follow recurrences. We have followed Emlet in these assumptions. We recognize that other charges within this heading may occur long after initial completed strokes, perhaps following recurrences, but these seem relatively insignificant. For the most part, these expenses follow closely first completed strokes: home modifications tend to be installed then and not subsequently altered, and most rehabilitation follows initial hospitalization, being judged then most timely and efficacious.

All subcategories of annual follow-on costs begin following discharge from neurological hospitalization, approximately 1 month after first stroke. The calculations for physician visits were described earlier. To obtain annual follow-on costs for recurrence hospitalization and nursing home care, we divided the total discounted costs in these categories by the total discounted

Table 4–15
Average Direct Costs per Patient: A Summary of Cost Components
for Completed Strokes
(Dollars)

Direct-Cost Category	First-Year Cost per Completed Stroke	Present-Valued Cost per Survivor of Initial Stroke	Average Annual Costs
Initial hospitalization			
Basic charges	1670		
Physician fees	184		
Procedures	71		
Subtotal	1925		
Initial survival costs[a]			
Inpatient rehabilitation		937	
Outpatient rehabilitation		555	
Home rehabilitation		846	
Vocational rehabilitation		82	
Medical equipment and appliances		353	
Paramedical expenses		1033	
Subtotal		3806	
Annual follow-on costs[b]			
Recurrence hospitalization			133
Nursing home care[c]			791
Physician visits			36
Subtotal			960

Note: All costs are in 1975 dollars.
[a]Assumed, following Emlet (1973), to occur overwhelmingly in conjunction with survival following first completed strokes.
[b]These costs begin in the year of the initial completed stroke.
[c]Calculated by dividing discounted (at 6 percent) future life-years into discounted costs.

years. This method ensures that the total present-valued costs obtained through our more laborious method of identifying precisely when these costs will occur for different groups also will be obtained by alternatively assuming that every year of stroke survivorship incurs the average costs shown in this part of table 4–15.

Direct Costs per Person and Total Direct Costs of Stroke

Direct costs per person and total direct costs incurred by stroke victims are displayed in table 4–16. The numbers there reflect all the separate compo-

Table 4–16

Present Value of Direct Costs for Stroke Patients of Varying Ages and Both Sexes, United States, 1975

Age at First Stroke	Hemorrhage		Infarction		Total Both Types of Stroke (Millions of Dollars)
	Per Person (Dollars)	Total (Millions of Dollars)	Per Person (Dollars)	Total (Millions of Dollars)	
Males					
0–14	5687	0.9	7624	1.5	2.4
15–24	5084	1.0	7173	2.2	3.2
25–34	5081	2.2	7169	3.8	6.0
35–44	5212	5.3	7296	9.5	14.8
45–54	5469	19.2	7543	45.3	64.5
55–64	7134	40.6	9817	200.2	240.8
65–74	7369	34.8	9611	369.7	404.5
75–84	7648	14.1	9469	319.3	333.4
85+	7690	6.3	8938	100.2	106.5
Total males	6765	124.4	9379	1051.7	1176.1
Females					
0–14	5847	0.9	7867	0.5	1.4
15–24	5212	0.9	7384	0.7	1.6
25–34	5227	2.1	7408	1.2	3.3
35–44	5386	5.2	7580	3.0	8.2
45–54	5673	11.4	7877	14.2	25.6
55–64	6523	38.3	8788	149.0	187.3
65–74	7256	25.4	9413	280.9	306.3
75–84	7575	20.1	9330	369.9	390.0
85+	7625	10.4	8824	143.7	154.1
Total females	6711	114.7	9151	963.2	1077.9
Total population	6740	239.1	9269	2014.9	2254.0

Notes: All costs are in 1975 dollars, discounted at 6 percent.

nents of direct costs shown in table 4–15 plus the estimated 4.5 percent of these costs required as insurance administration charges. It is seen in table 4–16 that the average first hemorrhagic stroke leads to direct costs per person of $6740 versus $9269 for a first infarctive stroke. The difference between the two derives from the greater survival of infarct victims, who therefore have greater costs for rehabilitation services, recurrences, nursing home care, and physician visits. (These differences in costs for the two types of stroke also will appear in table 4–18.) This difference in average per-person costs plus the far greater incidence of infarctive strokes relative to hemorrhages have led to even more significant differences in total direct costs. First infarctions in 1975 account for $2.015 billion in present-valued direct costs, while first

Table 4–17
Population Surviving 1975 First Transient Ischemic Attacks (TIAs)
without Completed Stroke

Years after Diagnosis	Persons Alive and Free of Stroke at Start of Interval
0	75,638
1/12	68,380
3/12	64,942
6/12	60,358
1	56,155
2	42,403
3	32,471
4	27,505
5	22,921
6	19,101
7	12,224
8	9,550
9	5,348
10	4,202

Source: Derived from data in Whisnant (1976).

hemorrhages account for only $.239 billion, approximately an eightfold difference.

For both types of stroke, direct costs per person are higher for those over 55 than for those under 55. This result occurs mainly because the older age groups have a greater likelihood of being placed in nursing homes following their initial hospitalizations. The average 50-year-old male hemorrhage victim is, for instance, estimated to incur a present-valued amount of $1037 in nursing home costs. In contrast, the 60-year-old male experiencing a hemorrhagic first stroke incurs an average of $2291—more than twice as much. A similar pattern prevails for infarcts. A 50-year-old woman having an infarctive first stroke can expect to generate $1349 in nursing home costs. For a 60-year-old woman, the comparable figure is $2289.

Direct Costs of Transient Ischemic Attacks (TIAs)

Hospitalization

The number of hospital discharges for transient ischemic attacks in 1975 reported by PAS survey is 40,904.[31] The survey covered approximately 42 percent of all discharges from U.S. hospitals. Dividing 40,904 by 0.42, we obtain an estimated total of 97,390 TIA discharges. Inhospital mortality need not be added to these discharges since TIAs, by definition, do not result in death. Of these 97,390, 13 percent, or 12,661, are estimated (in line with table 4–10) to be first cerebral events. Since our incidence figures estimated that 75,638 first TIAs occurred in 1975, we see that only 16.7 percent of these are hospitalized.

The average Blue Cross hospitalization bill for TIA admissions in Massachusetts from July 1976 through June 1977 was $1424. Adjusting for the difference between Massachusetts and national prices (division by 1.496) reduces this figure to $952. Adjustment for 18 months' inflation is achieved by division by 1.91, yielding $799. The average length of stay for TIAs with single diagnosis in PAS hospitals was 5.8 days. As for strokes, we take internist fee rates as a gauge for professional charges. These were $38.46 in 1975 for initial hospital care and $13.23 for each of an average 4.8 follow-up visits.

Special Procedures

Surgery in PAS hospitals was performed for 30.9 percent of single-diagnosis TIAs and for 20 percent of multiple-diagnosis TIAs. This reflects PAS classification of angiography as a surgical procedure. Even so, these data are at odds with those of Swanson (1977), who reported that 36 percent of single-diagnosis patients studied received angiography, while 71 percent of those with multiple-diagnosis did. We take as our best estimate of the angiography induced by TIAs to be the 36 percent reported by Swanson for single-diagnosis patients.

Professional fees for angiography are estimated from the California Relative Value Study to be $193 for unilateral studies and $247 for bilateral studies. Frequencies of unilateral and bilateral injections were found by Swanson (1977) for direct percutaneous injections to be 69 and 31 percent, respectively. Weighting accordingly, we find the average fee to be $210.

Vascular surgery was performed in 19 percent of the carotid TIA cases reported by Dyken (1977). The overall rate is 15.9 percent for operations we will assume to be endarterectomies. Specific studies ordered when patients were seen for TIA were tabulated by Dyken. These included complete blood count (92 percent of the cases), ECG (87 percent), chest roetgenogram (85 percent), serum electrolytes (83 percent), BUN (82 percent), urinalysis (81 percent), fasting blood sugar (77 percent), cholesterol (64 percent), skull roentgenogram (56 percent), serology (53 percent), EFG (51 percent), static brain scan (35 percent), triglycerides (31 percent), dynamic brain scan (29 percent), directional Doppler ultrasonic linear flow studies (26 percent), lumbar puncture (25 percent), 2-hour postprandial blood sugar (20 percent), ophthalmodynamometry (18 percent), serum lipoprotein electrophoresis (13 percent), serum electrophoresis (13 percent), glucose tolerance (10 percent), lupus erythamatosus preparation (10 percent), protein-bound iron (8 percent), prolonged ECG monitoring (8 percent), neuropsychological testing (6 percent), echoencephalography (A-scan) (5 percent), sickle-cell preparation (2 percent), cerebral blood flow (2 percent), and fluorescein circulation (1 percent).

Summing all professional fees charted for angiography, surgery, and special studies reveals that an average of $282 is added to the basic hospital bill. Since these fees are set in 1975 Massachusetts terms, division by 1.496 is needed to arrive at the national average of $189.

Adding together the average hospital bill ($799), average internist fees ($102), and other professional fees ($189), we calculate the average total costs of hospitalization for TIAs to be $1090.

*Discounting Costs of Subsequent Transient Ischemic
Attacks (TIAs) to Time of Initial Cerebrovascular
Disease (CVD) Incidence*

By reasoning given in the sections on the incidence and recurrence of TIAs (see table 4–10), we assume that 13 percent of all hospitalized TIA patients in 1975, or 12,661, had no prior history of TIA or completed stroke. Hospitalization costs for these TIAs were $13.8 million (that is, 12,661 × $1090). Thirty-three percent of all hospitalized TIAs, or 32,139, have had a prior stroke, and 54 percent, or 52,590, have had a prior TIA but not a prior stroke. These two groups comprise 87 percent of the hospitalized TIAs in any year.

We have further argued that the mean time lapse between first TIA and subsequent hospitalized TIA is 1 year for patients without prior stroke. Similarly, the mean time lapse between first stroke and subsequent hospitalized TIA is taken to be 1 year. In each case, therefore, the later TIA is presumed to occur on July 1, 1976. As for completed strokes, we assume that the decline in TIA incidence rates is counterbalanced by growth in the incident population. This assumption leads to the conclusion that persons with first CVD (either TIA or completed stroke) in 1975 will have just as many subsequent hospitalizations for TIAs as there were hospitalizations for TIAs in 1975 as subsequent cerebrovascular events. These hospitalizations for subsequent TIAs numbered 84,729 (that is, 87 percent of 97,390). Assuming them to occur on July 1, 1976, their present-valued costs (at 6 percent) amount to $87.1 million. Thirty-three eighty-sevenths of these costs ($33 million) occur after a completed cerebral infarction. Fifty-four eighty-sevenths of these costs ($54.1 million) are for hospitalized later TIAs that do not follow completed strokes.

Office Visits and Outpatient Care

Emlet (1971) estimated that patients with minimal functional impairment from stroke pay an average of two additional office visits per year for their CVD. In line with these data, we assume that TIA patients generally pay two additional office visits annually to check on their cerebrovascular condition. As for stroke, we estimate the cost of an average outpatient visit to be $11.

The population of post-TIA individuals paying these visits is estimated from the data provided by Whisnant (1976) for Rochester, Minnesota. Office visits occurring after completed stroke have been separately accounted. We therefore wish an estimate of the survival patterns of the 75,638 initial TIAs in 1975 for as long as they remain free from completed stroke. Whisnant's data provided in this form are applied to the 1975 first-TIA population to obtain the figures shown in table 4–17. This population is assumed to make two TIA-connected office visits annually. The summed and discounted costs for these visits come to $7.44 million at 6 percent.

Firm data on the frequency and costs of outpatient anticoagulant therapy are not available. Physician specialist consultants estimate that a decade ago roughly one-quarter of all patients seeking medical attention would be prescribed anticoagulants. Since then, antiplatelet-aggregating agents have been commonly used. In the hospital situation, Baker (1968) says only that anticoagulant therapy was administered "in some cases for the transient cerebral ischemic attacks." Dyken (1977) reports that anticoagulants were used for roughly 23 percent of the hospitalized TIA patients, while antiplatelet-aggregating agents were used for roughly 40 percent of the patients.

Our best estimate of outpatient anticoagulant use must be made on subjective interpretation of this evidence. We will assume that 12 percent of all persons with TIAs receive anticoagulant therapy at one time or another (recalling that many TIA patients do not even seek medical attention) and that this takes place in the first year following TIA onset. Total cost of the therapy in 1975 is estimated to be $105 (for three physician visits, monitoring, and the drug). The 9077 patients assumed to receive the therapy in 1975 thus incur total costs of $953,000. Dividing this figure by 75,638— the total number of first TIAs—yields an average cost of $13 per first TIA.

Direct Costs per Person of Strokes and
Transient Ischemic Attacks (TIAs)

The main components of direct costs are presented on a per-person basis in table 4–18 for hemorrhages, infarcts, all completed strokes, and TIAs. Initial

Table 4–18
Present Value of Direct Costs per Person for Stroke
Broken Down by Disease Category and Type of Cost
(Dollars)

	Hemorrhage	Infarct	Total Completed Stroke	Transient Ischemic Attack
Initial hospitalization	1925	1925	1925	182
Other, episodic, direct costs[a]	1659	2830	2665	13
Recurrence hospitalization[a]	412	567	546	1152[b]
Nursing home care[a]	2323	3396	3246	0
Physician visits[a]	131	152	149	98
Insurance administration[a]	290	399	384	65
Total direct costs[a]	6740	9269	8915	1510

[a]All costs occurring in subsequent years are discounted at 6 percent; all costs are in 1975 dollars.
[b]On expectation, $437 of the $1152 in costs of hospitalization for TIA recurrences are incurred following completed strokes.

hospitalization costs for completed first strokes are seen in the first line of table 4–18 to be tenfold greater than those for TIAs. This occurs because TIA victims are much less likely to be hospitalized and, when hospitalized, incur lower average costs. Other, episodic direct costs for hemorrhages are considerably lower, on average, than for infarcts, owing to greater survival for infarct patients. For TIAs, these charges are negligible, since the lack of lasting impairment precludes engaging rehabilitation services and the like.

TIAs tend to recur much more frequently than do completed strokes and to require hospitalizations. Recurrence hospitalization costs are therefore greater per TIA victim than per stroke victim. Average costs for nursing home care are greater for infarcts than for hemorrhages, owing to mortality differences and because hemorrhages tend to occur at younger ages, when persons are less likely to be admitted to nursing homes. We have assumed that all persons in nursing homes with CVD have had completed strokes. This misses the persons in the homes because of TIAs. We have accepted this exclusion for two reasons: first, because the National Nursing Home Survey does not distinguish between completed strokes and TIAs; and second, because the number of TIA admissions is likely to be small and for short stays. Discrepancies in charges for physician visits largely reflect mortality differentials.

Indirect Costs of Stroke

Work Incapacity Resulting from Stroke

To calculate earnings forgone because of stroke, we compare expectations at the age of stroke with those realized after stroke. Two population-based studies have examined the functional status of stroke survivors and have arrived at comparable results. Gresham (1979) reports on survivors in the Framingham study and Matsumoto (1973) surveys survivors in the Rochester, Minnesota population. Both studies report only on survivors at least 6 months beyond their first stroke. Gresham's group was composed of sixty-six men and eighty-two women whose mean ages at stroke were 64.3 years for the men and 66.7 years for the women. Neither study breaks its figures down by age at time of stroke.

Gresham found that 37 percent had no decrease in level of vocational function, as seen either in termination of work or incomplete resumption of homemaking activities. In Rochester, however, 36 percent of survivors were "working or able to work." Many of these, however, were aphasic (had speech difficulties).

Since stroke survivors represent an older population, much of their incapacity may result from causes other than stroke. We wish to know what proportion of vocational disability is attributable to stroke. A handle on this is found in Gresham, who reports that 49 percent of the survivors he studied showed stroke-related neurological deficits. These included motor deficits, sensory deficits, hemianopsia (blindness for one-half the field of vision), dysarthia (articulation difficulties), and dysphasia (speech impairment).

Calculating Value of Work by Stroke Survivors

Perhaps the best measure of vocational incapacity resulting from stroke is to be found in Gresham's comparison of stroke survivors with age- and sex-matched persons in the Framingham population. Whereas 37 percent of the stroke survivors had no decrease in vocational function, 64 percent of matched controls also were without decrease. This indicates that in terms solely of vocational function, stroke survivors perform at 58 percent (that is, $0.37 \div 0.64$) of the level of stroke-free but otherwise comparable individuals. It is noteworthy, however, that 65 percent of the stroke survivors who maintained their normal vocational status in fact were disabled either in activities of daily living, in mobility, or in decreased socialization outside the home (Gresham, 1975). This suggests that many of this group may have continued their previous vocational duties but with hardship or reduced efficiency. Loss owing to stroke may thus appear in the diminished abilities of a businessman who slurs his words and makes poorer decisions or in the additional time it takes to perform homemaking tasks. Unfortunately, we cannot reflect such losses in our analysis. The figure of 58 percent obtained in the Framingham study thus remains our best estimate of the proportion of normal vocational function (obtained by comparison with a matched stroke-free population) maintained by stroke survivors. We calculate poststroke earnings as 58 percent of earnings for comparable stroke-free individuals, but with the additional constraint that these earnings will accrue over a reduced lifespan. Our formula for the expected postmorbid earnings of a patient surviving at least 1 year after stroke is thus

$$PVPM = 0.58 \cdot \left[\sum_{n=l+1}^{85} P_{l+1,s}^{i}(n) \cdot E_s(n) \cdot Y_s(n) \cdot \left(\frac{1+\gamma}{1+r} \right)^{n-l} \right]$$

where all terms are as defined in chapter 2.

To maintain consistency with Gresham's data, expected earnings for stroke survivors accruing from 6 months to 1 year after stroke are estimated to be 0.58 of earnings for the comparable nonstroke population. For work performed within the first 6 months following first stroke, there are few data to indicate the appropriate weighting factor. Haerer (1975) reported that only 19.4 percent of non-TIA survivors of CVD were ambulatory without aid upon discharge from hospital. another 42.9 percent were ambulatory with aid, while others would regain functional ability over the course of the first 6 poststroke months. While this suggests that more than 19.4 percent could work in these months, we must recall that many of the healthier individuals will receive vocational therapy and will be advised to rest during this period. We accordingly assume that only 19 percent of normal work is performed by stroke survivors between the first and sixth months after stroke. We assume that no work is done during the first month after stroke.

Poststroke Earnings Expectations and
Total Forgone Earnings

We can now estimate complete postmorbid earnings expectations for all stroke patients. For patients in a particular age, sex, and diagnostic category, the expected earnings of a survivor accruing between 1 and 6 months after stroke, between 6 and 12 months after stroke, and from 1 year after stroke can be weighted, respectively, by the proportion of patients surviving at least 1 month, at least 6 months, and at least 1 year past the initial event. These figures, when summed, yield an estimate of average postmorbid earnings per patient for individuals in that category. If average postmorbid earnings are

Table 4-19
Forgone Earnings for Stroke Patients of Varying Ages and Both Sexes, United States, 1975

Age at First Stroke	Hemorrhage Per Person (Dollars)	Total (millions of Dollars)	Infarction Per Person (Dollars)	Total (millions of Dollars)	Total Both Types of Stroke (millions of Dollars)
Males					
0-14	92,953	14.4	73,771	14.7	29.1
15-24	177,964	34.0	147,279	45.8	79.8
25-34	195,306	83.8	160,719	85.7	169.5
35-44	161,999	165.9	132,787	172.4	338.3
45-54	106,994	375.2	87,003	522.5	897.7
55-64	41,016	233.4	32,798	668.9	902.3
65-74	4,747	22.4	4,018	154.5	176.9
75-84	458	0.8	401	13.5	14.3
85+	0	0.0	0	0.0	0.0
Total males	50,570	930.0	14,964	1,677.9	2,607.9
Females					
0-14	65,447	9.6	51,890	3.1	12.7
15-24	123,039	22.0	101,735	9.7	31.7
25-34	120,732	48.8	99,379	15.9	64.7
35-44	99,855	96.1	81,982	32.1	128.2
45-54	68,833	137.7	56,250	101.5	239.2
55-64	31,672	186.1	25,805	437.7	623.8
65-74	9,692	34.0	8,291	247.4	281.4
75-84	2,198	5.8	1,927	76.4	82.2
85+	0	0.0	0	0.0	0.0
Total females	31,596	540.1	8,776	923.7	1,463.8
Total population	41,429	1,470.1	11,968	2,601.6	4,071.7

Note: Forgone earnings are in 1975 dollars, discounted at 6 percent.

then subtracted from the earnings expectations of demographically matched stroke-free individuals, the result is an estimate of average forgone earnings per patient for people in that category.

Table 4-19 displays expected forgone-earnings results for both sexes, distinguishing by age and type of stroke. We note that for infarction, the less severe stroke type, the amounts of expected forgone earnings per stroke are less in every age and sex group than comparable figures for hemorrhages. For the first six age groups, the average forgone earnings per stroke are greater for men than for women, reflecting prevailing discrepancies in wage rates. (When the opportunity-cost approach is applied in valuing household labor, the forgone earnings of females rise from 56 percent of those of males, as seen in table 4-19, to 85 percent.) The greatest loss in expected earnings—

$195,306—occurs when a 30-year-old man suffers a hemorrhagic stroke.

Three columns in table 4–19 indicating totals show that the greatest indirect costs occur for strokes incident in the middle-age groups. At younger ages, the low levels of incidence reduce total forgone earnings; at older ages, limited-earnings capability has the same effect. For men, indirect-cost tables are greatest for ages 35 to 64; for women, these totals are greatest a decade later, from 45 to 74.

Calculation of forgone earnings brings out the importance of strokes occurring before the age of 55. Looking only at incidence figures, these strokes seem relatively unimportant, since only 8 percent of the first strokes in 1975 afflicted those under 55. However, 49 percent of all forgone earnings associated with stroke are for persons with first strokes occurring before the age of 55. Roughly one-seventh (14 percent) of all forgone productivity derives from first strokes incident on those over 65. Much of this total of $555 million loss appears as impaired homemaker function, which may necessitate the hiring of homemaker help from the general labor force.

Indirect Costs of Transient Ischemic Attacks (TIAs)

Insufficiency of Data on Transient Ischemic Attacks (TIAs)

Forgone earnings owing to TIAs stem wholly from productive time lost during morbidity, recovery, and treatment, and not from mortality. Considerably less time is lost to useful activity for TIAs than for nonfatal completed strokes. That significant time is lost, however, is indicated by the average TIA hospitalization of 5.8 days, to which convalescence must be added. Our hospitalization figures indicate that most TIAs are either treated on an outpatient basis or not treated at all. Many patients experiencing TIA will, however, take off time from work without consulting a physician. Still more time is lost in pursuing outpatient treatment, including anticoagulant therapy.

The literature is silent on the number of days lost from work as a result of the average TIA. Somewhat useful are case descriptions (for example, Toole, 1977), with minimal indications of their representativeness, however. This item is subject to more variance in estimation than any other component in cost estimations on stroke. Because of the paucity of data, we felt it necessary to conduct a limited survey of persons dealing with TIA patients to secure their best personal estimates. While agreement was far from complete, we have estimated on the basis of all information received that the average TIA occasions 4 days of vocational incapacity. This estimation leads to the calculation that 302,552 (that is, $4 \times 75,538$) otherwise productive days were lost in 1975 because of first TIAs.

Estimating Value of Work Loss as a Result of
Transient Ischemic Attacks (TIAs)

For subsequent TIAs, the analysis becomes more difficult because we do not wish to count the more frequent, less severe TIAs on a par with others. The estimate of 75,638 first prestroke TIAs in 1975 seems a good first approximation of the number of initial TIAs requiring work absence. This number excludes TIAs for which no medical attention was obtained. By and large, however, it seems likely that if medical attention is obtained, work is missed, and vice versa.

Among prestroke TIAs, we have estimated from Baker (1971)(see table 4–10) that for every hospitalized initial TIA there are 4.2 (that is, 0.54 ÷ 0.13) hospitalized subsequent TIAs. As a first approximation (in the absence of better data), we presume that the same ratio will hold for prestroke TIAs requiring work loss. That is, for every initial prestroke TIA requiring work loss (of which we estimate there were 75,638 in 1975), we estimate that there are 4.2 subsequent prestroke TIAs requiring work loss. The total of subsequent prestroke TIAs requiring work loss among the population with first prestroke TIAs in 1975 is thus estimated to be 314,189 (that is, 54/13 of 75,638). Since we estimate that the growth in the incidence population cancels the decline in the incidence rate, 314,189 is also our estimate of the number of subsequent work-loss TIAs of persons experiencing first CVD in 1975. Each such TIA causes 4 days of work loss, for a total of 1.26 million

Table 4–20
Total Forgone Earnings Owing to Incapacitation from
Transient Ischemic Attacks, United States, 1975
(Thousands of Dollars)

Age at TIA	Males	Females
0–14	0	0
15–24	48	8
25–34	248	35
35–44	715	84
45–54	1,975	711
55–64	5,317	1,723
65–74	2,000	2,057
> 75	119	660
Total[a]	10,422	5,277

Note: All figures are in 1975 dollars, discounted at 6 percent.
[a]Total for both sexes: $15,699,000.

days. These days are assumed to occur on average 1 year after incidence in 1976.

We calculate the forgone productivity of this time by assuming the same age and sex distribution for subsequent TIAs as for first TIAs. The results, which include forgone productivity both at incidence and 1 year later, are displayed in table 4–20, where it is seen that the indirect costs of TIAs amount to $15.7 million when discounted at 6 percent. This sum is roughly 0.4 percent of the comparable figure for completed strokes. This implies that whatever error is inherent in our estimate of forgone earnings owing to TIA, the error is minuscule when compared with total productivity forgone as a result of completed strokes.

Summary and Sensitivity Analysis

Direct and Indirect Costs

Table 4–21 presents the direct and indirect costs of hemorrhages and infarcts broken down by age and sex. Table 4–22 combines the direct, indirect, and total costs for the two diseases and compares them with the total costs of TIAs. The contrast between the direct and indirect costs is striking. We saw earlier (in table 4–19) that 51 percent of all indirect costs derive from strokes incident among those over 55. The direct costs associated with strokes incident in the same group amount, however, to 94 percent of all direct costs.

For societies intent on reducing the total economic burden of stroke, a number of lessons are apparent. First, the more evident direct costs of the disease give a misleading picture of its economic impact. Only when indirect costs are regarded does the importance of preventing strokes between the ages of 35 and 54 become clear. Second, neglect of indirect costs understates the importance of hemorrhages relative to infarcts. Regarding direct costs, hemorrhages account for only 11 percent of all direct costs of stroke. When indirect costs are also considered, hemorrhages are seen to be responsible for 27 percent of the total economic impact. This discrepancy arises because hemorrhages have greater short-term mortality than infarcts and are incident at generally younger ages. Third, we see that the economic importance of TIAs is small compared with that of completed strokes— barely one-fiftieth of the magnitude. This suggests that the main importance of TIAs arises from their nature as precursors of completed strokes. Fourth, the total economic burden of strokes incident in 1975 is seen to be $6.326 billion. Strokes in males account for $3.784 billion of this total, and strokes

Table 4–21
Present Value of Direct and Indirect Costs of Hemorrhagic and
Infarctive Strokes, by Age and Sex, United States, 1975
(Millions of Dollars)

Age at First Stroke	Hemorrhages		Infarcts	
	Direct Costs	Indirect Costs	Direct Costs	Indirect Costs
Males				
0–14	0.9	14.4	1.5	14.7
15–24	1.0	34.0	2.2	45.8
25–34	2.2	83.8	3.8	85.7
35–44	5.3	165.9	9.5	172.4
45–54	19.2	375.2	45.3	522.5
55–64	40.6	233.4	200.2	668.9
65–74	34.8	22.4	369.7	154.5
75–84	14.1	0.8	319.3	13.5
85+	6.3	0.0	100.2	0.0
Total males	124.4	930.0	1.051.7	1677.9
Females				
0–14	0.9	9.6	0.5	3.1
15–24	0.9	22.0	0.7	9.7
25–34	2.1	48.8	1.2	15.9
35–44	5.2	96.1	3.0	32.1
45–54	11.4	137.7	14.2	101.5
55–64	38.3	186.1	149.0	437.7
65–74	25.4	34.0	280.9	247.4
75–84	20.1	5.8	369.9	76.4
85+	10.4	0.0	143.7	0.0
Total females	114.7	540.1	963.2	923.7
Total population	239.1	1470.1	2014.9	2601.6

Note: All costs are in 1975 dollars, discounted at 6 percent.

in females account for $2.543 billion. Males have slightly higher direct costs, but indirect costs that are 78 percent higher than those for females.

Sensitivity Analysis for Stroke

While the conclusions found in the preceding section are potentially important for policy guidance, prudence argues that any policy utilization of any economic analysis should be based on recognition of possible inaccuracies. We examine the likely components of imprecision in our analysis of stroke and their consequences by means of sensitivity analyses addressed to six major possible sources of error: incidence, recurrence, mortality, direct costs, discounting, and indirect costs.

Incidence. The most critical component in estimating the economic costs of stroke is the calculation of incidence. The available data on incidence are plentiful relative to data used in other sections of this analysis, but they are vulnerable to many types of error. Possible errors include systematic biases introduced in estimating the rate of decline in incidence and in relying heavily on data from Rochester, Minnesota. The first type of error seems limited, because we have been able to base our estimates on recent time periods (1968 to 1976) and on comparisons with 1975 mortality data. Only if there had been a substantial shift in incidence rates within these time periods—occurring perhaps around 1972 and not affecting mortality figures—would our adjustments for declining incidence be significantly in error.

Geographic differences in incidence have been noted, in particular the higher incidence of strokes in the Southeast. Kuller's (1970) figures on the incidence of stroke in Georgia and North and South Carolina are 26 percent higher than the rates he found in Denver and Kansas. Age-adjusted rates for Miami were, however, 13 percent below those of Denver and Kansas. Taking into account the populations of the Southeast and of other regions whose mortality rates may differ from those of the North Central States (Soltero, 1978), it seems unlikely that our inability to measure regional differences could bias our rates downward by more than 10 percent.

In addition to these possible systematic errors, random errors in incidence estimation could occur for the younger age groups where available data are scanty. It is not impossible that our incidence estimates for, say, the 15- to 24-year-olds are off by 20 percent. This would occur if the Rochester, Minnesota data were idiosyncratic and if the relationship between incidence and mortality in those years was anomalous.

The consequences of these possible errors are readily seen. Any error in incidence estimation would simply bias all other costs but nursing home costs in the same proportion. Nursing home costs are an exception because their national total derives from direct measurement in a national survey, not from multiplying estimated per-case costs by estimated incidence. If, for example, we made a 5 percent underestimation of hemorrhage incidence, our indirect-cost calculations for hemorrhage strokes also would be 5 percent underestimates, while our direct-cost calculations would be biased downward by only 3.2 percent (since nursing home costs constitute 36 percent of all direct costs for hemorrhage victims).

Possible errors in estimating the incidence of strokes in younger persons may be larger proportionately, but (because so few strokes occur in these groups) they do not seriously affect disease totals. A 25 percent overestimation of infarctions for 15- to 24-year-old males would, for instance, lead to an overestimation of only 0.02 percent (1 part in 5000) of total direct costs and 0.35 percent of total indirect costs for infarctions.

Recurrence. Our estimates of recurrence rates were based on Framingham data. Marquardsen found a higher rate for females of 0.099 annually. This included third and subsequent strokes (second and subsequent recurrences). Using Matsumoto's finding that 44 of 184 recurrences were third or subsequent strokes, we can adjust Marquardsen's figure to capture second strokes only by multiplying 0.099 by 140/184. This is 0.075, which is higher by 13.4 percent than the rate of 0.066 calculated from the Framingham data. Should Marquardsen's estimated recurrence rates for females be correct, the total economic costs of all strokes would be increased by 0.2 percent.

Mortality. We noted in the section on mortality that our figures (from USDHEW, 1980) showed in certain age groups considerably better survival than the results of earlier studies (for example, Eisenberg, 1964; Shurtleff, 1974). We have relied exclusively on data from the National Survey of Stroke because they are both more extensive and more recent.

An indication of the variability in measuring mortality can be seen in the case of white male infarction victims. Eisenberg found a 1-year survival rate of 0.36, while we estimated from the National Survey of Stroke a figure of 0.619. Suppose, for the sake of illustration, that our numbers for survival in these age groups are 10 percent overestimates for all lengths of survival. If so, we would have overestimated by 10 percent the direct costs for rehabilitation, recurrences, and physician visits. Costs of initial hospitalization would not be affected, nor would the total (populationwide) expenditures on nursing homes. The total effect on direct costs would amount to an overestimation of $323 per person, or $12.8 million. At the same time, there would have been a counterbalancing effect, since overestimation of length of survival leads to an underestimation of indirect costs.

It seems, in sum, that possible errors in mortality estimation will not seriously bias overall cost estimates. This result derives partly from the insensitivity of initial hospitalization and nursing home costs to mortality figures, but more importantly, from the overall accuracy provided by the large sample size in the National Survey of Stroke.

Direct Costs. We judge that both the figures on hospitalization costs and Emlet's estimates for nonhospital costs could err by as much as 10 percent in either direction. This error could derive from variation in the limited data for gauging hospital charges, from systematic or random errors in Emlet's Delphi methods, from inaccuracies in the adjustment figures (used to calibrate procedure costs, to set all costs in 1975 figures, and to adapt regional rates to the national situation), and from our assumption that costs

Table 4–22
**Present Value of Direct, Indirect, and Total Costs of Completed Strokes
Compared with Total Costs of Transient Ischemic Attacks (TIAs),
by Age and Sex, United States, 1975**
(Millions of Dollars)

Age at First Stroke or TIA	Completed Strokes			TIAs
	Direct Costs	Indirect Costs	Total Costs	Total Costs
Males				
0–14	2.4	29.1	31.5	0.8
15–24	3.2	79.8	83.0	0.7
25–34	6.0	169.5	175.5	0.7
35–44	14.8	338.3	353.1	1.0
45–54	64.5	897.7	962.2	5.7
55–64	240.8	902.3	1143.1	18.7
65–74	404.5	176.9	581.4	26.1
75–84	333.4	14.3	347.7 ⎱	12.9
85+	106.5	0.0	106.5 ⎰	
All males	1176.1	2607.9	3784.0	66.7
Females				
0–14	1.4	12.7	14.1	0.2
15–24	1.6	31.7	33.3	0.1
25–34	3.3	64.7	68.0	0.1
35–44	8.2	128.2	136.4	0.2
45–54	25.6	239.2	264.8	3.0
55–64	187.3	623.8	811.1	9.6
65–74	306.3	281.4	587.7	24.8
75–84	390.0	82.2	472.2 ⎱	25.6
85+	154.1	0.0	154.1 ⎰	
All females	1077.9	1463.8	2541.7	63.5
Total population	2254.0	4071.7	6325.7	130.2

Note: All costs are in 1975 dollars, discounted at 6 percent.

will remain constant in 1975 real terms. Our estimates of physician-visit costs would seem to be subject to the same level of accuracy. Errors of these amounts would affect these categories of costs in all age and sex groups by an equal proportion.

Possible error of 10 percent should probably also be associated with the total estimate of nursing home costs. The total current estimate of nursing home costs seems relatively accurate because of the sound statistical structure and large sample size of the National Nursing Home Survey (NCHS, 1979). Error may, however, enter in disaggregating to the separate age and sex groups and in projecting into the future.

Our methods of disaggregation are somewhat makeshift and subject to imprecision; yet any error introduced thereby will mainly lead to assigning nursing home years to the wrong age and sex groups and will have limited impact on the overall estimates. Total present-valued nursing home costs would be affected by disaggregation error only in that some costs would be discounted over the wrong numbers of years. Even a large error of this type would have limited effect on the overall figures. Our discounting of future nursing home costs had the effect of reducing them from $955 million (undiscounted costs in 1975 prices) to $738 million. Had the discounting been in error by 50 percent, the total nursing home costs would then have been inaccurate by only 15 percent [that is, 50% (955 − 738) ÷ 738].

Perhaps more serious are possible errors in projecting future nursing home practices. We have implicitly assumed that nursing home committal policies will be the same in the future as in the past. Even, however, if these policies change, the aggregate effect will not be great. Suppose that each year the percentage of all types of stroke survivors admitted to nursing homes falls by 4 percent. Such a hypothetical trend would make our figures 11 percent overestimates of all nursing home costs.

Discounting. The choice of discount rate affects the present valuation of all future costs. Table 4–23 displays the effects of discounting the hospitalization costs for recurrences of infarctions at 2 and 10 percent—as well as at the 6 percent figure used in our base case. The table shows that the greatest proportional changes brought about by varying the discount rate occur for the youngest age groups—whose future recurrences will, on average, be discounted over the greatest number of years. The greatest absolute changes occur for persons with first strokes at ages between 55 and 74. The totals indicate that discounting at a rate of 2 percent would have increased the costs of recurrence hospitalization by $32.9 million, or 27 percent. Discounting at 10 percent would have decreased the estimated costs by 16 percent.

The same type of sensitivity analysis has been performed for all direct costs and all indirect costs of both types of completed strokes. These are shown in table 4–24. Direct costs are shown to be relatively insensitive to changes in the discount rate: increasing by 6 percent when a discount rate of 2 percent is used; decreasing by 4 percent when a discount rate of 10 percent is used. Indirect costs are considerably more sensitive to the choice of discount rate: increasing by 31 percent with a 2 percent discount rate; decreasing by 18 percent with a 10 percent discount rate.

Indirect Costs. Our base calculation of indirect costs presumed a discount rate of 6 percent, productivity growth of 1 percent, and market valuation of household labor. Table 4–25 displays the results of altering these suppositions: of discounting at 2, 6, and 10 percent; of taking productivity growth to be 0, 1, and 2 percent; and of regarding the opportunity-cost value of

Table 4–23
Sensitivity to the Discount Rate of Recurrence Hospitalization Costs
for Infarctive Stroke, by Age and Sex
(Thousands of Dollars)

Age at First Stroke	Discount Rate		
	2 Percent	*6 Percent*	*10 Percent*
Males			
0–14	378	183	119
15–24	421	223	150
25–34	638	365	252
35–44	1,315	818	588
45–54	4,885	3,324	2,506
55–64	32,536	24,198	19,256
65–74	34,516	28,304	24,132
75–84	16,471	14,530	13,064
85+	2,084	1,993	1,914
Total males	93,245	73,937	61,981
Females			
0–14	139	64	41
15–24	161	81	54
25–34	244	132	90
35–44	519	304	212
45–54	1,977	1,267	923
55–64	16,335	11,534	8,872
65–74	24,042	18,933	15,670
75–84	17,161	14,784	13,036
85+	2,398	2,286	2,189
Total females	62,976	49,385	41,086
Total population	156,221	123,322	103,067

Note: All costs are in 1975 dollars.

household labor. We see in the table that the indirect costs of stroke can be estimated as low as $3.19 billion and as high as $8.02 billion, depending on the analytic assumptions underlying those calculations. The difference between the two figures is large ($4.83 billion) and bears an important message to the reader: that while we have in all cases sought to make the most reasonable and defensible assumptions, alternative choices could have led to quite different results.

This sensitivity-analysis finding shows the imprecision in the current state of the analytic art. The variations evident in table 4–25 are not, however, as serious as they may seem. For the most part, we are interested in comparative analyses of diseases. Analyses of all diseases vary in much the same way depending on the assumptions made, as the sensitivity analyses elsewhere in this book show. The comparative economic costs of the conditions

Table 4–24
Sensitivity of Total Stroke Costs to the Choice of Discount Rate by Type of Completed Stroke
(Billions of Dollars)

		Hemorrhages	Infarctions	Total Completed Stroke
Direct costs discounted at	2%	0.26	2.14	2.39
	6	0.24	2.01	2.25
	10	0.23	1.94	2.17
Indirect costs discounted at	2%	2.02	3.32	5.34
	6	1.47	2.60	4.07
	10	1.17	2.17	3.34
Total costs discounted at	2%	2.28	5.46	7.73
	6	1.71	4.61	6.32
	10	1.40	4.11	5.51

Note: All costs are in 1975 dollars.

studied are therefore much less sensitive than the absolute costs to the assumptions varied in table 4–25.

Indirect costs also would be critically affected by data on the decrease in work capacity of stroke survivors. Based on Gresham (1979), we estimated that the earnings of stroke survivors were 58 percent of those of matched individuals without stroke. Gresham's study, however, was of predominantly older individuals, leaving open the possibility that the 50-year-old male stroke survivor could work at a rate as high as 70 percent of that of his stroke-free counterpart. Under this hypothesis, that group's expected postmorbid earnings would rise by $150 million—an increase of 21 percent—and expected forgone earnings would drop by the same amount.

Transient Ischemic Attacks (TIAs)

Data on TIAs are generally inferior to those for completed strokes. Errors in our estimated incidence rates will affect calculated forgone earnings but not hospitalization costs, which were based on PAS figures and on observed charges. In estimating the timing and sequencing of TIAs, we were on particularly shaky ground. Table 4–10 was derived from the published data of Baker and Marshall, with the gaps in their work (for example, the final degree of freedom in table 4–10) supplied by our subjective estimation. The data are not fully satisfactory: Baker's are restricted to selected American males; and Marshall's to British experience. If our estimates of the proportions of prestroke and poststroke TIAs are off, this will have only minimal

Table 4–25
Sensitivity of Total Indirect Costs of Stroke to the Discount Rate,
Productivity Growth Factor, and Mode of Valuing Household Labor
(Billions of Dollars)

			Rate of Productivity Growth		
			0 Percent	1 Percent	2 Percent
Market-value approach	Discount rate	2%	4.94	5.34	5.81
		6	3.84	4.07	4.33
		10	3.19	3.34	3.50
Opportunity-cost approach	Discount rate	2%	6.80	7.36	8.02
		6	5.28	5.60	5.96
		10	4.37	4.58	4.81

Note: All costs are in 1975 dollars.

impact on prestroke TIA costs and none at all on poststroke TIA costs. If we had, for instance, supposed that only 1 percent (instead of 3 percent) of hospitalized TIAs were initial TIAs but subsequent to a cerebral infarction, total costs for prestroke TIAs would increase by only $120,000.

We assumed, largely on the basis of evidence from Marshall, that TIAs as subsequent cerebrovascular events followed first events by 1 year. Suppose instead that this interval is 2 years. The subsequent hospitalized TIAs, of which there were 84,729 (that is, $97,390 \times 0.87$), occasioned costs of $92.4 million, which have a present value of $82.2 million when discounted at 6 percent back to 1975. This amount is $4.9 million less than our estimate with an assumed average interval of 1 year.

In estimating forgone earnings owing to TIA, we noted an extreme lack of data and had to estimate the average number of workdays lost per TIA by a limited poll of experts. One isolated expert thought our consensus figure of 4 days was too low by a factor of 5. Should we have indeed erred by this amount, we would have underestimated TIA indirect costs by $78.5 million. This is only 1.2 percent of total CVD costs.

Conclusions from the Sensitivity Analysis

We gain from the sensitivity analysis an overall sense of how sound our calculations are. We have not exhaustively examined all possible sources of analytical imprecision but have concentrated on the most salient and critical. The sensitivity analysis has been useful in identifying the most important sources of error. These are (1) *systematic misestimation of incidence rates* (the entire analysis will be affected if the data from Rochester, Minnesota are unrepresentative, if regional variation is stronger than has usually been assumed, or if incidence rates have varied idiosyncratically between 1969 and 1975); (2) *direct costs* (the literature on costs of stroke care is woefully incomplete, leaving open the possibility of serious estimation error); and (3) *work rates of stroke survivors* (the few studies on the occupational status of stroke survivors have not specifically addressed the status of younger survivors, for whom the potential impact on future productivity is largest.

Notwithstanding these factors, the major message we take from the sensitivity analysis is that the ultimate likely impact of possible errors does not cripple our study. Leaving aside the variation in the economic parameters (discount rate, productivity growth, mode of valuing household labor), we are reassured by the sensitivity analysis to find that errors in stroke-specific data are extremely unlikely to bias our estimates of the total national impact of stroke by more than 15 percent (in either direction). This is found for several reasons: (1) because possible errors in many phases of the analysis (for example, the breakdown of strokes by types, the estimation of recurrence rates, the measurement of mortality, the treatment of TIAs) do not have significant impact on the totals; (2) because the errors will run in both directions and thus partially cancel one other; and (3) because the most critical data for our analysis (for example, incidence rates, nursing home charges) tend to have been the most diligently gathered.

Notes

1. N.O. Borhani, Epidemiology of stroke, in N.O. Borhani and J.S. Meyer (eds.), *Medical Basis for Comprehensive Community Stroke Programs* (National Institutes of Health, 1968), p. 25.

2. Ibid.

3. J.F. Kurtzke, Epidemiology of cerebrovascular disease, in R.G. Siekert (ed.), *Cerebrovascular Survey Report* (Rochester, Minn.: Whiting Press, 1976), p. 230.

4. Ibid., p. 218.

5. Ibid., p. 231.

6. U.S. Department of Health, Education and Welfare, *National Survey of Stroke*, NIH Pub. No. 80–2069, p. 12

7. C.M. Wylie, Rehabilitative care of stroke patients, *Journal of the American Medical Association* 196(1966):1118.

8. M.L. Dyken, P.M. Conneally, A.F. Hearer, et al., Cooperative study of hospital frequency and character of transient ischemic attacks. I: Background, organization, and clinical survey, *Journal of the American Medical Association* 237(1977):882–886.

9. J.F. Kurtzke, *Epidemiology of Cerebrovascular Disease* (New York: Springer-Verlag, 1969), p. 66.

10. Dyken et al., Cooperative study of hospital frequency, p. 885.

11. Ibid., p. 883.

12. Ibid., p. 885.

13. R.N. Baker, Prospective study of transient ischemic attacks, in J. Moossy and R. Janeway (eds.), *Cerebral Vascular Diseases: Seventh Conference* (New York: Grune and Stratton, 1971).

14. Kurtzke, *Epidemiology of Cerebrovascular Disease*, note 14, p. 67.

15. J.P. Whisnant, A population study of stroke and TIA, in F.J. Gillingham, C. Mawdsley, and A.E. Williams (eds.), *Stroke* (Edinburgh: Churchill Livingstone, 1976), p. 32; H.R. Karp, A. Heyman, S. Heyden, et al., Transient cerebral ischemia. Prevalence and prognosis in biracial rural community, *Journal of the American Medical Association* 225(1973):125–128.

16. W.S. Fields, R.D. Remington, and J.S. Meyer, Progress report of the joint study of extracranial arterial occlusion, in J. Moossy and R. Janeway (eds.), *Cerebral Vascular Diseases: Seventh Conference* (New York: Grune and Stratton, 1971).

17. Baker, Prospective study of transient ischemic attacks, p. 168.

18. Ibid.

19. J.F. Kurtzke, Epidemiology of cerebrovascular disease," in R.G. Siekert (ed.), *Cerebrovascular Survey Report* (Rochester, Minn.: Whiting Press, 1976).

20. J.P. Whisnant, A population study of stroke and TIA, p. 33.

21. Ibid.

22. Baker, Prospective study of transient ischemic attacks, p. 168.

23. A.B. Ford and S. Katz, Prognosis after stroke. I: A critical review, *Medicine* 45(1966):223–246.

24. N. Matsumoto, J.P. Whisnant, L.T. Kurland, et al., Natural history of stroke in Rochester, Minnesota, 1955–1969: An extension of a previous study, 1945–1954, *Stroke* 4(1973):20–29. Also shown in unpublished data on recurrence from the Framingham Heart Study.

25. H. Eisenberg, J.T. Morrison, P. Sullivan, et al., CVAs, incidence and survival rates in a defined population, Middlesex County, Connecticut, *Journal of the American Medical Association* 189(1964):887.

26. Commission on Professional and Hospital Activities. *Length of Stay in PAS Hospitals by Diagnosis: United States: 1975* (Ann Arbor, Mich., 1976), pp. 95–97.

27. From *Medical Economics* (October 13, 1975):106.

28. California Medical Association, *1974 Revision of the 1969 California Relative Value Studies*, 1974; S.A. Minter and M.E. Scovell, *Medicaid Fee Schedule—Service and Procedure Codes Effective January 1, 1974*, Massachusetts Department of Public Welfare, 1974.

29. Single and multiple diagnoses are not differentiated in these figures.

30. National Center for Health Statistics, Prevalence of chronic circulatory conditions, *Vital and Health Statistics Series* 10(94).

31. Commission on Professional and Hospital Activities, *Length of Stay in PAS Hospitals*.

5 Cancer

Although not as violent as motor vehicle trauma and in numbers of people damaged or killed not as deadly as cardiovascular diseases, cancer is perhaps the most frightening of the four afflictions considered in this study. Cancer is not a single disease but a family of diseases that result when the controlled growth processes of body cells are disrupted, with changes in cell function that at present are mostly irreversible. These altered cells—a new type of tissue or *neoplasm*—reproduce themselves, invading surrounding tissues and usurping the space and nutrients that normal cells require to survive. Cells from the malignant neoplasm may break away from their site of origin and spread to regional lymph nodes, to adjacent organs or tissues, or to both. Eventually the malignancy may *metastasize* (spread) to more distant body tissues. Metastasis is a stealthy process: a solitary, undetected cancer cell has the potential to migrate through the blood or lymph systems to distant tissues, there to spread cancer anew.

Epidemiology

Cancer occurs worldwide in all races, but incidence and mortality rates vary greatly depending on geographic area, race, age, and sex. Cancer of the digestive, respiratory, and reproductive systems accounts for 69 percent of cancers in males and 77 percent of cancers in females.[1] Colon and rectal cancer (14 percent of all cancers in 1975[2]) occur at the same rate in both sexes until age 55, when they become more common in men. Women have high rates of breast and cervical cancer—almost half of all cancer in women. In men, colon and lung cancers account for more than 50 percent of the cancers, and men are 4 times more likely than women to contract lung cancer (this ratio is decreasing as more women become smokers).

Although people may contract the disease at any age, the majority of cases occur among patients over 65 years of age. In 1975, for example, 52 percent of the 660,680 newly diagnosed cases were in this age category; this was 57 percent of all new cases in males and 48 percent of all new cases in females.[3] The relatively old age at onset of cancer may be due in part to (1) the long period of latency between the time of exposure to risk factors and the appearance of clinical symptoms, and (2) the longer life expectancies that advances in medicine have achieved, especially in the control of infectious diseases (people live long enough for a precancerous condition to become actively malignant).

Although many aspects of cancer remain unexplained, evidence increasingly points to environmental factors (including diet) as major influences in the development of human cancers. It is estimated, for example, that cigarette smoking is a major causative agent in 80 percent of lung cancers.[4] Other environmental agents linked to the incidence of lung cancer include air pollution, airborne asbestos particles, and coal and radon gasses. The introduction each year of thousands of new chemical compounds and the widespread use of food additives and pesticides have led some experts to predict an increase in the incidence of cancer.

Therapy and Management

Despite their common tendencies toward uncontrolled proliferation and metastasis, cancers vary widely in body location, behavior, and response to therapy. Some malignancies, such as basal cell epithelioma (a type of skin cancer), are easy to detect, grow slowly, rarely spread, and can be excised by surgery. Other tumors, such as those in the pancreas, commonly lurk undetected only to reveal themselves too late as stubborn, swift killers.

Once the pathologist has confirmed a diagnosis of cancer by microscopic examination of suspect tissue, the attending physician must determine the stage of the disease. To classify the stage of advancement of many cancers, oncologists generally use two types of descriptive staging systems. (Leukemias, being a systemic disease, are an exception; they are classified by cell type and degree of malignancy.) The first system—TNM—defines the primary tumor (T), the extent of lymph node spread (N), and the extent of distant metastases (M).[5] A single, small (3-cm) primary tumor with no lymph node involvement and no metastases will thus be graded as $T_1N_0M_0$. As it grows and spreads, it may be upgraded to $T_2N_2M_1$ and so on. The other type of system is used for such cancers as Hodgkin's disease and non-Hodgkin's lymphomas, with the degree of clinical involvement divided into three or four subcategories, sometimes with subgroups.[6] Such staging systems give physicians a common point of reference as they ponder possible prognoses and therapies and, in the literature, as they compare therapies used in different treatment centers. For our purposes, we use a simplified system (along the lines of the TNM system), referring to cancers as local, regional, or distant: localized cancers are restricted to the site of origin; regional cancers have spread to regional lymph nodes or to adjacent organs; distant cancers have metastisized beyond the adjacent region.

After cancer's stage of advancement is determined, curative or palliative therapies must be chosen. This may require only a few diagnostic tests or a whole battery of radiological, laboratory, or surgical procedures and consultations among specialists. In general, one or more of three treatment modalities are used: surgery, radiation, or drugs. Just as cancers vary widely in their behavior and severity, they differ in their responses to treatment. Treatment tends, therefore, to be trial-and-error, with major emphasis on surgery and supervoltage radiotherapy. Breast cancer, for example, has usually been treated by radical mastectomy. However, as female patients urge physicians to investigate less mutilating treatment, newer approaches are being tested using combinations of surgery, radiation, and chemotherapy.

Use of chemotherapy remains limited. In contrast to many antibiotics used against infectious diseases, there is no truly broadspectrum anticancer drug. The line between therapeutic benefit and toxicity is narrow, and oncologists continue to refine the delicate dosage balances required. Chemotherapy has been most successful in treating pediatric cancers and lymphomas, where drugs have been used instead of surgery or radiation. Chemotherapy also has been used satisfactorily in a combined treatment modality (with surgery and radiation) for cancers of the male and female reproductive systems.[7]

As the repertoire of treatments becomes more sophisticated, costs rise. However, although physicians are learning better how to manage the disease, their knowledge of the causes and mechanisms of cancer remains limited. Breakthroughs, such as those heralding the age of antibiotics, elude researchers. As we shall see, the 660,680 new cases of cancer diagnosed in 1975 will generate more than $23 billion in total lifelong economic costs. The high incidence of cancer and its direct and indirect costs are enormously expensive. As long as medical treatment remains costly and uncertain, the vast total costs of cancer oblige us to find alternative approaches to the disease. Education and screening of populations at risk may help to avert cases or at least to permit early detection with greater likelihood of cure. The strong environmental connection for many cancers underscores the need for health-care research findings to be linked to policies for reducing the exposure of populations to potential carcinogens. With cure for cancer still problematic, we need to develop social and environmental techniques to prevent cancer or at least reduce its incidence and mortality.

Incidence

In contrast to the other disease and injury categories we examine in this book, our analysis of cancer incidence has benefited from an excellent data base in the Third National Cancer Survey. The ideal incidence study would (1) rely on a probability sample of the national population, (2) include all forms of neoplasms, (3) reflect standard diagnostic criteria, and (4) limit the cases to first manifestations of the disease—a perfect study that has yet to be performed. The Third National Cancer Survey (TNCS) is a reliable real-world approximation of the ideal, fulfilling three of the ideal criteria and sampling at least 10 percent of the nation's population. We compared the TNCS data with those from the New York State Cancer Registry and found no significant differences in their incidence data.[8] Recognizing the importance of the TNCS to our incidence estimates, we shall review briefly its salient features.

The Third National Cancer Survey

The TNCS is the latest of three surveys which the National Cancer Institute (NCI) has undertaken since 1937. The survey was compiled from information abstracted from physician reports, hospital records, clinic and laboratory reports, and death certificates with cancer-incidence data classified by patient age, sex, histologic cell type, and anatomic site. Conducted in the 3-year period from 1969 to 1971, it surveyed seven standard metropolitan statistical areas—Atlanta, Birmingham, Dallas–Ft. Worth, Detroit, Minneapolis–St. Paul, Pittsburgh, and San Francisco–Oakland—and two states—Colorado and Iowa. Their combined populations were 10.3 percent of the total U.S. population and represented 10.4 percent of all whites, 9.9 percent of all blacks, and 10.8 percent of all other races combined.[9] The age groups surveyed closely reflected the national age distribution—the maximum difference between any age group surveyed and its national counterpart was 5 percent (that for 55- to 64-year-olds).[10]

During the study period, 181,027 newly diagnosed primary cases of cancer were report in the survey areas (60,543 cases in 1969, 60,360 in 1970, and 60,124 in 1971). The average annual incidence of cancer in the survey population was roughly 29 per 10,000 population. The age-adjusted incidence rate (adjusted to conform with the 1970 national population distribution) was 30 per 10,000. From this rate, we estimated that 610,000 new cases of cancer were diagnosed in 1970 in the U.S. population. In subsequent paragraphs, we explain our method for calculating from this the incidence for 1975.

The TNCS findings show differences in cancer incidence between the sexes and among races and ages. On average, men have a higher age-specific incidence rate, and among men, cancer occurs more often in blacks (the opposite is true for women). Age patterns of cancer incidence vary between the sexes because of differences in the ages at which specific types of cancer occur. Women, for example, have high rates of breast and uterine cancer; the incidence of these malignancies is high by age 40. Incidence of reproductive-system cancers in men, by contrast, begins to rise in later years and increases rapidly with age. Cancers of the large intestine (colon and rectum) occur at the same rate in both sexes until age 55, after which their incidence in men increases.

Some find fault with the TNCS because it excluded the northeastern United States from its sample. The inclusion of this highly industrialized, densely populated sector would valuably aid those seeking industrial and environmental factors in cancer etiology. We focus instead on incidence and costs. It is possible to adjust incidence figures to reflect the somewhat older average median age of populations in the Northeast. The major effect of excluding this area is that we may underestimate the total direct costs of cancer because the regional health-care costs tend to be higher than the national average.[11] Consensus exists, however, that the incidence figures in the TNCS are reliable and representative of national trends. We have no qualms in relying on that survey as a valid data base for estimating national cancer incidence.[12]

The Nine Diagnostic Categories

The TNCS coded tumor type and site according to the American Cancer Society *Manual of Tumor Nomenclature and Coding* (1968). Carcinomas in situ (tumors that grow to the size of a pinhead but no larger and do not penetrate the surrounding tissue) and nonmelanotic skin cancers were not included in the incidence data, but all anatomic sites are included. We have used the same general classification system. For simplicity, we grouped cancers occurring at each anatomic site into nine diagnostic categories representing seven major physiological systems and two generic disease groups. Table 5–1 lists these categories and component sites.

Calculation of the 1975 National Cancer Incidence Estimates

The TNCS groups incidence data by sex and by 5-year age intervals (birth to 4 years, 5 to 9, . . . , 80 to 84, 85 or older) for the individual sites listed in table 5–1. Following the age groupings in the incidence sections of the other disease chapters, we regrouped the ages into eight groups: 0 to 14 years, 15 to 24, 25 to 34, 35 to 44, . . . , 65 to 74, and 75 or older. Our next step was to convert the 1970 incidence rates into 1975 values. To find this value, for example, for males aged 55 to 64, we calculate

$$IR_i(55\text{--}64) = \frac{a_i \cdot P(55\text{--}59) + b_i \cdot P(60\text{--}64)}{P(55\text{--}59) + P(60\text{--}64)}$$

Table 5-1
The Nine Diagnostic Categories and Component Anatomic Sites

1. *Digestive system*
   Esophagus
   Stomach
   Small intestine
   Colon
   Rectosigmoid junction
   Rectum
   Liver
   Gallbladder and other
     biliary glands
   Pancreas
   Other parts of
     digestive system

2. *Respiratory system*
   Lung
   Larynx
   Other parts of
     respiratory
     system

3. *Buccal cavity*
   Lip
   Tongue
   Salivary glands
   Gum and mouth
   Nasopharynx
   Tonsil
   Other parts of
     pharynx

4. *Reproductive system*
   Male
   Prostate
   Testis
   Breast
   Penis
   Other parts of
     genital system
   Female
   Breast
   Cervix uteri
   Corpus uteri
   Uterus, not otherwise
     specified (NOS)
   Ovary
   Vagina
   Vulva
   Other parts of genital system

5. *Urinary system*
   Bladder
   Kidney and renal
     pelvis
   Other parts of
     urinary system

6. *Nervous system*
   Brain
   Other parts of
     nervous system

7. *Leukemias*
   Acute lymphocytic
     leukemia
   Chronic lymphocytic
     leukemia
   Other lymphocytic
     leukemia
   Acute granulocytic
     leukemia
   Chronic granulocytic
     leukemia
   Other granulocytic
     leukemia
   Monocytic leukemia
   Other leukemias

8. *Lymphomas*
   Lympho- and
     reticulum
     cell
     sarcoma
   Hodgkin's
     disease
   Multiple
     myeloma

9. *Other sites*
   Bones and joints
   Soft tissue
   Skin melanomas
   Eye and orbit
   Endocrine system
   Thyroid
   Other endocrine glands
   Unknown primary sites

where IR_i = 1975 incidence rate for cancer site i for males aged 55 to 64

a_i = 1970 incidence rate from the TNCS for site i for males aged 55 to 59

b_i = 1970 incidence rate from the TNCS for site i for males aged 60 to 64

$P(55 \text{ to } 59)$ = number of males aged 55 to 59 in the 1975 U.S. population

$P(60 \text{ to } 64)$ = number of males aged 60 to 64 in the 1975 U.S. population

The 1975 incidence rates for males and females in our other age categories were calculated analogously. No secular changes were made in the age-specific incidence rates. Applying the 1970 incidence estimates from the TNCS to the 1975 population,[13] we estimated that 660,680 cases of cancer were newly diagnosed in that year: 331,821 in males and 328,859 in females. Table 5-2 summarizes the distribution of these cases by age, sex, and diagnostic category.

Summary of Incidence Results

Sex. In 1975, males and females had approximately the same overall incidence of cancer. The affected sites, however, differed, as shown below:

	New Cases in 1975		Percent of Total Incidence	
System	Males	Females	Males	Females
Digestive	87,939	80,472	27	24
Respiratory	79,563	20,326	24	6
Reproductive	60,724	154,034	18	47

Age. The incidence data confirm that the risk of developing cancer increases sharply with age. If we consider all cancers together, they fit accurately the exponential functions: For males:

$$IR_l \sim .504 \exp .081l \quad r^2 = .984$$

where the domain of the function is $l = \{8,20,30,40,\ldots,80 \text{ years}\}$; and for females:

$$IR_l \sim .776 \exp .071l \quad r^2 = .963$$

where the domain of the function is the same as for males.

Table 5–2

Annual Incidence of Cancer, by Age, Sex, and Diagnostic Type, United States, 1975

Age	1975 U.S. Population (in Thousands)ᵃ	Digestive System Incidence Rateᵇ	Incidence	Respiratory System Incidence Rate	Incidence	Buccal Cavity Incidence Rate	Incidence	Reproductive System and Breast Incidence Rate	Incidence
Male									
0–14	27,365	0.053	145	0.029	79	0.021	57	0.029	79
15–24	20,357	0.148	301	0.063	128	0.059	120	0.403	820
25–34	15,355	0.500	768	0.249	382	0.165	253	0.673	1,033
35–44	11,153	2.009	2,241	2.409	2,687	0.745	831	0.780	870
45–54	11,491	8.418	9,673	10.486	12,049	2.618	3,008	1.742	2,002
55–64	9,345	22.611	21,130	27.005	25,236	5.973	5,582	10.306	9,631
65–74	6,027	47.788	28,802	43.848	26,427	7.199	4,339	36.086	21,749
75+	3,145	79.105	24,879	39.983	12,575	8.047	2,531	78.029	24,540
Total male	104,238		87,939		79,563		16,721		60,724
Female									
0–14	26,284	0.032	84	0.020	53	0.021	55	0.036	95
15–24	19,913	0.088	175	0.044	88	0.044	88	0.587	1,169
25–34	15,580	0.410	639	0.145	226	0.121	189	3.916	6,101
35–44	11,671	1.758	2,052	0.913	1,066	0.312	364	13.010	15,184
45–54	12,280	6.224	7,643	3.244	3,984	1.058	1,299	27.598	33,890
55–64	10,435	15.035	15,689	5.318	5,549	1.877	1,959	37.226	38,845
65–74	7,847	31.146	24,440	6.126	4,807	1.763	1,383	42.758	33,552
75+	5,382	55.276	29,750	6.396	4,553	2.794	1,504	46.819	25,198
Total female	109,392		80,472		20,326		6,841		154,034
Total	213,630		168,411		99,889		23,562		214,758

Source: Derived from data presented in the *Third National Cancer Survey*, Tables 19D, 19F.

ᵃBased on resident population, all races, July 1, 1975, from *Current Population Reports*, Series p-25, Number 614, Table 1.

ᵇIncidence rates are presented per 10,000 population.

These exponential functional forms suggest that disproportionately higher incidence rates should apply to individuals 65 years of age or older, and as a consequence, the majority of total cancer cases should involve patients in this age group. We find that for men and women together, 52 percent of all cancers occur in people over 65. This trend is similar to that for the incidence of stroke, which is also highest among older people, but contrasts to that of coronary heart disease, which is highest in middle-aged individuals, and to that of motor vehicle injuries, which have their highest incidence among young adults.

It is important to note that while the majority of cancer cases occur in people older than 65, 48 percent of all cancers do occur in younger persons. As we will show, this latter group generates the greatest economic costs.

Severity. While the Third National Cancer Survey provides details on the incidence of cancer cases by anatomic site, it gives no data on the stage of

Urinary System		Nervous System		Leukemias		Lymphomas		Other Sites		All Sites	
Incidence Rate	Incidence	Incidence Rate[b]	Incidence	Incidence Rate	Incidence	Incidence Rate	Incidence	Incidence Rate	Incidence	Incidence Rate	Incidence
0.100	274	0.248	679	0.442	1,210	0.168	460	0.220	602	1.31	3,585
0.077	157	0.173	352	0.279	568	0.591	1,203	0.497	1,012	2.29	4,661
0.208	319	0.283	435	0.239	367	0.714	1,096	0.949	1,497	3.98	6,150
0.821	916	0.428	477	0.405	452	0.978	1,091	1.475	1,645	10.05	11,210
3.188	3,663	0.976	1,122	0.900	1,034	1.901	2,184	2.801	3,219	33.03	37,954
7.686	7,183	1.468	1,372	2.221	2,076	3.696	3,454	5.234	4,891	86.20	80,555
16.530	9,963	1.755	1,058	5.112	3,081	6.086	3,668	8.716	5,253	173.13	104,340
25.191	7,923	0.957	301	10.526	3,310	8.734	2,747	14.498	4,560	265.07	83,366
	30,398		5,796		12,098		15,903		22,679		331,821
0.077	202	0.260	683	0.343	902	0.086	226	0.245	644	1.12	2,944
0.045	90	0.136	271	0.155	309	0.416	828	0.745	1,484	2.26	4,502
0.107	167	0.225	351	0.159	248	0.413	643	1.484	2,312	6.98	10,876
0.383	447	0.335	391	0.279	326	0.622	726	1.998	2,332	19.61	22,888
1.125	1,382	0.632	776	0.566	695	1.308	1,606	2.945	3,616	44.70	54,891
2.571	2,683	1.037	1,082	1.260	1,315	2.481	2,589	4.085	4,263	70.89	73,974
4.949	3,883	1.189	933	2.822	2,214	4.500	3,531	7.097	5,569	102.35	80,312
8.036	4,325	0.533	287	5.920	3,186	6.106	3,286	11.860	6,383	143.74	78,472
	13,179		4,774		9,195		13,435		26,603		328,859
	43,577		10,570		21,293		29,338		49,282		660,680

progression of the disease (severity of the disease) at time of diagnosis. Since this information is necessary for our analysis of cancer mortality and for our cost analysis, we supplemented the TNCS incidence data with sex-specific information on the progression of the disease at diagnosis (local stage, regional stage, or distant stage, as defined in the beginning of the chapter). The basis for this was data published in *Recent Trends in Survival of Cancer Patients, 1960 to 1971*,[15] a supplement to *End Results in Cancer*.[16] These data include a numerical breakdown of cancer incidence at each anatomic site by stage of advancement. Table 5–3 presents this breakdown according to the tumor site and the sex of the patient.

Mortality and Life Expectancy

Invariably, cancer patients have higher mortality rates and lower life expectancies than their healthy counterparts in the general population.

Table 5–3

**Distribution of Cancer Incidence, by Stage of Advancement,
Tumor Site, and Sex of Patient**

(Percent)

	Male			Female		
Anatomical site	*Local*	*Regional*	*Distant*	*Local*	*Regional*	*Distant*
Buccal cavity	34.0	46.0	20.0	39.0	43.0	18.0
Digestive system						
Esophagus	33.3	21.4	45.2	32.9	29.1	38.0
Stomach	16.3	31.5	52.2	22.0	28.6	49.5
Colon	43.8	25.0	31.2	42.1	28.4	29.5
Rectum	46.8	25.5	27.7	48.9	25.5	25.5
Liver	36.1	14.0	50.0	28.4	16.0	55.7
Gallbladder	25.3	44.2	30.5	20.0	35.8	44.2
Pancreas	14.1	16.3	69.6	17.4	14.1	68.5
Respiratory system						
Lung	19.1	27.0	53.9	19.1	23.6	57.3
Larynx	58.8	30.9	10.3	51.6	38.1	10.3
Reproductive system						
Male genitals						
Testis and penis	45.7	24.5	29.8	—	—	—
Prostate	63.2	14.7	22.1	—	—	—
Female genitals						
Cervix	—	—	—	44.9	43.0	11.2
Corpus uteri	—	—	—	81.4	8.3	10.3
Ovary	—	—	—	24.0	8.3	67.7
Vulva	—	—	—	59.2	30.6	10.2
Vagina	—	—	—	45.7	38.3	16.0
Breast	No information on staging			45.9	43.9	10.2
Urinary system						
Kidney	42.7	20.8	36.5	47.9	19.8	32.3
Bladder	82.7	11.2	6.1	80.2	11.5	8.3
Nervous system	89.7	9.3	1.0	91.8	6.2	2.1
Other sites						
Bone	43.6	40.4	16.0	29.4	48.9	21.7
Soft tissue	55.9	19.4	24.7	58.2	19.8	22.0
Thyroid	39.0	40.0	21.0	53.5	32.3	14.1
Eye and orbit	80.4	11.3	8.3	85.3	9.5	5.3
Melanomas	70.5	14.7	14.7	78.4	13.4	8.3

Source: Computed from data in Axtell and Myers (1974).

Note: No figures are presented for leukemias and lymphomas, since these cancers are not staged.

Although specific mortality rates and survival patterns depend on the site of the cancer and its stage of advancement, cancer patients on average experience a 3-year relative survival rate (RSR) of 0.45 and a 5-year relative survival rate of 0.39.[17] The average prognosis for men is worse than that for women, the former having a 3-year RSR of 0.37 compared with 0.53 for the latter.[18] Although the excess mortality owing to cancer is greatest during the first 3 to 7 years past diagnosis, our data indicate that the period of time during which the mortality of cancer patients exceeds that of a demographically matched population extends, in most cases, to at least 15 years.

The survival probabilities we computed for cancer patients do not differentiate between mortality associated with the initial cancer and that resulting from other complicating conditions (for example, subsequent heart attack, infectious disease). To control for such confounding factors in the development of mortality statistics is beyond current epidemiological capability. We shall therefore attribute all excess mortality to cancer.

Available Data

Data from population-based studies avoid the problems of selectivity biases associated with hospital-based studies or those which select exclusively from a specific group (for example, members of a group medical plan). No long-term population-based study of cancer patients has been done. The TNCS, while providing excellent incidence data, has few direct mortality data. We turned instead to the work of the End Results Group of the National Cancer Institute. Supported in part by the National Cancer Institute (U.S. Public Health Service), the End Results Group coordinated a national cooperative program for evaluating the end results of cancer therapy in more than 100 hospitals. The extent to which the institutions participating in the End Results Survey are representative is unknown, but they do represent a broad experience and as such give us a foundation for examining survival trends.

In its fourth report (Axtell, Cutler, and Meyers, 1972) the group analyzed the survival of white cancer patients diagnosed between 1940 and 1969 (the survival data for other races were analyzed separately). Fifteen-year survival curves for 1940–1949 and 1950–1959 were carried out to 15 years after diagnosis. Ten-year survival data were presented for the 219,493 cancers diagnosed from 1955 to 1964. Five-year survival rates for patients diagnosed from 1965 to 1969 were not available. Follow-up data were reported, however, in the 1974 supplement to that report, *Recent Trends in Survival of Cancer Patients* (Axtell and Meyers, 1974).

As a further check on the validity of survival rates we have derived from these studies—which were not population-based—we compared them with the incidence and mortality data reported by the Surveillance, Epidemiology, and End Results (SEER) Project of the Biometry Branch of the National Cancer Institute (Young, Asire, and Pollack, 1978). Although not a random population sample, the SEER Project participants represented just over 10 percent of the total U. S. population and were fairly representative with respect to age. We found no significant disparities between the survival and mortality trends described in the SEER report (Young, Asire, and Pollack,

1978) and those we have derived from interpolating and extrapolating the End Results data.

The End Results Group developed three measures of survival: the observed survival rate, the median survival rate, and the relative survival rate. The latter was the basis for our estimates of survival rate. The relative survival rate is the ratio of the patients' survival rate to the expected rate for their age- and sex-matched peers in the general population in the same period of observation. Because it adjusts for "normal" mortality, it allows meaningful comparisons of the survival experience of patient groups that differ by age at diagnosis, sex, and period of observation. By comparing relative survival rates, we thus can gauge the differences in mortality associated with specific forms of cancer in patient groups with different "normal" mortality expectations. Relative survival rates in the End Results data are reported for 1, 3, 5, and, in some cases, 10 and 15 years after initial diagnosis, enabling us to disaggregate along these dimensions. These data are presented for both sexes and various age intervals, dependent on the specific type of cancer. (For example, lung cancer data are given for the following age groups: (1) younger than 45, (2) 45 to 54 years, (3) 55 to 64 years, (4) 65 to 74 years, and (5) older than or equal to 75 years.) Data of this sort form the basis for imputing the relative survival rates for 15-year period starting from the year of onset.

Determinants of Mortality

Age, tumor site, and tumor-stage severity are the three major variables in the survival experience of cancer patients, with tumor stage being the most crucial. The End Results data show that, other factors being equal, older cancer patients have shorter survival expectations than younger patients with identical cancers. This trend is more pronounced for males than for females. Tumors in less accessible, more hidden sites are more likely to be diagnosed at more advanced stages and hence are more dangerous. As one would expect, cancers that have progressed to regional or distant stages are significantly more life-threatening than localized tumors. For example, 69 percent of pancreatic cancers are diagnosed at the distant stage, giving the patient a poor prognosis for survival.[19] Breast cancers, however, are diagnosed at the local stage 45 percent of the time.[20] In the aggregate, therefore, breast cancer patients have significantly better survival prognoses than age- and sex-matched patients with pancreatic cancer.

Relative Survival Rates by Cancer Site and Stage

We used the End Results survival data to calculate the relative survival rates for cancer patients 1, 3, 5, 10, and 15 years past diagnosis. Then extrapolating from these figures, we determined survival rates for the missing years. Tables 5–4 through 5–8 display these 15-year relative survival rates for male and female patients with cancers in the nine diagnostic categories and at the three stages of advancement.

Summary of Relative Survival Rates (RSR)

The clearest trend in the relative survival rates (RSR) is that the stage of advancement is the most important factor in determining the likelihood that a patient will survive for a specified number of years past diagnosis. As we shall see, however, there are wide variations in the survival rates for patients with cancers at the same stage of advancement but located in different sites. Equally marked differences are evident among patients who have cancers at the same site and same stage of advancement but who are at opposite ends of the 15-year- postdiagnosis period. The relative survival rates, as displayed in tables 5–4 through 5–8 are summarized in the following paragraphs.

Digestive System. Table 5–4 presents the relative survival rates for the seven sites that constitute the digestive system. Of the seven, patients with cancers of the esophagus, pancreas, and liver experience the highest mortality during the initial year following diagnosis. The first-year RSRs for these three sites diagnosed at the local stage are, for men, 0.39, 0.33, and 0.19, respectively, and for women, 0.37, 0.30, and 0.24, respectively. The relative survival rates decrease rapidly in future years; 5 years past diagnosis, the RSRs for these same three sites are 0.04, 0.05, and 0.12, respectively, for men and 0.08, 0.04, and 0.21, respectively, for women. If digestive system cancers diagnosed at the distant stage are considered, the situation becomes even bleaker. At best, we can expect an RSR of 0.07 five years past diagnosis (for colon cancer); in most cases, the expectation is substantially worse.

The sites with the most favorable prognoses are the localized cancers of the colon and rectum. Men are found to have a first-year RSR of approximately 0.81, while women have an even higher RSR of about 0.88. Patients with these cancers also have relatively favorable long-term prognoses. Fifteen years past diagnosis, men have RSRs of 0.62 and 0.55 for colon and rectum cancers, respectively, and women have corresponding RSRs of 0.67 and 0.59.

Respiratory System. Table 5–5 displays the relative survival rates for the respiratory system. Of the two sites in this category—the lung and the larynx—patients with larynx cancer have the better prognosis. One year past diagnosis, a patient with localized larynx cancer has a RSR of at least 0.92. For patients with localized lung cancer, the prognosis is less encouraging, with a relative survival rate of 0.60 or 0.71, depending on the sex of the

Table 5-4
Relative Survival Rates of Cancer Patients for Up to 15 Years Past Diagnosis, by Sex, Diagnostic Category, and Stage: Digestive System

Years	Esophagus			Stomach			Colon			Rectum			Liver			Gallbladder			Pancreas		
	L	R	D	L	R	D	L	R	D	L	R	D	L	D	R	L	R	D	L	R	D
Male																					
1	0.39	0.34	0.11	0.67	0.47	0.15	0.81	0.77	0.26	0.81	0.79	0.39	0.19	0.11	0.04	0.55	0.29	0.14	0.33	0.25	0.06
2	0.08	0.07	0.07	0.56	0.34	0.09	0.80	0.62	0.19	0.78	0.61	0.08	0.18	0.08	0.03	0.29	0.20	0.10	0.21	0.14	0.04
3	0.07	0.04	0.02	0.44	0.21	0.02	0.78	0.56	0.12	0.75	0.46	0.06	0.17	0.05	0.02	0.23	0.10	0.06	0.08	0.03	0.01
4	0.06	0.04	0.02	0.42	0.18	0.02	0.75	0.48	0.10	0.71	0.36	0.04	0.15	0.05	0.02	0.21	0.07	0.06	0.07	0.03	0.01
5	0.06	0.03	0.01	0.40	0.14	0.01	0.71	0.42	0.07	0.57	0.31	0.02	0.12	0.05	0.01	0.15	0.07	0.05	0.05	0.02	0.01
6	0.04	0.03	0	0.39	0.13	0.01	0.70	0.37	0.07	0.65	0.26	0.02	0.10	0.03	0	0.18	0.06	0.05	0.05	0.02	0.01
7	0.04	0.02	0	0.38	0.12	0.01	0.69	0.34	0.07	0.63	0.22	0.02	0.07	0.03	0	0.18	0.06	0.05	0.04	0.02	0.01
8	0.03	0.02	0	0.37	0.12	0.01	0.67	0.34	0.07	0.61	0.22	0.02	0.05	0.02	0	0.18	0.05	0.05	0.04	0.01	0.01
9	0.02	0.02	0	0.36	0.11	0.01	0.66	0.33	0.07	0.59	0.21	0.02	0.02	0.01	0	0.17	0.05	0.05	0.03	0.01	0.01
10	0.02	0.02	0	0.35	0.10	0.01	0.65	0.33	0.07	0.57	0.21	0.02	0	0	0	0.17	0.04	0.05	0.03	0.01	0.01
11	0.02	0.02	0	0.35	0.10	0.01	0.64	0.33	0.07	0.57	0.21	0.02	0	0	0	0.17	0.04	0.05	0.03	0.01	0.01
12	0.02	0.02	0	0.35	0.10	0.01	0.64	0.33	0.07	0.57	0.21	0.02	0	0	0	0.17	0.04	0.05	0.03	0.01	0.01
13	0.02	0.02	0	0.34	0.10	0.01	0.63	0.33	0.07	0.56	0.21	0.02	0	0	0	0.17	0.04	0.05	0.03	0.01	0.01
14	0.02	0.02	0	0.34	0.10	0.01	0.63	0.33	0.07	0.56	0.21	0.02	0	0	0	0.17	0.04	0.05	0.03	0.01	0.01
15	0.02	0.02	0	0.34	0.10	0.01	0.62	0.33	0.07	0.55	0.21	0.02	0	0	0	0.17	0.04	0.05	0.03	0.01	0.01
Female																					
1	0.37	0.25	0.17	0.64	0.44	0.16	0.87	0.84	0.34	0.88	0.83	0.32	0.24	0.17	0.12	0.43	0.32	0.08	0.30	0.30	0.09
2	0.24	0.19	0.09	0.58	0.32	0.10	0.81	0.70	0.22	0.80	0.68	0.19	0.23	0.08	0.07	0.39	0.20	0.07	0.17	0.17	0.06
3	0.11	0.11	0.01	0.51	0.20	0.03	0.80	0.58	0.10	0.75	0.54	0.06	0.22	0.03	0.02	0.34	0.07	0.01	0.04	0.04	0.03
4	0.10	0.10	0.01	0.47	0.17	0.03	0.77	0.52	0.09	0.70	0.45	0.05	0.21	0.02	0.01	0.31	0.06	0.01	0.04	0.04	0.02
5	0.08	0.08	0	0.43	0.13	0.02	0.74	0.50	0.07	0.67	0.39	0.04	0.20	0	0	0.27	0.04	0	0.04	0.04	0.01
6	0.08	0.08	0	0.41	0.13	0.02	0.73	0.48	0.07	0.66	0.34	0.04	0.18	0	0	0.25	0.04	0	0.04	0.04	0.01
7	0.08	0.07	0	0.40	0.13	0.02	0.72	0.45	0.07	0.65	0.30	0.04	0.15	0	0	0.23	0.03	0	0.04	0.04	0.01
8	0.07	0.07	0	0.37	0.12	0.02	0.71	0.43	0.07	0.63	0.27	0.04	0.12	0	0	0.21	0.03	0	0.04	0.04	0.01
9	0.07	0.07	0	0.37	0.12	0.02	0.70	0.40	0.07	0.62	0.27	0.04	0.10	0	0	0.19	0.02	0	0.04	0.04	0.01
10	0.07	0.07	0	0.35	0.12	0.02	0.69	0.38	0.07	0.61	0.27	0.04	0.05	0	0	0.17	0.02	0	0.04	0.04	0.01
11	0.07	0.07	0	0.35	0.12	0.02	0.69	0.38	0.07	0.61	0.27	0.04	0.05	0	0	0.17	0.02	0	0.04	0.04	0.01
12	0.07	0.07	0	0.35	0.12	0.02	0.68	0.37	0.07	0.60	0.27	0.04	0.05	0	0	0.17	0.02	0	0.04	0.04	0.01
13	0.07	0.07	0	0.35	0.12	0.02	0.68	0.37	0.07	0.60	0.27	0.04	0.05	0	0	0.17	0.02	0	0.04	0.04	0.01
14	0.07	0.07	0	0.35	0.12	0.02	0.67	0.37	0.07	0.59	0.27	0.04	0.05	0	0	0.17	0.02	0	0.04	0.04	0.01
15	0.07	0.07	0	0.35	0.12	0.02	0.67	0.37	0.07	0.59	0.27	0.04	0.05	0	0	0.17	0.02	0	0.04	0.04	0.01

patient. Again, if the cancer is more advanced, the prognosis is worse: for distant lung cancer, the relative survival rate 1 year past diagnosis is 0.12 and 0.16 for men and women, respectively, and after 5 years, there is virtually no chance of survival for patients of either sex.

Buccal Cavity. As we see in table 5–5, patients with cancers at this site have a better prognosis than most other cancer patients. The relative survival rates for localized cancers 1 year past diagnosis are 0.83 for men and 0.90 for women. After 5 years, these rates drop to 0.53 and 0.62, respectively.

Urinary System. In the local stage, both sites, kidney and bladder, have similar prognoses, with 1-year relative survival rates of 0.82 and 0.90 for male and female kidney cancers, respectively, and of 0.88 and 0.87 for corresponding bladder cancers. When the stage is more advanced, kidney cancer patients have a better moderate-term prognosis than bladder cancer patients. However, after 15 years, the prognoses are similar, with RSRs of 0.16 and 0.22 for regional kidney cancer and corresponding RSRs of 0.15 and 0.14 for regional bladder cancer.

Nervous System. As indicated in table 5–5, the relative survival rates for this category of cancer are slightly lower than those observed on average for all cancers. For men with localized cancer, the relative survival rates are 0.46 and 0.28 at 1 and 5 years past diagnosis, respectively. The corresponding rates for women are 0.48 and 0.36. However, the decrease in survival rates that a patient can expect if the cancer is diagnosed at a more severe state of development is not as pronounced as it is in other cancers.

Reproductive System. The relative survival rates for cancers of the male genitals are unusually high. Local testis and penis cancers, for example, have 1-year RSRs of 0.98 and 0.96, respectively. Even at 15 years, the RSRs are still substantial—0.75, and 0.62 for these two sites. However, although cancers of the third genital site, the prostate, are also considered mild, patients with these cancers have less favorable survival prognoses than patients with cancers of the other two sites.

Like the case of cancers of the male genitals, the relative survival rates of cancers of the female genitals are high in comparison with those of other cancers. This is especially so for localized cancers. Female breast cancers also follow this trend, although when allowed to advance beyond the local stage, they become especially deadly. For instance, while localized breast cancer has RSRs of 0.99 and 0.84 for 1 and 5 years past diagnosis, respectively, these values drop dramatically to 0.56 and 0.10 for regional breast cancer.

Table 5-5
Relative Survival Rates of Cancer Patients for Up to 15 Years Past Diagnosis, by Sex, Diagnostic Category, and Stage: Respiratory System, Buccal Cavity, Urinary System, and Brain and Nervous System

| | Respiratory System | | | | | | Buccal Cavity | | | Urinary System | | | | | | Brain and Nervous System | | |
| | Lung | | | Larynx | | | | | | Kidney | | | Bladder | | | | | |
Years	L	R	D	L	R	D	L	R	D	L	R	D	L	R	D	L	R	D
Male																		
1	0.60	0.40	0.12	0.93	0.79	0.51	0.83	0.70	0.44	0.82	0.76	0.25	0.88	0.57	0.28	0.46	0.38	0.18
2	0.39	0.20	0.06	0.89	0.62	0.25	0.70	0.50	0.29	0.79	0.59	0.14	0.80	0.33	0.16	0.39	0.31	0.18
3	0.36	0.12	0.02	0.85	0.48	0.21	0.61	0.40	0.19	0.77	0.48	0.06	0.75	0.29	0.08	0.31	0.23	0.18
4	0.30	0.10	0.02	0.82	0.40	0.19	0.55	0.35	0.14	0.71	0.43	0.06	0.72	0.27	0.05	0.30	0.22	0.15
5	0.29	0.09	0.01	0.80	0.38	0.17	0.53	0.32	0.13	0.66	0.40	0.05	0.70	0.25	0.02	0.28	0.21	0.12
6	0.27	0.08	0	0.77	0.36	0.17	0.51	0.29	0.13	0.63	0.36	0.05	0.68	0.23	0	0.26	0.20	0.12
7	0.25	0.07	0	0.74	0.33	0.17	0.50	0.27	0.13	0.60	0.32	0.05	0.67	0.22	0	0.25	0.18	0.12
8	0.22	0.07	0	0.70	0.31	0.17	0.48	0.24	0.13	0.57	0.28	0.05	0.65	0.20	0	0.23	0.17	0.12
9	0.20	0.06	0	0.67	0.28	0.17	0.47	0.22	0.13	0.54	0.24	0.05	0.64	0.19	0	0.22	0.15	0.12
10	0.18	0.06	0	0.64	0.26	0.17	0.45	0.19	0.13	0.51	0.20	0.05	0.62	0.17	0	0.20	0.14	0.12
11	0.17	0.05	0	0.63	0.26	0.17	0.44	0.18	0.13	0.49	0.19	0.05	0.61	0.17	0	0.20	0.14	0.12
12	0.17	0.05	0	0.61	0.25	0.17	0.42	0.17	0.13	0.47	0.18	0.05	0.60	0.16	0	0.20	0.14	0.12
13	0.16	0.05	0	0.60	0.25	0.17	0.41	0.15	0.13	0.46	0.17	0.05	0.60	0.16	0	0.19	0.13	0.12
14	0.16	0.05	0	0.58	0.24	0.17	0.39	0.14	0.13	0.44	0.16	0.05	0.59	0.15	0	0.19	0.13	0.12
15	0.15	0.05	0	0.57	0.24	0.17	0.38	0.13	0.13	0.42	0.16	0.05	0.59	0.15	0	0.19	0.13	0.12

Females

1	0.71	0.50	0.16	0.92	0.78	0.50	0.90	0.74	0.50	0.90	0.80	0.28	0.87	0.41	0.11	0.48	0.42	0.20
2	0.39	0.23	0.08	0.88	0.63	0.24	0.80	0.54	0.35	0.80	0.62	0.15	0.82	0.25	0.07	0.43	0.37	0.20
3	0.36	0.20	0.03	0.83	0.54	0.20	0.69	0.41	0.25	0.72	0.46	0.06	0.78	0.15	0.05	0.38	0.32	0.20
4	0.30	0.14	0.01	0.78	0.46	0.18	0.64	0.36	0.19	0.70	0.43	0.06	0.77	0.14	0.03	0.36	0.29	0.17
5	0.29	0.13	0.01	0.73	0.40	0.16	0.62	0.33	0.18	0.69	0.40	0.06	0.76	0.14	0	0.34	0.25	0.15
6	0.27	0.11	0	0.72	0.40	0.16	0.60	0.31	0.18	0.66	0.37	0.06	0.74	0.14	0	0.32	0.24	0.15
7	0.25	0.10	0	0.71	0.39	0.16	0.58	0.29	0.18	0.62	0.34	0.06	0.71	0.14	0	0.31	0.22	0.15
8	0.22	0.08	0	0.70	0.37	0.16	0.55	0.28	0.18	0.59	0.31	0.06	0.69	0.14	0	0.29	0.21	0.15
9	0.20	0.07	0	0.69	0.36	0.16	0.53	0.26	0.18	0.55	0.28	0.06	0.66	0.14	0	0.28	0.19	0.15
10	0.18	0.05	0	0.68	0.34	0.16	0.51	0.24	0.18	0.52	0.25	0.06	0.64	0.14	0	0.26	0.18	0.15
11	0.17	0.05	0	0.67	0.32	0.16	0.51	0.24	0.18	0.51	0.24	0.06	0.64	0.14	0	0.26	0.17	0.15
12	0.17	0.05	0	0.66	0.29	0.16	0.50	0.23	0.18	0.50	0.24	0.06	0.64	0.14	0	0.26	0.16	0.15
13	0.16	0.04	0	0.64	0.26	0.16	0.50	0.23	0.18	0.50	0.23	0.06	0.63	0.14	0	0.25	0.16	0.15
14	0.16	0.04	0	0.63	0.23	0.16	0.49	0.22	0.18	0.49	0.23	0.06	0.63	0.14	0	0.25	0.15	0.15
15	0.15	0.04	0	0.62	0.19	0.16	0.49	0.21	0.18	0.49	0.22	0.06	0.63	0.14	0	0.25	0.15	0.15

Source: Derived from data in *End Results in Cancer*, Report No. 4 (1972).

Table 5-6
Relative Survival Rates of Cancer Patients for Up to 15 Years
Past Diagnosis, by Sex, Diagnostic Category, and Stage:
Reproductive System

	Male Reproductive													
	Male Genitals										*Female*			
	Testis			*Penis*			*Prostate*			*Breast*			
Years	L	R	D	L	R	D[a]	L	R	D	L	R	D	
1	0.98	0.89	0.51	0.96	0.76		0.92	0.90	0.65	0.99	0.93	0.47	
2	0.95	0.78	0.36	0.85	0.62		0.85	0.80	0.43	0.95	0.83	0.19	
3	0.92	0.68	0.26	0.77	0.58		0.79	0.71	0.33	0.91	0.70	0.17	
4	0.90	0.67	0.24	0.72	0.51		0.73	0.63	0.24	0.87	0.62	0.13	
5	0.89	0.66	0.22	0.71	0.44		0.68	0.57	0.19	0.84	0.56	0.10	
6	0.87	0.64	0.22	0.70	0.43		0.63	0.51	0.19	0.81	0.52	0.10	
7	0.85	0.62	0.22	0.70	0.42		0.59	0.46	0.19	0.78	0.48	0.10	
8	0.84	0.60	0.22	0.69	0.40		0.54	0.40	0.19	0.76	0.43	0.10	
9	0.82	0.58	0.22	0.69	0.39		0.50	0.35	0.19	0.74	0.39	0.10	
10	0.80	0.56	0.22	0.68	0.38		0.45	0.29	0.19	0.73	0.35	0.10	
11	0.79	0.55	0.22	0.67	0.36		0.43	0.27	0.19	0.72	0.34	0.10	
12	0.78	0.55	0.22	0.66	0.34		0.41	0.25	0.19	0.71	0.33	0.10	
13	0.77	0.54	0.22	0.64	0.31		0.39	0.23	0.19	0.70	0.31	0.10	
14	0.76	0.54	0.22	0.63	0.29		0.37	0.21	0.19	0.69	0.30	0.10	
15	0.75	0.53	0.22	0.62	0.26		0.35	0.19	0.19	0.68	0.29	0.10	

Source: Derived from data in *End Results in Cancer*, Report No. 4 (1972).
[a]No data available.

Lymphomas. The 1-year RSR for forms of this disease, which are almost always found in the distant stage, ranges for men from 0.83 for Hodgkin's disease to 0.41 for reticulum cell sarcoma, and for women, from 0.82 to 0.52 for these same diseases.

Leukemias. Under the acute leukemias, the lymphocytic leukemia patients have a better short-term prognosis than corresponding granulocytic patients. However, both types have almost no statistical chance of surviving past 10 years. For chronic leukemias, approximately the same relative survival trend is observed for lymphocytic as for granulocytic patients over the short term (1 year). Ten years past diagnosis, however, the chronic lymphocytic patient has a RSR of 0.20, while the chronic granulocytic patient has a RSR of only 0.02. In the case of monocytic leukemias, the RSR for the first year is significantly worse for women (0.10) than for men (0.32). Ten years past diagnosis, however, the survival experiences are equally dismal, with both sexes experiencing virtually no chance of survival.

Other Sites. Bone cancers have moderate to low survival rates. For local bone cancer, the RSR 1 year past diagnosis is 0.76 and 0.78 for men and

Genitals														
						Female Reproductive								
Cervix Uteri			*Corpus Uteri*			*Ovary*			*Vulva*			*Vagina*		
L	R	D	L	R	D	L	R	D	L	R	D	L	R	D
0.96	0.80	0.42	0.96	0.81	0.34	0.91	0.80	0.43	0.92	0.67	0.38	0.88	0.74	0.40
0.90	0.64	0.20	0.92	0.65	0.29	0.85	0.61	0.29	0.86	0.60	0.30	0.79	0.58	0.30
0.83	0.53	0.13	0.89	0.53	0.26	0.81	0.44	0.17	0.83	0.55	0.24	0.74	0.51	0.17
0.80	0.48	0.11	0.87	0.47	0.23	0.78	0.35	0.14	0.79	0.52	0.24	0.69	0.43	0.13
0.78	0.44	0.10	0.85	0.47	0.21	0.76	0.32	0.12	0.75	0.50	0.24	0.65	0.36	0.10
0.76	0.43	0.10	0.84	0.47	0.21	0.74	0.30	0.12	0.74	0.48	0.24	0.63	0.34	0.10
0.75	0.43	0.10	0.83	0.47	0.21	0.71	0.29	0.12	0.73	0.46	0.24	0.61	0.33	0.10
0.74	0.42	0.10	0.82	0.47	0.21	0.68	0.28	0.12	0.73	0.44	0.24	0.59	0.30	0.10
0.73	0.42	0.10	0.81	0.47	0.21	0.66	0.26	0.12	0.72	0.42	0.24	0.57	0.27	0.10
0.72	0.41	0.10	0.80	0.47	0.21	0.64	0.25	0.12	0.71	0.40	0.24	0.56	0.25	0.10
0.72	0.40	0.10	0.80	0.47	0.21	0.64	0.25	0.12	0.71	0.40	0.24	0.56	0.25	0.10
0.71	0.39	0.10	0.80	0.47	0.21	0.63	0.25	0.12	0.70	0.40	0.24	0.55	0.25	0.10
0.71	0.38	0.10	0.80	0.47	0.21	0.63	0.24	0.12	0.70	0.40	0.24	0.55	0.25	0.10
0.70	0.37	0.10	0.80	0.47	0.21	0.62	0.24	0.12	0.69	0.40	0.24	0.55	0.25	0.10
0.70	0.36	0.10	0.80	0.47	0.21	0.62	0.24	0.12	0.68	0.40	0.24	0.54	0.25	0.10

women, respectively, dropping at 5 years to 0.44 and 0.52, respectively. Cancers of the soft tissue have better survival prognoses than bone cancers, provided the stage of development is local. The 1-year RSR for these cancers is 0.90 for men and 0.94 for women. At 5 years past diagnosis, the RSR drops to 0.66 for men and 0.63 for women.

Thyroid carcinoma, in terms of relative survival rates, is one of the milder forms of cancer. In the local stage, it has a 5-year RSR of approximately 0.98; even at 15 years, the RSR is still a high 0.90 for men and 0.94 for women. Even when the stage is more severe, the prognosis remains fairly good. In the regional stage, for example, the 5-year relative survival rate is 0.85 for both sexes. The relative survival rates for cancers of the eye and orbit are also high. RSRs for men with localized cancer range from 0.99 one year past diagnosis to 0.86 five years out. Corresponding figures for women are similar—0.96 and 0.82 one and five years past diagnosis, respectively. Both sexes have a 15-year RSR of about 0.77.

Melanomas show a marked dichotomy regarding survival rates. If we confine our attention to cancers at the local stage, the prognosis is good for both men and women. The RSR 15 years past diagnosis is high for both sexes—0.63 for men and 0.71 for women. Melanomas at the distant stage are

Table 5-7
Relative Survival Rates of Cancer Patients for Up to 15 Years Past Diagnosis, by Sex, Diagnostic Category, and Stage: Lymphomas and Leukemias

| | Lymphomas[a] | | | | Leukemias[a] | | | | |
| | | | | | Acute | | Chronic | | |
Years	Reticulum Cell Sarcoma	Lympho-sarcoma	Hodgkin's Disease	Myeloma	Lymphocytic	Granulocytic	Lymphocytic	Granulocytic	Monocytic
Male									
1	0.41	0.65	0.83	0.59	0.82	0.21	0.73	0.62	0.32
2	0.32	0.45	0.70	0.36	0.54	0.12	0.59	0.37	0.19
3	0.22	0.40	0.62	0.30	0.15	0.06	0.57	0.26	0.10
4	0.19	0.36	0.56	0.21	0.10	0.04	0.49	0.17	0.08
5	0.16	0.32	0.52	0.16	0.05	0.03	0.40	0.14	0.06
6	0.15	0.29	0.46	0.11	0.04	0.03	0.33	0.10	0.05
7	0.14	0.26	0.40	0.07	0.03	0.02	0.28	0.06	0.04
8	0.13	0.22	0.34	0.04	0.02	0.01	0.23	0.04	0.04
9	0.12	0.19	0.27	0.03	0.01	0	0.20	0.02	0.03
10	0.12	0.16	0.20	0.03	0	0	0.18	0.02	0.02
11	0.12	0.15	0.19	0.03	0	0	0.15	0.02	0.02
12	0.12	0.15	0.18	0.03	0	0	0.13	0.02	0.02
13	0.11	0.15	0.16	0.03	0	0	0.12	0.02	0.02
14	0.11	0.15	0.15	0.03	0	0	0.10	0.02	0.02
15	0.11	0.15	0.14	0.03	0	0	0.10	0.02	0.02

Female									
1	0.52	0.69	0.82	0.52	0.78	0.18	0.84	0.53	0.10
2	0.38	0.50	0.70	0.29	0.53	0.11	0.70	0.37	0.07
3	0.24	0.44	0.65	0.26	0.24	0.06	0.58	0.33	0.04
4	0.22	0.38	0.60	0.22	0.16	0.02	0.50	0.23	0.03
5	0.20	0.32	0.56	0.16	0.07	0	0.45	0.14	0.02
6	0.18	0.29	0.51	0.11	0.06	0	0.39	0.11	0.02
7	0.17	0.27	0.45	0.07	0.04	0	0.34	0.08	0.01
8	0.16	0.24	0.39	0.05	0.03	0	0.30	0.06	0.01
9	0.15	0.22	0.32	0.04	0.01	0	0.26	0.04	0.01
10	0.14	0.19	0.25	0.04	0	0	0.22	0.03	0
11	0.14	0.18	0.24	0.04	0	0	0.19	0.02	0
12	0.14	0.17	0.23	0.04	0	0	0.17	0.02	0
13	0.14	0.17	0.22	0.04	0	0	0.15	0.01	0
14	0.14	0.16	0.21	0.04	0	0	0.14	0.01	0
15	0.14	0.16	0.20	0.04	0	0	0.14	0	0

Source: Derived from data in *End Results in Cancer*, Report No. 4 (1972).
[a]These cancers are unstaged.

Table 5–8
Relative Survival Rates of Cancer Patients for Up to 15 Years Past Diagnosis, by Sex, Diagnostic Catogory, and Stage: Other Sites

	Bone			Soft Tissue			Thyroid			Eye and Orbit			Melanoma		
	L	R	D	L	R	D	L	R	D	L	R	D[a]	L	R	D
Male															
1	0.76	0.71	0.31	0.90	0.58	0.28	0.99	0.96	0.48	0.99	0.94		0.96	0.89	0.27
2	0.62	0.53	0.20	0.81	0.52	0.19	0.99	0.91	0.44	0.96	0.89		0.91	0.73	0.20
3	0.58	0.47	0.09	0.73	0.45	0.10	0.98	0.86	0.40	0.90	0.85		0.86	0.53	0.12
4	0.51	0.42	0.08	0.68	0.37	0.10	0.98	0.85	0.37	0.87	0.82		0.81	0.53	0.11
5	0.44	0.37	0.08	0.66	0.28	0.09	0.98	0.84	0.34	0.86	0.79		0.75	0.53	0.10
6	0.44	0.34	0.08	0.66	0.28	0.09	0.96	0.82	0.34	0.85	0.74		0.73	0.49	0.10
7	0.43	0.31	0.08	0.66	0.27	0.09	0.94	0.81	0.34	0.83	0.67		0.71	0.45	0.10
8	0.43	0.27	0.08	0.66	0.27	0.09	0.92	0.79	0.34	0.82	0.59		0.68	0.41	0.10
9	0.42	0.24	0.08	0.66	0.27	0.09	0.91	0.78	0.34	0.80	0.49		0.66	0.37	0.10
10	0.41	0.21	0.08	0.66	0.27	0.09	0.90	0.76	0.34	0.79	0.38		0.64	0.36	0.10
11	0.41	0.21	0.08	0.66	0.27	0.09	0.90	0.76	0.34	0.79	0.38		0.64	0.35	0.10
12	0.41	0.21	0.08	0.66	0.27	0.09	0.90	0.76	0.34	0.78	0.38		0.64	0.35	0.10
13	0.41	0.21	0.08	0.66	0.27	0.09	0.90	0.76	0.34	0.78	0.38		0.63	0.35	0.10
14	0.41	0.21	0.08	0.66	0.27	0.09	0.90	0.76	0.34	0.77	0.38		0.63	0.35	0.10
15	0.41	0.21	0.08	0.66	0.27	0.09	0.90	0.76	0.34	0.77	0.38		0.63	0.35	0.10
Female															
1	0.78	0.78	0.32	0.94	0.66	0.47	0.98	0.94	0.56	0.96	0.87		0.99	0.90	0.31
2	0.64	0.61	0.21	0.84	0.46	0.17	0.98	0.90	0.53	0.92	0.76		0.95	0.73	0.25
3	0.58	0.50	0.09	0.69	0.40	0.11	0.97	0.88	0.49	0.88	0.68		0.91	0.53	0.19
4	0.53	0.42	0.08	0.63	0.38	0.08	0.97	0.86	0.48	0.85	0.61		0.88	0.46	0.17
5	0.52	0.38	0.06	0.63	0.36	0.06	0.97	0.85	0.46	0.82	0.56		0.85	0.39	0.14
6	0.51	0.37	0.06	0.62	0.36	0.06	0.96	0.85	0.46	0.81	0.56		0.83	0.38	0.14
7	0.50	0.36	0.06	0.62	0.36	0.06	0.95	0.84	0.46	0.81	0.56		0.81	0.37	0.14
8	0.48	0.34	0.06	0.62	0.36	0.06	0.95	0.84	0.46	0.80	0.56		0.78	0.36	0.14
9	0.47	0.33	0.06	0.62	0.36	0.06	0.94	0.83	0.45	0.79	0.56		0.76	0.35	0.14
10	0.46	0.32	0.06	0.62	0.36	0.06	0.94	0.83	0.46	0.79	0.56		0.74	0.34	0.14
11	0.46	0.32	0.06	0.62	0.36	0.06	0.94	0.82	0.46	0.79	0.56		0.73	0.34	0.14
12	0.46	0.32	0.06	0.62	0.36	0.06	0.94	0.82	0.46	0.79	0.56		0.72	0.33	0.14
13	0.46	0.32	0.06	0.62	0.36	0.06	0.94	0.82	0.46	0.78	0.56		0.71	0.33	0.14
14	0.46	0.32	0.06	0.62	0.36	0.06	0.94	0.82	0.46	0.78	0.56		0.71	0.33	0.14
15	0.46	0.32	0.06	0.62	0.36	0.06	0.94	0.82	0.46	0.78	0.56		0.71	0.33	0.14

Source: Derived from data in *End Results in Cancer*, Report No. 4 (1972).
[a]No data available.

significantly more lethal, with RSRs 5 years past diagnosis of only 0.10 for men and 0.14 for women.

Survival Probabilities

Using these relative survival rates, we computed cumulative survival probabilities for cancer patients in each age, sex, and diagnostic group. The

mathematical relationship is illustrated below for a 60-year-old male patient
with localized lung cancer:

$$P_{60,M}^{L,L}(60 + K) = \sigma_M^{L,L}(K) \cdot P_{60,M}^{GP}(60 + K)$$

where $P_{60,M}^{GP}(60 + K)$ = probability that a man in the general population at
age 60 will survive to age $60 + K$

$\sigma_M^{L,L}(K)$ = relative survival rate K years past diagnosis for a
male with local lung cancer

$P_{60,M}^{L,L}(60 + K)$ = probability that a man with local lung cancer
diagnosed at age 60 will survive to age $60 + K$

This formula may be applied for successive years past 60. The results of the
computations are shown in detail in table 5–9 for our particular lung cancer
patient.

When the difference between 99 years and the age at diagnosis exceeds
15 years—the maximum period for which relative survival rate data have
been gathered—we assume that survival beyond the fifteenth year follows the
conditional probabilities of survival for the U.S. general population (given in
most recent life tables). In practice, this is tantamount to assuming that the
relative survival rate for the fifteenth year past diagnosis remains constant for
any year following the fifteenth (that is, the RSR value remains constant for
years 15, 16, 17, 18, and so forth past diagnosis). Epidemiological proof that
some particular time following diagnosis does not yet exist. We have
observed that the empirical relative survival rates for certain cancers show a
small increase after a long period elapses following diagnosis. This paradox
can be explained as a consequence of the selection effect briefly discussed in
chapter 2. Epidemiologists and other medical experts we interviewed agreed
that once a long period, such as 15 years, has elapsed since the onset of the
disease, it is reasonable to assume that the survival experience of cancer
patients parallels that of persons in the general population.

Life Expectancies

We can illustrate the excess mortality that a disease causes by comparing the
average life expectancy of a patient diagnosed as having that disease with
that of his age- and sex-matched peers in the general population. The
estimated life expectancies of people in the general population and of cancer
patients are presented in tables 5–10 to 5–13. Tables 5–10 to 5–12 present

Table 5–9

Calculation of the Cumulative Probabilities of Survival from Age 60 to Age 85 of a 60-Year-Old Male Localized Lung Cancer Patient

Age	Relative Survival Rate	×	Cumulative Probability of Survival for the General Population[a]	=	Cumulative Probability of Survival for Localized Lung Cancer Patient
60	1.0		1.0000		1.0000
61	0.60		0.9773		0.5864
62	0.39		0.9532		0.3717
63	0.36		0.9279		0.3340
64	0.30		0.9012		0.2704
65	0.29		0.8734		0.2533
66	0.27		0.8444		0.2280
67	0.25		0.8142		0.2036
68	0.22		0.7830		0.1723
69	0.20		0.7504		0.1501
70	0.18		0.7166		0.1290
71	0.17		0.6816		0.1159
72	0.17		0.6457		0.1098
73	0.16		0.6089		0.0974
74	0.16		0.5712		0.0914
75	0.15		0.5328		0.0799
76	0.15		0.4940		0.0741
77	0.15		0.4550		0.0683
78	0.15		0.4162		0.0624
79	0.15		0.3778		0.0567
80	0.15		0.3405		0.0511
81	0.15		0.3044		0.0457
82	0.15		0.2701		0.0405
83	0.15		0.2380		0.0357
84	0.15		0.2086		0.0313
85	0.15		0.1823		0.0273

[a]After 15 years past diagnosis, the assumption is made that a patient having cancer will experience the same conditional probability of survival as his age- and sex-matched peers in the general population. On an operational basis, this is tantamount to keeping the relative survival rate at a constant value for each year past the fifteenth.

life expectancy by age and sex for each of the specific cancer sites. These life expectancies were found by averaging the life expectancies that were initially computed both by site and stage. From these three tables it can be seen that patients with cancers of the digestive system (except colon and rectum) and the lung and patients with leukemias, reticulum cell sarcomas, and myelomas experience the shortest life expectancy. Patients with cancers of the reproductive system, colon, rectum, urinary system, other systems, and Hodgkin's disease experience significantly longer life expectancies. Table 5–13 aggregates the cancers into the nine diagnostic categories by patient age and sex and by stage of advancement of the tumor. As we observed from the 15-year survival rates (tables 5–4 to 5–8), the major determinants of life expectancies

Table 5–10
Life Expectancies for Patients with Cancers of the Respiratory, Digestive, Urinary, and Nervous Systems and of the Buccal Cavity and for the General Population, by Age and Sex
(Years)

Age	Respiratory System		Digestive System							Urinary		Buccal Cavity	Nervous System	General Population
	Lung	Larynx	Esophagus	Stomach	Colon	Rectum	Liver	Gallbladder	Pancreas	Bladder	Kidney			
Male														
0–14	3.3	28.5	1.1	6.3	24.3	20.8	0.5	5.2	1.0	32.6	16.1	25.9	12.4	62.2
15–24	2.8	23.6	1.0	5.2	20.0	17.2	0.5	4.3	0.9	26.8	13.4	21.4	10.3	50.7
25–34	2.4	19.7	0.9	4.4	16.6	14.3	0.5	3.6	0.8	22.2	11.3	17.8	8.6	41.6
35–44	2.0	15.8	0.8	3.6	13.1	11.4	0.5	2.9	0.6	17.6	9.2	14.2	7.0	32.5
45–54	1.6	12.1	0.7	2.8	9.9	8.7	0.5	2.3	0.5	13.2	7.2	10.8	5.4	23.9
55–64	1.3	8.8	0.6	2.1	7.0	6.3	0.4	1.7	0.4	9.4	5.4	7.8	3.9	16.4
65–74	1.0	6.0	0.5	1.5	4.7	4.3	0.3	1.2	0.3	6.3	3.8	5.3	2.8	10.5
75+	0.7	3.9	0.4	1.0	2.9	2.8	0.3	0.8	0.3	3.9	2.5	3.4	1.8	6.1
All	1.2	8.3	0.5	1.7	5.6	5.2	0.4	1.3	0.4	7.6	5.3	7.6	5.9	40.6
Female														
0–14	3.4	30.5	3.4	9.0	29.4	26.7	1.6	3.4	1.6	37.3	22.3	32.2	17.8	69.7
15–24	3.0	25.7	2.9	7.6	24.6	22.4	1.4	2.9	1.4	31.2	18.8	27.0	15.0	58.0
25–34	2.6	21.8	2.5	6.4	20.7	18.8	1.2	2.5	1.2	26.2	15.9	22.7	12.7	48.3
35–44	2.3	17.9	2.1	5.3	16.8	15.3	1.1	2.1	1.0	21.2	13.0	18.5	10.4	38.8
45–54	1.9	14.2	1.7	4.2	13.1	12.0	1.0	1.7	0.8	16.5	10.3	14.5	8.2	29.8
55–64	1.6	10.7	1.3	3.1	9.7	8.9	0.9	1.4	0.7	12.2	7.8	10.8	6.1	21.5
65–74	1.3	7.5	1.0	2.2	6.6	6.2	0.7	1.1	0.5	8.2	5.5	7.4	4.3	14.1
75+	1.0	4.8	0.7	1.5	4.1	3.9	0.6	0.8	0.4	5.1	3.6	4.7	2.7	8.2
All	1.5	11.2	1.2	2.3	7.3	6.9	0.8	1.0	0.5	9.1	7.6	10.6	8.9	45.1

Table 5-11
Life Expectancies for Patients with Cancer of the Reproductive System and for the General Population, by Age and Sex
(Years)

| | Male Reproductive | | | | Female Reproductive | | | | | | | |
| | Male Genitals | | | | Female Genitals | | | | | | | |
Age	Penis	Testes	Prostate	Male GP	Cervix	Corpus Uteri	Ovary	Vulva	Vagina	Breast	Female GP
0–14	31.6	38.7	23.2	62.2	34.6	50.2	18.2	39.3	26.6	33.5	69.7
15–24	26.6	32.3	19.8	50.7	29.0	41.8	15.3	32.8	22.3	28.2	58.0
25–34	22.6	27.2	17.0	41.6	24.4	35.0	12.9	27.5	18.8	23.9	48.3
35–44	18.5	22.0	14.2	32.5	19.8	28.2	10.5	22.3	15.4	19.6	38.8
45–54	14.6	17.2	11.5	23.9	15.4	21.8	8.3	17.3	12.1	15.5	29.8
55–64	11.0	12.6	9.0	16.4	11.4	15.8	6.2	12.7	9.0	11.7	21.5
65–74	7.7	8.6	6.7	10.5	7.8	10.5	4.3	8.6	6.3	8.2	14.1
75+	4.9	5.3	4.5	6.1	4.8	6.3	2.8	5.3	4.0	5.3	8.2
All	9.6	24.1	6.2	40.6	14.5	15.4	6.9	10.6	8.2	11.8	45.1

of cancer patients are (1) the stage of advancement of the tumor at diagnosis, (2) tumor site, and (3) patient age at diagnosis. Of these three, the first is most crucial and emphasizes the importance of cancer-management strategies that focus on prevention and early detection of cancer.

Direct Costs of Cancer

Use of a single umbrella term *cancer* to describe a complex group of diseases obscures the wide variation in incidence, mortality, life expectancies, and especially costs of medical treatment. It is possible, nevertheless, to estimate these costs, referring to the data on incidence and survival probabilities described earlier and by supplementing them with two sets of cost data that were developed with the Third National Cancer Survey.

As in the other chapters, the direct costs of cancer include costs of hospital and physician care, drugs, physical therapy, private nursing, medical equipment and prosthetics, and nursing home and attendant care. The cost data gathered with the TNCS are a comprehensive, although short-term description of the direct financial dimensions of cancer treatment. Although they apply only to the first 2 years following diagnosis, they were a useful basis for the treatment-cost model we used to estimate short- and long-term costs.

Data Sources

As part of the Third National Cancer Survey, a random sample of 10 percent of the individuals diagnosed during the 3-year study was selected. Of that sample group, about 8500 patients or surviving relatives were interviewed. Using a detailed questionnaire, the Patient Interview Book (PIB), the interviewers gathered data about costs for nonhospital medical services, (for example, costs for physicians, drugs, and special nursing care. These data constitute one of the few broad sources of cost information available.[21]

In addition, Joseph Scotto and Leonard Chiazze followed 6332 newly diagnosed patients from the same 10 percent sample over a 2-year period to establish hospitalization and payment patterns for inpatient care.[22] The Scotto-Chiazze study is unique because it provides complete hospital admissions and expenditure data for patients with specific cancers from the time of first admission until the end of a 2-year follow-up period.

Because the Scotto-Chiazze data play such an important part in our analysis, we highlight their significant results in subsequent paragraphs. Scotto-Chiazze found that the mean number of admissions for all patients combined over a 2-year follow-up period was 1.8, varying only slightly

Table 5-12
Life Expectancies for Patients with Leukemias, Lymphomas, and
Other Cancers and for the General Population, by Age and Sex
(Years)

	Leukemias						Lymphomas
	Acute		Chronic				
						Reti-cullum	
	Lympho-	Granu-locy-	Lympho-	Granu-locy-	Mono-	Cell	Lympho-
Age	*cytic*	*tic*	*cytic*	*tic*	*cytic*	*Sarcoma*	*sarcoma*
Male							
0–14	1.8	0.5	9.3	2.8	2.0	7.7	11.1
15–24	1.8	0.5	8.1	2.6	1.7	6.5	9.4
25–34	1.8	0.5	7.2	2.4	1.6	5.5	8.0
35–44	1.7	0.5	6.3	2.2	1.4	4.4	6.6
45–54	1.7	0.5	5.4	2.0	1.2	3.5	5.3
55–64	1.7	0.5	4.4	1.8	1.0	2.6	4.1
65–74	1.6	0.5	3.5	1.6	0.9	1.9	3.1
75+	1.4	0.4	2.6	1.3	0.7	1.3	2.2
All	1.7	0.5	3.6	1.8	0.9	2.9	4.4
Female							
0–14	1.9	0.4	13.0	2.0	0.3	10.7	13.1
15–24	1.9	0.4	11.4	2.0	0.3	9.1	11.3
25–34	1.9	0.4	10.0	2.0	0.3	7.7	9.7
35–44	1.9	0.4	8.7	2.0	0.3	6.4	8.2
45–54	1.9	0.4	7.4	1.9	0.3	5.1	6.7
55–64	1.9	0.4	6.1	1.9	0.3	3.9	5.3
65–74	1.8	0.4	4.9	1.8	0.3	2.9	4.0
75+	1.6	0.3	3.6	1.6	0.3	2.0	2.9
All	1.9	0.4	4.8	1.8	0.3	3.7	5.0

among different geographic areas (1.7 to 2.0). The number of admissions was related to age at time of diagnosis, with younger patients admitted more frequently than older patients. Patients under 65 years of age at time of diagnosis averaged 1.9 admissions, compared with 1.7 admissions for patients 65 and over. The length of stay for all admissions combined averaged 15.6 days per admission. Length of stay decreased sequentially, with first admissions averaging about 17.4 days, second admissions averaging 13.9 days, and subsequent admissions averaging 12.8 days. Average lengths of stay per admission were 23.4 percent longer for patients under 65 (14.1 days). Total hospitalization per patient during the 2-year follow-up period averaged 28.2 days for all patients.[23]

The Scotto-Chiazze study also provides data on the distribution of total hospitalization days by site and stage of disease, age of the patient, and admission (that is, first admission, second admission, all admissions during

					Other Cancers		
Hodg-kin's Dis-ease	Mye-loma	Bone	Soft Tissue	Thy-roid	Eye and Orbit	Melan-oma	General Population
12.3	3.5	18.4	28.1	45.7	44.6	33.0	62.2
10.7	3.1	15.2	23.0	37.4	36.6	27.2	50.7
9.4	2.8	12.7	19.0	30.8	30.3	22.6	41.6
8.1	2.6	10.1	14.9	24.2	24.0	17.9	32.5
6.8	2.3	7.8	11.1	17.9	18.0	13.5	23.9
5.6	2.0	5.6	7.8	12.5	12.7	9.6	16.4
4.4	1.7	3.9	5.1	8.1	8.4	6.4	10.5
3.2	1.4	2.6	3.1	4.9	5.2	4.0	6.1
7.7	1.8	11.2	10.9	19.2	16.8	13.2	40.6
17.3	4.1	22.2	31.8	58.3	52.8	44.0	69.7
14.9	3.7	18.6	26.6	48.6	44.0	36.9	58.0
13.0	3.3	15.7	22.3	40.5	36.8	31.0	48.3
11.1	2.9	12.8	18.1	32.6	29.7	25.1	38.8
9.2	2.5	10.0	14.1	25.1	22.9	19.6	29.8
7.5	2.2	7.5	10.3	18.2	16.7	14.4	21.5
5.8	1.8	5.2	7.0	12.0	11.1	9.8	14.1
4.1	1.5	3.3	4.3	7.1	6.7	6.1	8.2
10.2	1.9	12.4	14.0	28.9	22.9	19.1	45.1

the first 2 years), as well as data on the average daily payments depending on the same four variables. Cancers of the digestive system accounted for the greatest proportion of total days of hospitalization (31.35 percent), followed by cancers of the respiratory system (16.29 percent), breast (11.4 percent), female genitals (8.87 percent), and male genitals (6.55 percent). The average daily hospital payment in 1970 dollars for all cancers combined was about $90. If we do not disaggregate by stage of the disease, the highest daily payment for all admissions was observed for patients with thyroid cancers ($108), followed by bone cancers ($106), esophogeal cancers ($98), leu-kemias ($97), and lymphomas ($94). The lowest daily payment was observed for patients with prostate cancers ($82).[24]

Using the Scotto-Chiazze data, we estimated hospitalization costs for patients during the first and second years following diagnosis and projected future annual costs for surviving patients. The scope of the data permitted us

Table 5-13
Life Expectancies for Cancer Patients, by Age, Sex, Diagnostic Category, and Tumor Stage, and for the General Population
(Years)

Age	Respiratory				Digestive				Urinary				Buccal			
	L	*R*	*D*	*All*	*L*	*R*	*D*	*All*	*L*	*R*	*D*	*All*	*L*	*R*	*D*	*All*
Male																
0–14	11.0	3.9	0.2	3.3	12.9	8.9	1.0	6.9	30.3	12.4	3.4	17.8	40.6	23.5	6.5	25.9
15–24	17.7	5.3	0.6	6.3	26.1	13.2	2.1	14.2	29.9	9.6	2.2	23.0	33.4	19.5	5.4	21.4
25–34	11.1	3.5	0.3	3.5	22.6	10.5	1.7	11.4	24.8	8.2	1.9	19.0	27.7	16.4	4.5	17.8
35–44	10.3	3.3	0.4	3.5	17.1	7.8	1.3	8.5	19.3	7.0	1.7	14.3	21.9	13.1	3.5	14.2
45–54	8.5	2.8	0.4	3.0	12.1	5.5	0.9	5.8	14.6	5.6	1.3	10.8	16.4	10.1	2.7	10.8
55–64	6.1	2.1	0.3	2.1	8.5	4.1	0.7	4.2	10.5	4.2	1.0	8.1	11.7	7.4	1.9	7.8
65–74	4.0	1.5	0.3	1.4	5.9	3.0	0.5	3.0	7.1	3.0	0.7	5.7	7.8	5.2	1.3	5.3
75+	2.6	1.1	0.2	1.0	3.7	2.1	0.4	1.9	4.4	2.1	0.5	3.6	4.8	3.4	0.9	3.4
All	5.4	1.9	0.3	1.9	7.1	3.5	0.6	3.5	8.7	3.7	0.9	6.9	11.5	7.3	1.9	7.6
Female																
0–14	28.5	10.2	6.0	17.0	16.8	8.9	0.9	7.3	36.6	17.8	4.5	22.9	50.9	24.5	10.1	32.2
15–24	10.4	3.6	0.3	3.0	32.1	18.3	2.6	18.0	33.7	13.8	3.4	22.9	42.6	20.6	8.5	27.0
25–34	14.5	4.7	0.5	4.7	27.6	14.5	2.2	14.8	29.4	10.9	2.6	21.0	35.7	17.5	7.1	22.7
35–44	10.8	3.7	0.4	3.4	22.5	11.9	1.9	12.1	23.4	9.5	2.3	16.3	29.0	14.3	5.8	18.5
45–54	8.5	3.1	0.4	2.8	17.6	9.5	1.5	9.6	18.6	7.2	1.7	13.4	22.6	11.3	4.5	14.5
55–64	6.6	2.6	0.3	2.3	12.8	7.1	1.2	7.0	13.9	5.3	1.3	10.3	16.6	8.6	3.4	10.8
65–74	4.4	2.0	0.3	1.6	8.6	4.9	0.8	4.7	9.6	3.7	0.9	7.2	11.3	6.1	2.3	7.4
75+	2.8	1.4	0.3	1.1	5.3	3.2	0.6	3.0	6.0	2.3	0.6	4.6	6.9	4.0	1.5	4.7
All	6.2	2.4	0.3	2.1	9.6	5.4	0.9	5.3	11.3	4.7	1.2	8.5	16.3	8.4	3.3	10.6

Age	Nervous				Leu-kemia	Lymph-omas	Reproductive				Other Cancers				General Population
	L	R	D	All			L	D	R	All	L	R	D	All	
Male															
0–14	12.8	9.0	7.7	12.4	1.6	10.7	49.1	36.6	15.6	36.6	39.1	18.0	8.5	28.2	62.2
15–24	10.6	7.5	6.3	10.3	1.4	9.7	44.9	32.2	13.2	32.3	32.7	22.1	8.4	25.0	50.7
25–34	8.9	6.3	6.2	8.6	1.5	8.3	37.3	26.8	11.1	27.0	29.0	21.6	7.4	23.3	41.6
35–44	7.2	5.1	4.1	7.0	2.1	6.2	28.2	20.6	9.2	20.9	23.1	17.6	5.9	18.8	32.5
45–54	5.5	4.0	3.1	5.4	2.4	4.5	15.8	12.0	7.0	13.0	17.3	12.9	4.4	14.1	23.9
55–64	4.1	3.0	2.2	3.9	2.7	3.4	10.9	8.0	5.1	9.1	12.2	9.1	3.3	10.0	16.4
65–74	2.8	2.1	1.4	2.8	2.1	2.4	7.9	6.1	3.6	6.7	7.9	5.9	2.1	6.4	10.5
75+	1.9	1.4	0.9	1.8	1.7	1.8	5.3	4.4	2.4	4.5	4.8	3.5	1.2	3.9	6.1
All	6.1	4.3	3.4	5.9	2.0	4.1	8.5	7.4	3.9	7.3	17.2	13.0	4.5	14.0	40.6
Female															
0–14	18.4	11.7	10.6	17.8	1.5	14.4	45.4	21.4	9.0	20.4	49.4	30.9	10.6	38.0	69.7
15–24	15.5	9.9	8.9	15.0	0.9	14.0	40.8	21.1	7.3	24.4	47.2	37.7	16.7	40.1	58.0
25–34	13.1	8.5	7.4	12.7	1.2	11.3	34.8	18.0	5.9	23.5	40.4	34.0	16.3	35.6	48.3
35–44	10.7	7.0	6.0	10.4	1.9	8.0	28.4	14.6	4.9	19.5	31.5	25.5	11.7	27.7	38.8
45–54	8.4	5.7	4.6	8.2	2.8	5.8	22.4	11.7	4.1	15.8	24.0	19.0	8.3	20.9	29.8
55–64	6.3	4.4	3.4	6.1	2.7	4.4	16.6	9.1	3.2	12.0	17.3	13.4	5.6	14.9	21.5
65–74	4.4	3.2	2.3	4.3	2.7	3.2	11.2	6.7	2.2	8.3	11.6	8.9	3.8	10.0	14.1
75+	2.8	2.2	1.4	2.7	2.0	2.3	6.8	4.5	1.5	5.2	6.9	5.2	2.1	5.9	8.2
All	9.2	6.1	5.1	8.9	2.2	4.9	17.1	9.5	3.3	12.3	25.3	21.2	9.2	22.2	45.1

not only to estimate specific component costs, but also to differentiate these estimates by site, stage, and age of the patient (less than 65, 65 and older). Scotto and Chiazze did not disaggregate their data by sex. We followed their lead, because the literature suggests that there is little or no difference between the sexes in the treatment of cancer. We adjusted our estimates for changes in cancer-treatment procedures (for example, increased use of chemotherapy) that have taken place between 1970 and 1975. We incorporated this change by increasing hospital-related drug expenses by 50 percent.[25] In like manner, we adjusted the distribution of nursing home days among the first and subsequent years past diagnosis.

Probably because of their respective sources, the Scotto-Chiazze data have been found to be more reliable predictors of absolute cost levels than the PIB data.[26] We thus use the PIB data in our model primarily to indicate the *relative* distribution of costs by component categories (with special emphasis on non-hospital-related costs).[27] The data for hospital costs from Scotto-Chiazze and for nonhospital medical expenditures from the PIB survey enabled us to develop a model of cancer-treatment costs without first having to identify and speculate on costs for a variety of individual cancer-treatment protocols. This eliminated the need for several intermediate calculations, but makes our results no less representative.

Direct-Cost Components

The direct-cost components were developed in two stages. In the first stage, we used hospital-payment data obtained from Scotto-Chiazze, as mentioned earlier, to calculate average hospitalization costs during the first and second years following diagnosis and to project estimates of those costs during any subsequent year. Included in the calculations was the conversion of the 1970 payment data to more realistic estimates of 1975 hospital costs. First, we upgraded all payments by 20 percent to reflect the general relationship between payments and actual costs,[28] Then we converted these results from 1970 to 1975 price levels using the standard hospital price indices.[29] In the second stage, information from the PIB survey on the proportional distribution of hospital and nonhospital costs enabled us to estimate selected nonhospital expenditures (that is, costs of physician services, private nursing, nursing home and attendant care, drugs, physical therapy, special equipment and prosthetics, and other miscellaneous services) as a percentage of the hospitalization costs developed during the first stage.

Hospital Costs. The data from Scotto-Chiazze provided information on length of stay during first and second admissions, total length of stay during all admissions occurring over the first 2 years, and hospital per-diem charges (adjusted to 1975 levels) specific to first, second, and all admissions. These data were disaggregated by site, stage, and age of the patient. Using the data and assuming that any admissions past the first would be distributed uniformly over the time from the conclusion of the first admission to the end of the second year, we estimated the proportion of hospital costs in each of the first 2 years past diagnosis. If we let

α = length of stay per patient during first admission

γ = total length of stay per patient for all admissions during the first 2 years

d_1 = per-diem cost during first admission

d' = per-diem cost averaged over all admissions during the first 2 years

we have

a = costs per patient of first admission = αd_1

b = costs per patient of *subsequent* admission past the first = $\gamma d' - \alpha d_1$

And finally,

$$C_{H,1} = \text{average first-year hospital costs per patient} = a + \left(\frac{365 - \alpha}{730 - \alpha}\right) \cdot b$$

$$C_{H,2} = \text{average second-year hospital costs per patient} = \left(\frac{365}{730 - \alpha}\right) \cdot b$$

To obtain a rough estimate of the average annual hospital costs for cancer patients surviving to the third, fourth, or any subsequent year past diagnosis, we assumed that these costs would best be approximated by the costs occurring during the first 2 years that exceeded the costs of the first and second admissions.[30] Our assumption implicitly recognizes that a patient who has multiple hospitalizations during the first 2 years and survives is likely to require frequent hospitalizations and thus generate high annual hospital costs in the future. Notice that if we let

β = length of stay per patient during second admission

d_2 = per-diem cost during second admission

$C_{H,n}$ = average annual hospital costs per surviving patient for each year past the second we have

$C_{H,n} \sim$ total hospital costs per patient during the first 2 years $-$ costs per patient of first and second admissions

$\sim \gamma d' - (\alpha d_1 + \beta d_2)$

As an example, if we apply this model in the case of a patient under 65 years of age with localized lung cancer, we find that average hospitalization costs during the first and second years past diagnosis, as well as the average annual costs during subsequent years, are

$$C_{\text{Hospital, 1}}^{\text{Lung, Local}} = \$3891$$

$$C_{\text{Hospital, 2}}^{\text{Lung, Local}} = \$916$$

$$C_{\text{Hospital, } n}^{\text{Lung, Local}} = \$817$$

All these costs are in 1975 dollars.

Nonhospital Costs. To estimate the costs of other treatment components, we used the PIB data to derive a proportional distribution of total medical expenditures among the different treatment components (for example, hospital, physician, drugs, private nursing, and so forth). This *relative* distribution of expenditures combined with our prior estimates of average hospitalization costs per patient (derived from Scotto-Chiazze) was sufficient to produce first-order estimates of the costs of non-hospital-related treatment. As for hospitalization costs, we estimated nonhospital costs for each subcategory of cancer patients.

For each cancer site, we let

$E_{\text{K}}^{\text{PIB}}$ = total expenditures on treatment component K reported by PIB patients

$\sum_{\text{K}} E_{\text{K}}^{\text{PIB}}$ = total overall treatment expenditures reported by PIB patients

$P_{\text{K}}^{\text{PIB}}$ = proportion of total expenditures allocated to treatment component K by PIB patients

then, by definition, we have

$$P_{\text{K}}^{\text{PIB}} = \frac{E_{\text{K}}^{\text{PIB}}}{\sum_{\text{K}} E_{\text{K}}^{\text{PIB}}} \qquad \text{for every K}$$

To estimate average costs per patient, let

$C_{K,1}$ = average first-year costs per patient for treatment component K

$C_{K,2}$ = average second-year costs per patient for treatment component K

$C_{K,n}$ = average annual costs per surviving patient for treatment component K during each year past the second

Using estimates developed earlier from the Scotto-Chiazze data for $C_{H,1}$, $C_{H,2}$, and $C_{H,n}$, we assume the relationship

$$\frac{P_K^{P\,IB}}{P_H^{P\,IB}} = \frac{C_{K,1}}{C_{H,1}} = \frac{C_{K,2}}{C_{H,2}} = \frac{C_{K,n}}{C_{H,n}}$$

holds for every K. It follows for each treatment component K that

$$C_{K,1} = \frac{P_K^{P\,IB}}{P_H^{P\,IB}} \cdot C_{H,1}$$

$$C_{K,2} = \frac{P_K^{P\,IB}}{P_H^{P\,IB}} \cdot C_{H,2}$$

$$C_{K,n} = \frac{P_K^{P\,IB}}{P_H^{P\,IB}} \cdot C_{H,n}$$

This approach allows us to estimate for each subcategory of cancer patients the average costs per patients of each treatment component.

Returning to the example of a localized lung cancer patient under 65 years of age, we find proportionality factors for treatment expenditures that range from approximately 0.599 for hospital costs to 0.286 for physician charges to 0.001 for expenditures for physical therapy. Since average first-year hospital costs per patient for individuals in this group are estimated to be $3891, the average physician charges during the first year would be

$$\frac{0.286}{0.599} \times \$3891 = \$1858$$

Similar estimates of the costs of treatment components accruing during the first, second, and subsequent years past diagnosis are summarized in table 5–14.

Table 5–14
Average Annual Direct Costs per Patient with Lung Cancer[a]
(Dollars)

	First Year	Second Year	Any Year Past the Second[b]
Hospital	3891	916	817
Physician	1858	437	390
Nursing home and attendant care[c]	259	259	259
Drugs	195	46	41
Physical therapy	5	1	1
Special equipment and prosthetics	65	15	14
Others (including private nursing)	130	31	27
Total	6403	1705	1549

[a]Cost estimates apply to a localized lung cancer patient under 65 years of age.

[b]Cost estimates apply only to patients *surviving* past the second year.

[c]Average annual nursing home/attendant-care costs are assumed to be the same for each year past diagnosis.

The annual costs of the various treatment components may be summed to give average total costs per patient per year. Accordingly, we define

$F_l^{i,j}$ = average first-year costs for a patient of age l at diagnosis ($l < 65$ or $l > 65$) with cancer at site i and stage j

$S_l^{i,j}$ = average second-year costs for a patient of age l at diagnosis ($l < 65$ or $l > 65$) with cancer at site i and stage j

$AC_l^{i,j}$ = average annual costs for patients surviving past the second year of age l at diagnosis ($l < 65$ or $l > 65$) with cancer at site i and stage j

From the table, we see that in the case of the localized lung cancer patient, these values become

$$F_{<65}^{\text{Lung, Local}} = \$6403$$

$$S_{<65}^{\text{Lung, Local}} = \$1705$$

$$AC_{<65}^{\text{Lung, Local}} = \$1549$$

Average Costs per Patient

For people in each incidence category (age, sex, diagnosis), total direct costs per patient include the direct costs accumulating over the entire lifetime of that patient (as indicated by his survival probabilities), with all future costs discounted back to the year of incidence (1975). In accordance with the discussion on direct costs in chapter 2, we model the present value of average direct costs for a patient of given cancer type, sex, and age at diagnosis as

$$PVC = F_l^{i,j} + \frac{S_l^{i,j} \cdot P_{l,s}^{i,j}(l+1)}{1+r} + \sum_{n=l+2}^{99} \frac{P_{l,s}^{i,j}(n) \cdot AC_l^{i,j}}{(1+r)^{n-l}}$$

or equivalently,

$$PVC = F_l^{i,j} + \frac{S_l^{i,j} \cdot P_{l,s}^{i,j}(l+1)}{1+r} + AC_l^{i,j} \left(\sum_{n=l+2}^{99} \frac{P_{l,s}^{i,j}(n)}{(1+r)^{n-l}} \right)$$

where $F_l^{i,j}$, $S_l^{i,j}$, and $AC_l^{i,j}$ are defined earlier and

$PVC =$ present value of average direct costs accruing over a patient's lifetime and discounted back to the year of incidence (1975)

$r =$ discount rate

$P_{l,s}^{i,j}(n) =$ probability of a patient of sex s with cancer at site i and stage j surviving to age n, given a diagnosis of cancer at age l

Applying this model to the example of a localized lung cancer patient—a 60-year-old male at the time of initial diagnosis—and discounting future costs at 6 percent, we have

$$PVC = F_{<65}^{L,L} + \frac{S_{<65}^{L,L} \cdot P_{60,M}^{L,L}(61)}{1.06} + AC_{<65}^{L,L} \left[\sum_{n=62}^{99} \frac{P_{60,M}^{L,L}(n)}{(1.06)^{n-60}} \right]$$

Since

$$F_{<65}^{L,L} = \$6403$$

$$S_{<65,M}^{L,L} = \$1705$$

$$AC_{<65}^{L,L} = \$1549$$

$$P_{60,M}^{L,L}(61) = 0.5878$$

and

$$\sum_{n=62}^{99} \frac{P_{60,M}^{L,L}(n)}{(1.06)^{n-60}} = 2.0501$$

then the costs for this patient are

$$PVC = \$6403 + \frac{\$1705(0.5878)}{1.06} + \$1549(2.0501) = \$10,524$$

Hence, for all patients in this particular cancer category (males between the ages of 55 to 64 who are diagnosed as having localized lung cancer), this result is a first-order estimate of the average total direct costs per patient. Corresponding estimates have been computed for each age and sex cohort; there are 109 possible site and stage combinations and thus 109 possible per-patient cost estimates. To conform with our incidence analysis, these estimates are aggregated into one of nine groups, where each group represents one of the nine diagnostic categories. For each diagnostic category, a weighted average of the individual site and stage costs produces an overall average for total direct costs per patient. The weights applied coincide with the proportion of individuals of that age and sex in the general group who had cancers at a particular site and stage. We may illustrate this procedure by working through a specific example. Since cancers of the respiratory system—lung and larynx cancers—may be diagnosed at the local, regional, or distant stages, there are six possible site and stage combinations within this general category. If we consider, for instance, 60-year-old male patients with cancer of the respiratory system, our incidence estimates indicate that 88.6 percent will have lung cancer and 11.4 percent will have larynx cancer. Within the lung cancer group, roughly 19.1 percent will have localized cancers; 27 percent, regional; and 53.9 percent, distant. From our previous numerical example, local lung cancer patients who are 60 years of age generate about $10,524 in lifelong direct costs (discounted at 6 percent); similar estimates for regional and distant lung cancer are $7659 and $6112, respectively. Weighting these costs by the proportion of patients at each stage, we obtain average direct costs of $7373 (that is, $0.191 \times \$10,524 + 0.27 \times \$7659 + 0.539 \times \$6112$) for a typical lung cancer patient of that age and sex. A corresponding estimate for a larynx cancer patient is $18,173. Again, weighting by the overall proportions of lung and larynx patients, we calculate $8604 (that is, $0.886 \times \$7373 + 0.114 \times \$18,173$) as the average direct cost for a 60-year-old male respiratory system cancer patient. (To incorporate insurance administration costs, this result should be multiplied by a factor of 1.045, yielding overall direct costs of $8994 per patient. This result is applicable to all such patients between the ages of 55 and 64.)

Table 5–15
Present Value of Direct Costs per Cancer Patient, by Age, Sex, and Diagnostic Category, United States, 1975
(Dollars)

Age	Digestive	Respiratory	Buccal Cavity	Reproductive	Urinary	Nervous	Leukemias	Lymphomas	Cancers of Other Sites
Males									
0–14	5,488	8,231	16,731	16,396	9,098	16,916	9,409	15,711	15,785
15–24	11,276	10,952	16,396	15,969	13,661	16,657	8,633	16,648	12,317
25–34	10,986	9,189	16,019	16,912	13,201	16,370	8,653	15,633	9,159
35–44	11,186	9,633	15,343	13,966	11,952	15,850	9,703	14,380	8,535
45–54	10,510	9,628	14,349	13,647	11,012	15,079	10,414	12,824	10,468
55–64	8,340	8,994	13,068	11,954	10,370	7,728	11,196	11,362	9,156
65–74	7,875	7,484	10,085	9,215	9,416	9,064	10,186	9,768	10,698
75+	7,341	7,005	8,583	7,030	7,960	8,270	9,534	8,132	10,096
Females									
0–14	5,172	16,018	16,861	15,920	8,958	18,660	9,340	17,319	19,524
15–24	10,721	8,341	16,631	15,920	11,156	18,449	7,809	19,116	8,671
25–34	11,351	10,027	16,312	16,912	12,205	18,158	8,234	17,995	7,569
35–44	11,615	9,380	15,782	13,966	11,086	17,669	9,301	15,327	7,708
45–54	11,480	9,134	14,995	12,394	11,241	16,943	10,806	13,680	9,555
55–64	9,987	8,925	13,894	11,591	10,739	10,975	10,947	12,327	9,303
65–74	8,669	7,411	10,432	9,477	10,068	10,123	11,248	10,616	11,730
75+	7,921	6,942	8,912	6,920	8,265	9,100	9,534	8,011	9,614

Note: All costs are in 1975 collars, discounted at 6 percent and include insurance administration costs.

Similar estimates for patients in each of the other incidence categories are shown in table 5–15. They substantiate several expected trends. First, the present value of average direct costs per patient decreases with age. In some cases, this may not be immediately apparent, since the figures in table 5–15 reflect the aggregation process across sites and stages described earlier. However, if reference is made to the initial site- and stage-specific estimates, we can see clearly that the direct costs decrease monotonically with age. Second, the per-patient costs for men in a particular incidence category are smaller than the corresponding costs for women. This difference is primarily a consequence of the higher relative survival rates for women. Finally, nervous system cancers, followed by the lymphomas, generate the largest lifetime costs per patient.

Total Direct Costs by Cost Components

Since the per-capita annual cost components that were estimated earlier derived from the annual costs of hospital, physician, nursing home, drugs, special equipment and prosthetics, and other categories, we can disaggregate the total present-valued direct costs by these dimensions. The results are presented in table 5–16. Hospital and physician costs represent over 85 percent of the total treatment costs.

we find higher, excluding insur. admin.

Insurance Administration Costs

Insurance administration costs are 4.5 percent of the treatment costs of cancer. These costs are created by the administrative expenditures that insurance companies and government agencies incur in reimbursing the patients' direct expenses for treatment. The insurance administration costs associated with the incidence of cancer in 1975 amounted to $275.9 million, or 4.5 percent of total treatment costs.

Summary of Total Direct Costs

Multiplying the cost estimates in table 5–15 by the corresponding number of patients in each incidence category yields the total direct costs generated by patients in each category. Then summing these results over the various categories, we obtain an estimate of the present value of total direct costs for all cancer patients during their lifetimes (see table 5–17).

Women generate slightly more total direct costs than men, primarily because of their higher survival rates following diagnosis. The sensitivity of

Table 5–16
Present Value of Total Direct Costs of Cancer, by Cost Component and Diagnostic Category, United States, 1975
(Millions of Dollars)

	Hospital	Physician	Attendant and Nursing Home Care	Drugs	Special Equipment and Prosthetics	Others	Total Treatment Costs	Insurance Administration	Total
Digestive	806.0	346.2	167.7	37.4	7.3	14.4	1379.0	62.0	1441.0
Respiratory	452.9	245.4	45.0	21.6	5.3	21.5	791.7	35.6	827.3
Buccal cavity	122.4	101.0	17.2	8.8	4.0	21.3	274.7	12.4	287.1
Reproductive	1218.9	614.2	191.2	56.9	13.3	46.2	2140.7	96.3	2237.1
Urinary	242.8	125.6	21.5	9.4	1.3	3.3	403.9	18.2	422.1
Nervous	76.1	38.5	15.3	2.1	0.5	4.0	136.5	6.1	142.6
Leukemias	117.8	59.3	18.5	5.5	1.3	4.4	206.7	9.3	216.1
Lymphomas	188.5	95.0	29.6	8.8	2.1	7.1	331.1	14.9	346.0
Other sites	268.1	135.1	42.1	12.5	2.9	10.2	470.9	21.1	492.0
All cancers	3493.5	1760.3	548.1	163.0	38.0	132.4	6135.3	275.9	6411.2

Note: All costs are in 1975 dollars, discounted at 6 percent.

Table 5-17
Present Value of Total Direct Costs of Cancer, by Age, Sex, and Diagnostic Category, United States, 1975
(Millions of Dollars)

Age	Digestive	Respiratory	Buccal Cavity	Reproductive	Urinary	Nervous	Leukemias	Lymphomas	Cancers of Other Sites	All
Male										
0–14	0.8	0.6	1.0	1.3	2.5	11.5	11.4	7.2	9.3	45.6
15–24	3.4	1.4	2.0	13.1	2.1	5.9	4.9	20.0	12.5	65.3
25–34	8.4	3.5	4.1	17.5	4.2	7.1	3.2	17.1	13.7	78.8
35–44	25.1	25.9	12.8	12.1	10.9	7.6	4.4	15.7	14.0	128.5
45–54	101.7	116.0	43.2	27.3	40.3	16.9	10.8	28.0	33.7	417.9
55–64	176.2	227.0	72.9	115.1	74.5	13.5	23.2	39.2	44.8	786.5
65–74	226.8	197.8	43.8	200.4	93.8	9.6	31.4	35.8	56.2	895.6
75+	182.6	88.1	21.7	172.5	63.1	2.5	31.6	22.3	46.0	630.4
Total males	725.0	660.3	201.3	559.4	291.5	74.5	120.8	185.5	230.2	3048.5
Females										
0–14	0.4	0.9	0.9	1.5	1.8	12.7	8.4	3.9	12.6	41.2
15–24	1.9	0.7	1.5	18.6	1.0	5.0	2.4	15.8	12.9	59.8
25–34	7.3	2.3	3.1	103.2	2.0	6.4	2.0	11.6	17.5	155.3
35–44	23.8	10.0	5.7	212.1	5.0	6.9	3.0	11.1	18.0	295.6
45–54	87.7	36.4	19.5	420.0	15.5	13.1	7.5	22.0	34.6	656.4
55–64	147.3	49.5	27.2	429.0	28.8	11.9	14.4	31.9	39.7	780.7
65–74	211.9	35.6	14.4	318.0	39.1	9.4	24.9	36.6	65.3	755.3
75+	235.7	31.6	13.4	174.4	37.4	2.6	32.6	27.5	61.4	616.4
Total females	716.0	167.0	85.7	1677.7	130.6	68.1	95.3	160.5	261.8	3362.7
Total population	1441.0	827.3	287.1	2237.1	422.1	142.6	216.1	346.0	492.0	6411.2

Note: All costs are in 1975 dollars discounted at 6 percent.

total costs to age at diagnosis is reflected in the disproportionately larger costs associated with cancer patients under the age of 65 compared with those of patients 65 years of age and over. For instance, men under 65 account for about 50 percent of the total male-related direct costs but represent only 44 percent of the male incidence population. Women under 65, while constituting 52 percent of the female incidence, generate over 59 percent of total female-related costs.

If we compare the major diagnostic groups, cancers of the reproductive system have the highest direct costs, accounting for approximately 35 percent of total direct costs. Of these direct costs, about 75 percent are for cancers of the female reproductive system, reflecting our inclusion of breast cancer in that group. Direct costs associated with cancers of the reproductive system are followed in order of magnitude by costs of digestive system cancers (22 percent) and of respiratory system cancers (13 percent).

Indirect Costs of Cancer

Forgone Productivity

To calculate earnings forgone as a result of cancer, we compared earnings expectations of the patient at the time of initial cancer diagnosis with those realized after diagnosis. We examined unpublished data gathered through the PIB survey (referred to in the Direct Cost section) to determine the functional status of cancer survivors.[31] The survey focuses on individuals who were employed prior to their cancer diagnosis and presumably would have remained employed at their regular jobs if they had not been afflicted by the disease. Using these data along with information from the mortality analysis, we estimated the mean number of weeks during the first year that a previously employed patient with cancer would be out of work. This is expressed in table 5–18. From these results, we then calculated the fraction of potential first-year productivity lost by cancer patients. In addition, the data enable us to estimate the proportion of cancer patients who were working before illness who survive and return to work 1 year after diagnosis.

It is not possible, with available data, to estimate losses resulting from cancer that are caused by possible diminished capabilities of cancer victims after they return to work. We assume therefore that patients who return to work function at essentially full predisease capacity. This is reasonable, since cancer survivors, like heart attack survivors but unlike those suffering from debilitating impairments such as stroke or spinal cord injury, do not appear to suffer the types of physical disabilities that would limit on-the-job performance.[32]

Table 5–18
Mean Number of Weeks during the First Year that a
Surviving Cancer Patient Loses from Work

Cancer Site	Number of Weeks Lost from work
Digestive system	
Esophagus	16.8
Stomach	26.6
Colon	17.4
Rectum	21.4
Pancreas	17.6
Respiratory system	
Lung	19.9
Larynx	16.0
Buccal cavity	17.4
Reproductive system	
Female breast	17.2
Female genital system:	
Cervix	14.2
Uterus	15.2
Ovary	22.3
Male genital system:	
Prostate	14.9
Urinary system	
Bladder	13.0
Kidney	19.4
Nervous system	23.6
Lymphomas	
Lymphosarcoma and reticulum cell sarcoma	23.8
Hodgkin's disease	19.2
Leukemias	
Acute lymphocytic	21.0
Acute granulocytic	23.6
Chronic lymphocytic	17.2
Chronic granulocytic	14.7
Monocytic	5.0
Other sites	
Thyroid	5.9
Bones and joints	23.3
Melanomas	11.9

Calculating Value of Work

Using the TNCS PIB data and incorporating mortality/survival information, we estimate by age, sex, and cancer type (1) the fraction of potential first-year productivity actually generated by cancer patients ($\alpha^i_{l,s}$) and (2) the proportion of previously employed cancer patients (including both previously employed patients and those engaged in homemaking activities) who survive and return to work 1 year after diagnosis ($\beta^i_{l,s}$). Incorporating these two parameters, we model the expected postmorbid earnings of a cancer patient as

$$PVPM = [\alpha^i_{l,s} \cdot Y_s(l) \cdot E_s(l)]$$

$$+ \left\{ \beta^i_{l,s} \cdot \left[\sum_{n=l+1}^{85} P^i_{l+1,s} \cdot Y_s(n) \cdot E_s(n) \cdot \left(\frac{1+\gamma}{1+r} \right)^{n-l} \right] \right\}$$

where all other parameters are as defined in chapter 2. The first term on the right side of the equation represents average first-year earnings, and the second term represents the present value of average earnings generated in subsequent years by cancer patients. It is important to recognize that the value of $\beta^i_{l,s}$ in the preceding equation reflects the multiplication of the values of two implicit parameters, the first being the proportion of cancer patients of that class who survive at least 1 year past diagnosis, and the second, the fraction of those survivors who were also working before illness who actually return to work 1 year later. The second parameter provides our best estimate of the proportion of normal vocational function maintained by cancer survivors relative to that of a matched cancer-free population. It enables us to estimate postdiagnosis earnings for such survivors as a proportion of the earnings for comparable cancer-free individuals, but with the full realization that these earnings will accrue over a reduced lifespan.

Applying our model to the example of a 60-year-old male local lung cancer patient, we can compute his postmorbid earnings. Notice that for an individual in this category the following relationships hold:

$$\alpha^L_{60,M} = 0.4079$$

$$\beta^L_{60,M} = 0.5878$$

$$E_M(60) = 0.6850$$

$$Y_M(60) = \$13,413$$

Also, if $r = 6\%$ and $\gamma = 1\%$, as we assume, we have

$$\sum_{n=61}^{85} P^{\text{L,L}}_{61,\text{M}}(n) \cdot Y_{\text{M}}(n) \cdot E_{\text{M}}(n) \left(\frac{1.01}{1.06}\right)^{n-60} = \$29,281$$

Thus, combining terms, it follows that

$$PVPM = (0.4079) \cdot (0.6850) \cdot (13413) + (0.5878) \cdot (29281) = \$20,959$$

For all patients in the incidence category defined to include male local lung cancer patients between the ages of 55 and 64, this result constitutes a first-order estimate of the average postmorbid earnings per patient.

Postdiagnosis Earnings Expectations

Using the model just described, we estimated average postmorbid earnings for cancer patients of different ages, sexes, and diagnostic types and combined and averaged them to yield results for each of the nine diagnostic categories. Subtracting a cancer patient's postmorbid earnings from the estimate of his expected future earnings had he not contracted the disease (that is, the earnings estimate for a person free of cancer), we find the estimated net forgone earnings owing to the disease. Table 5–19 displays the forgone earnings per patient for each diagnostic category. We see, for example, that male leukemia patients aged 15 to 24 and 25 to 34 have the greatest forgone earnings, the 15- to 24-year-olds forgoing $214,126, and the 25- to 34-year-olds, $225,631. In general, males have greater forgone earnings than females, thus reflecting their higher average wages and their poorer survival possibilities. Regardless of sex and cancer type, forgone earnings are greatest for patients in the 15- to 34-year age group and decrease thereafter. Despite the large fraction of cancer patients over 65 years old, young and middle-aged cancer patients forgo the largest proportion of earnings.

Total Forgone Earnings

As for direct costs, we multiply the forgone earnings per capita displayed in table 5–19 by the corresponding number of patients in each incidence category to find the total forgone earnings accruing to patients in each category. Then summing these results over the various categories, we obtain an estimate of the present value of total forgone earnings sustained by all

Table 5–19
Forgone Earnings per Patient Owing to Cancer, by Age, Sex, and Diagnostic Category
(Dollars)

Age	Digestive	Respiratory	Buccal Cavity	Reproductive	Urinary	Nervous	Leukemias	Lymphomas	Other Sites
Male									
0–14	117,720	125,255	79,022	70,642	96,474	106,653	120,674	112,778	73,458
15–24	159,551	193,819	125,473	110,889	118,241	176,190	214,126	171,488	111,356
25–34	172,638	218,299	129,638	111,520	123,322	187,604	225,631	175,645	100,256
35–44	143,847	174,505	103,289	80,906	102,943	152,612	176,356	147,275	77,451
45–54	95,982	110,636	63,463	44,468	64,150	97,490	106,376	94,913	47,747
55–64	34,690	40,718	21,368	15,348	21,024	35,392	33,643	33,474	16,337
65–74	3,740	4,524	2,314	1,549	2,192	3,873	3,752	3,697	1,894
75+	373	408	198	136	187	348	309	320	172
Females									
0–14	83,372	71,126	51,143	66,296	63,580	69,854	92,189	75,815	42,672
15–24	103,735	143,589	78,126	84,784	89,017	112,018	148,838	105,840	45,604
25–34	101,095	131,338	73,465	69,656	79,471	107,813	141,117	102,216	36,759
35–44	82,148	108,813	58,857	53,832	66,491	87,807	110,834	88,864	32,262
45–54	54,208	72,978	37,955	33,498	41,775	58,736	68,458	60,531	22,421
55–64	24,334	32,487	16,322	14,013	17,828	26,244	29,403	26,882	10,429
65–74	7,095	9,507	4,614	3,945	4,968	7,571	7,891	7,736	2,985
75+	1,456	1,972	870	722	952	1,577	1,505	1,523	620

Note: All figures are in 1975 dollars, discounted at 6 percent.-

Table 5-20
Present Value of Total Forgone Earnings Owing to Cancer, by Age, Sex, and Diagnostic Category, United States, 1975
(Millions of Dollars)

Age	Digestive	Respiratory	Buccal Cavity	Reproductive	Urinary	Nervous	Leukemias	Lymphomas	Cancers of Other Sites	All
Male										
0–14	17.1	9.9	4.5	5.6	26.4	6.1	158.1	51.9	44.2	323.8
15–24	48.0	24.8	15.1	90.9	18.6	21.1	121.6	206.3	112.7	659.1
25–34	132.6	83.4	32.8	115.2	39.4	47.5	82.8	192.5	150.1	876.2
35–44	322.4	468.9	85.8	70.4	94.3	126.8	79.7	160.7	127.4	1536.4
45–54	928.4	1333.1	190.9	89.0	235.0	293.3	110.0	207.3	153.7	3540.6
55–64	732.0	1027.6	119.3	147.9	151.0	197.6	69.8	116.6	78.7	2640.4
65–74	107.7	119.6	10.0	33.7	21.8	16.8	11.6	13.6	9.9	344.7
75+	8.3	5.1	3.3	3.3	1.5	0.9	1.0	0.9	0.8	24.3
Total males	2297.5	3072.3	458.9	556.0	588.0	710.0	634.7	948.7	677.6	9945.5
Females										
0–14	7.0	3.8	2.8	6.3	12.8	3.8	83.2	17.1	27.5	164.3
15–24	18.2	12.6	6.9	99.1	8.0	9.9	46.0	87.6	67.7	356.0
25–34	64.6	29.7	13.9	425.0	13.3	20.4	34.0	65.7	85.0	752.4
35–44	168.6	116.0	21.4	817.8	29.7	32.0	36.1	64.5	75.2	1361.3
45–54	415.1	290.8	49.3	1111.8	57.7	76.3	47.6	97.2	81.1	2226.8
55–64	381.8	180.3	32.0	544.3	47.8	51.4	38.7	69.6	44.5	1390.3
65–74	173.4	45.7	6.4	132.4	19.3	10.5	17.5	27.3	16.6	449.0
75+	43.3	9.0	0.5	18.2	4.1	2.8	4.8	5.0	4.0	92.0
Total females	1271.9	687.8	134.0	3154.8	192.8	206.6	308.8	434.1	401.5	6792.3
Total population	3569.4	3760.1	592.9	3710.8	780.8	916.6	943.5	1382.9	1079.1	16,737.8

Note: All costs are in 1975 dollars, discounted at 6 percent.

members of the incidence population over their lifetimes. These estimates are shown in table 5–20, disaggregated by age, sex, and diagnostic type.

The age-related distribution of forgone earnings reflects the rapid reduction with age of forgone earnings per capita. Cancer patients aged 65 and over account for only 5.5 percent of forgone-earnings losses, while they constitute over 52.3 percent of total incidence. Men account for 59.4 percent of total cancer incidence, and they generate a disproportionately large proportion of forgone earnings.

Respiratory, reproductive, and digestive system cancers account for the largest part of total forgone earnings, generating 22.5, 22.2, and 21.3 percent of earnings losses, respectively—almost two-thirds of the total forgone earnings resulting from cancer. For men, the respiratory system cancers generate almost 31 percent of total forgone earnings; for women, cancers of the reproductive system (including breast cancer) account for almost 47 percent of total forgone earnings. The lymphomas and the leukemias generate the highest forgone earnings per capita—about $47,135 and $44,308 per patient, respectively (obtained by dividing total forgone earnings for each diagnostic type by total incidence). For all the cancer sites combined, the average forgone earnings per capita are $25,334.

Summary and Sensitivity Analysis

Direct, Indirect, and Total Costs

Table 5–21 presents the direct and indirect costs of the various cancers broken down by age, sex, and diagnostic category. Table 5–22 combines the direct, indirect, and total costs for the nine disease categories. From these tables emerges a comprehensive picture of the economic costs associated with cancer. The total costs associated with the incidence of cancer in 1975 are approximately $23.149 billion. This corresponds to an average loss per patient of $35,038—$9,704 direct and $25,334 indirect.

Table 5–22 shows that roughly 84 percent of all costs are sustained by patients under the age of 65. In contrast, individuals of this age account for only 48 percent of total incidence. This implies a disproportional shifting of total costs onto patients in the younger and middle-aged groups. If we examine the breakdown of costs by sex, approximately 56 percent of all costs are associated with male patients, who constitute slightly more than 50 percent of the incidence. For both sexes, the 45 to 54 age cohort occasions the largest costs, accounting for about 30 and 28 percent of the total costs for males and females, respectively.

For the incidence population as a whole, approximately 28 percent of the total costs are direct. In contrast, for patients 65 and older, approximately 76

Table 5–21
Present Value of Total Direct and Indirect Costs of Cancer, by Age, Sex, and Diagnostic Category
(Millions of Dollars)

Age	Digestive		Respiratory		Buccal		Reproductive	
	Direct	In-direct	Direct	In-direct	Direct	In-direct	Direct	In-direct
Male								
0–14	0.8	17.1	0.6	9.9	1.0	4.5	1.3	5.6
15–24	3.4	48.0	1.4	24.8	2.0	15.1	13.1	90.9
25–34	8.4	132.6	3.5	83.4	4.1	32.8	17.5	115.2
35–44	25.1	322.4	25.9	468.9	12.8	85.8	12.1	70.4
45–54	101.7	928.4	116.0	1733.1	43.2	190.9	27.3	89.0
55–64	176.2	732.0	227.0	1027.6	72.9	119.3	115.1	147.8
65–74	226.8	107.7	197.8	119.6	43.8	10.0	200.4	33.7
75+	182.6	8.3	88.1	5.1	21.7	0.5	172.5	3.4
Total males	725.0	2297.5	660.3	3072.3	201.3	458.9	559.4	556.0
Females								
0–14	0.4	7.0	0.9	3.8	0.9	2.8	1.5	6.3
15–24	1.9	18.2	0.7	12.6	1.5	6.9	18.6	99.1
25–34	7.3	64.6	2.3	29.7	3.1	13.9	103.2	425.0
35–44	23.8	168.6	10.0	116.0	5.7	21.4	212.1	817.8
45–54	87.7	415.1	36.4	290.7	19.5	49.3	420.0	1111.8
55–64	147.3	381.8	49.5	180.3	27.2	32.0	429.9	544.3
65–74	211.9	173.4	35.6	45.7	14.4	6.4	318.0	132.4
75+	235.7	43.3	31.6	9.0	13.4	1.3	174.4	18.2
Total females	716.0	1271.9	167.0	687.8	85.7	134.0	1677.7	3154.8
Total population	1441.0	3,569.3	827.3	3760.1	287.1	592.9	2237.1	3710.8

Note: All costs are in 1975 dollars, discounted at 6 percent.

percent of the societal costs of cancer are direct. This age-dependent relationship between total direct and total indirect costs is perhaps best explained by reviewing the analogous relationship between per-capita costs. Tables 5–15 and 5–19 show that while average direct costs are somewhat smaller for older patients, the average indirect costs of older patients are orders of magnitude less than those of patients of middle age. Indirect costs per patient for younger patients are substantially larger than the per-capita estimates of direct costs; the opposite is true for older patients. This occurs because in most cases the most significant portion of direct costs is produced during the year of incidence and hence will accrue to all patients regardless of age, while most indirect costs, in the form of forgone earnings, are sustained in future years and will accrue predominantly to younger patients who have longer life expectancies. Only 30 percent of all indirect costs derive from cancers incident among those over 55. The direct costs associated with cancers incident in the same age group, however, amount to 70 percent of all direct costs.

Urinary		Nervous		Leukemias		Lymphomas		Cancer of Other Sites	
Direct	In-direct	Direct	In-direct	Direct	In-direct	Direct	In-direct	Direct	In-direct
2.5	26.4	11.5	6.1	11.4	158.1	7.2	51.9	9.3	44.2
2.1	18.6	5.9	21.1	4.9	121.6	20.0	206.3	12.5	112.7
4.2	39.4	7.1	47.5	3.2	82.8	17.1	192.5	13.7	150.1
10.9	94.3	7.6	126.8	4.4	79.7	15.7	160.7	14.0	127.4
40.3	235.0	16.9	293.3	10.8	110.0	28.0	207.3	33.7	153.7
74.5	151.0	13.5	197.6	23.2	69.8	39.2	116.6	44.8	78.7
93.8	21.8	9.6	16.8	31.4	11.6	35.8	13.6	56.2	9.9
63.1	1.5	2.5	0.9	31.6	1.0	22.3	0.9	46.0	0.8
291.5	588.0	74.5	710.0	120.8	634.7	185.5	948.7	230.2	677.6
1.8	12.8	12.7	3.8	8.4	83.2	3.9	17.1	12.6	27.5
1.0	8.0	5.0	9.9	2.4	46.0	15.8	87.6	12.9	67.7
2.0	13.3	6.4	20.4	2.0	34.0	11.6	65.7	17.5	85.0
5.0	29.7	6.9	32.0	3.0	36.1	11.1	64.5	18.0	75.2
15.5	57.7	13.1	76.3	7.5	47.6	22.0	97.2	34.6	81.1
28.8	47.8	11.9	51.4	14.4	38.7	31.9	69.6	39.7	44.5
39.1	19.3	9.4	10.5	24.9	17.5	36.6	27.3	65.3	16.6
37.4	4.1	2.6	2.8	32.6	4.8	27.5	5.0	61.4	4.0
130.6	192.8	68.1	206.6	95.3	308.8	160.5	434.1	261.8	401.5
422.1	780.8	142.6	916.6	216.1	943.5	346.0	1382.9	492.0	1079.1

Table 5–21 shows that in 1975 the reproductive system cancers (which include breast cancers) were the costliest category, accounting for about 26 percent of all cancer costs. Estimated costs of $5.948 billion were associated with the incidence of cancers of this type. The reproductive system, along with the digestive and respiratory systems, generated approximately two-thirds of the total societal costs of cancer. For all categories of cancers, except those of the male reproductive system, indirect costs outweighed direct costs by large margins.

Sensitivity Analysis

As in the previous chapters, we examine the likely components of imprecision in our analysis of cancer and their consequences by means of sensitivity analyses addressed to five major possible sources of error: incidence, mortality, direct costs, discounting, and indirect costs.

Table 5-22
Present Value of Direct, Indirect, and Total Costs of Cancer,
by Age and Sex
(Millions of Dollars)

	All Cancers		
Age	Direct Costs	Indirect Costs	Total Costs
Males			
0–14	45.6	323.8	369.4
15–24	65.3	659.1	724.4
25–34	78.8	876.2	955.0
35–44	128.5	1536.4	1664.9
45–54	417.9	3450.6	3,958.5
55–64	786.5	2,640.4	3,426.9
65–74	895.6	344.7	1,240.3
75+	630.4	24.3	654.7
All males	3,048.5	9945.5	12,994.0
Females			
0–14	41.2	164.4	205.6
15–24	59.8	356.0	415.8
25–34	155.3	752.5	907.8
35–44	295.6	1361.3	1,656.9
45–54	656.4	2226.8	2,883.2
55–64	780.7	1390.3	2,171.0
65–74	755.3	499.0	1,204.3
75+	616.4	92.0	708.4
All females	3362.7	6792.3	10,155.0
Total population	6,411.2	16,737.8	23,149.0

Note: All costs are in 1975 dollars, discounted at 6 percent.

Incidence. Probably the most critical component in estimating the economic costs of cancer is the calculation of incidence. The data source used—the Third National Cancer Survey (TNCS)—is unique because it is a statistical sample of approximately 10 percent of the national population. Consequently, the incidence rates resulting from the TNCS are considered accurate for 1970. Since we used these rates to estimate 1975 incidence rates and have not adjusted for possible secular changes, biases may result. More recent data from cancer registries and from the SEER data indicate that incidence rates have not changed significantly. While some rates, for example, lung cancer in women, have increased moderately, they have been offset by declines in others, such as stomach cancer, thus leaving the overall incidence rates for cancer fairly constant from 1970 to 1975.

The consequence of a possible error in overall incidence estimation would bias all the costs proportionately, since the costs per person are simply multiplied by the incidence to arrive at total costs. We feel that the maximum possible error in estimation of 1975 incidence rates is 3 percent, so if an error of this magnitude was actually present, then our cost estimates would err by the same 3 percent.

Mortality. We have relied exclusively on the End Results report (Axtell, Cutler, and Myers, 1972) for data on mortality. The possible errors in estimation of the relative survival rates were approximately 10 percent. While an underestimate in the relative survival rates for a specific cancer would lead to an underestimate of the life expectancy associated with that cancer, that error would not seriously bias overall cost estimates. If the life expectancy is underestimated, the direct costs will be underestimated (since the patient would generate treatment costs over a longer period than we used in the analysis), and correspondingly, forgone earnings will be overestimated (since the patient would have earned more than he is being assigned in the analysis). To check the effect of a 10 percent error in estimating the relative survival rates, the present-value costs and forgone earnings for a 60-year-old male local lung cancer patient were computed using different survival streams. The following table summarizes the results:

Relative Survival Rates	Direct Cost	Forgone Earnings	Total Cost
If 10% overestimate	$10,567	$34,196	$44,763
If correct as is	10,998	32,353	43,351
If 10% underestimate	11,428	30,517	41,945

From the table we can see, for example, that if we have underestimated the relative survival rates by 10 percent, the original direct-cost estimate should be increased by 4 percent, the estimate of forgone earnings decreased by 6 percent, and the estimate of total costs decreased by only 3 percent. Similarly, if we have overestimated the relative survival rates by 10 percent, the estimate of total costs should be increased by only 3 percent.

Direct Costs. We judge that estimates of *payments* made to hospitals and recorded by the TNCS are extremely reliable. However, these payments were adjusted by 20 percent to reflect costs more accurately. If this adjustment was incorrect, then we have overestimated total direct costs by 20 percent, but total costs (direct plus indirect) were then overestimated by only 6 percent. A number of other assumptions were made that could impart errors to our costs estimates. First, it was necessary to estimate from data in the TNCS's personal interview booklets relative proportions that were then applied against the hospital data to estimate the other cost elements (physician, nursing home, and the like). We judge that these proportions could be off by up to 10 percent. However, this would result in, at most, a 5 percent error in total direct costs, since hospital costs represent approximately half of all such costs. Second, it was necessary to estimate cost flows over the lifetime of a patient from the 2-year cost information collected by the TNCS. We had to estimate the costs generated in the incident year and in subsequent years. Our methodology for doing this resulted in unique first- and second-year costs (which summed to the 2-year cost total estimated by the TNCS) and constant cost flows after 2 years. Errors could exist in our estimation of the magnitudes of either the first-, second-, or third- and subsequent-year costs.

We analyzed the problem as follows. First, we judged that the maximum possible error in any one of these cost components was approximately 20 percent. Then, as a test example, we ran a series of one-variable sensitivity analyses on the total direct cost of respiratory system cancers where we varied first-year costs, second-year costs, and third- and subsequent-year costs by 20 percent. In addition, we also performed a sensitivity analysis in which second- as well as third- and subsequent-year costs were varied simultaneously at the 20 percent level. The results are persented below:

Cost Components Varied	Percentage of Variation from Original Values (in 000,000)				
	−20%	−10%	0%	+10%	+20%
First-year costs	706	767	828	887	948
Second-year costs	815	821	828	833	839
Third- and subsequent year costs	794	811	828	844	860
Second-, third-, and subsequent-year costs	783	805	828	850	873

Notice that the maximum possible error in total direct costs is 15 percent when first-year costs are increased by 20 percent without adjusting second-, third-, or subsequent-year cost estimates. Since we feel that first-year costs could err by at most 5 percent, the actual error in total costs would be only about 3 percent. The most likely source of a 20 percent error was in the estimate of third- and subsequent-year costs, owing to the admittedly arbitrary nature of the algorithm used to estimate those costs (see section on Direct Costs). The resulting change in direct costs in that eventuality would be approximately 4 percent. If we also had erred by as much as 20 percent in the second-year costs along with the third- and subsequent-year costs— because the TNCS data may not have been as representative of the second year past diagnosis as it was of the first year—the composite error in total direct costs would be only 5 percent.

Two special sensitivities were performed on respiratory system direct costs that we feel are especially enlightening. For the extremely hypothetical case where patient costs are thought to be generated only during the first year past diagnosis (in other words, second- and subsequent-year costs are zero), we found that total direct costs would be reduced by 27 percent. This means that first-year costs account for 73 percent of our correct total—a formidable proportion. Second, if we were to assume that costs are generated in the first and second years past diagnosis but end thereafter (essentially, third- and subsequent-year costs set to zero), total direct costs would be reduced by 20 percent. This indicates that second-year costs contribute 7 percent (27 percent minus 20 percent) and third- and subsequent-year costs contribute 20 percent to our current estimate of total direct costs of respiratory cancers.

Discounting. The choice of discount rate affects the present valuation of all future costs. Table 5–23 displays the effects of discounting of the direct costs of the respiratory cancers at 2 and 10 percent—as well as at the 6 percent figure used in our original analysis. The table shows that the greatest

Table 5–23
Sensitivity to the Discount Rate of Total Direct Costs
for Respiratory Cancers, by Age and Sex
(Thousands of Dollars)

Age	2 Percent	6 Percent	10 Percent
Males			
0–14	732	622	583
15–24	1,763	1,341	1,180
25–34	3,994	3,359	3,085
35–44	29,079	24,769	22,692
45–54	126,225	111,007	102,742
55–64	236,335	217,206	205,396
65–74	198,018	189,270	183,192
75+	86,365	84,290	82,693
Total males	682,511	631,866	601,563
Females			
0–14	1,348	849	688
15–24	810	702	661
25–34	2,689	2,168	1,958
35–44	11,223	9,568	8,816
45–54	39,386	34,824	32,470
55–64	51,939	47,394	44,736
65–74	35,798	34,091	32,947
75+	31,042	30,246	29,640
Total females	174,234	159,843	151,916
Total population	856,745	791,709	753,479

Note: All costs are in 1975 dollars.

proportional changes brought about by varying the discount rate occur for the youngest age groups, whose future costs will, on average, be discounted over the greatest number of years. The greatest absolute changes occur for persons with respiratory cancers at ages between 45 and 64. The totals indicate that discounting at a rate of 2 percent would have increased the costs of respiratory system cancer by $65 million, or 8 percent. Discounting at 10 percent would have decreased the estimated costs by 5 percent.

The same type of sensitivity analysis has been performed for all direct costs. Table 5–24 presents these results. Note that direct costs increase by about 16 percent when a 2 percent discount rate is used and decrease by 10 percent when a discount rate of 10 percent is used.

For indirect costs, the effect of a choice of discount rate is more important because these costs are more sensitive to the rate. This can be seen in table 5–25, where indirect costs increase by 47 percent when a discount rate of 2 percent is used and decrease by 24 percent when the discount rate is 10 percent.

Indirect Costs. Our original calculation of indirect costs presumed a discount rate of 6 percent, annual productivity growth of 1 percent, and market valuation of household labor. Table 5–26 displays the results of altering these suppositions: of discounting at 2, 6, and 10 percent; of taking productivity growth to be 0, 1, and 2 percent; and of using the opportunity-cost value of household labor. We see in the table that the indirect costs of cancer can be estimated as low as $11.98 billion and as high as $35.52 billion—depending on the analytic assumptions underlying those calculations. The difference between the two figures is large ($23.54 billion), and

Table 5–24
Total Direct Costs for Cancers in the Nine Diagnostic Categories, Discounted at 2, 6, and 10 percent
(Millions of Dollars)

	2 Percent	6 Percent	10 Percent
Digestive system	1595	1441	1354
Respiratory system	896	828	788
Buccal cavity	349	287	253
Reproductive system	2680	2237	1957
Urinary system	505	422	375
Nervous system	183	142	125
Leukemia	233	216	205
Lymphomas	398	346	315
Others	564	492	431
All cancers	7428	6411	5803

Note: All costs are in 1975 dollars.

Table 5-25
Total Indirect Costs for Cancers in the Nine Diagnostic Categories,
Discounted at 2, 6, and 10 percent.
(Millions of Dollars)

	2 Percent	6 Percent	10 Percent
Digestive	4770	3569	2866
Respiratory	4927	3760	3048
Buccal	838	593	457
Reproductive system	5590	3711	2736
Urinary system	1139	781	599
Nervous system	1259	917	725
Leukemia	1850	944	605
Lymphomas	2334	1383	959
Other sites	1818	1079	750
All cancers	24,525	16,737	12,745

Note: All costs are in 1975 dollars.

while we have in all cases sought to make the most reasonable and defensible assumptions, alternative choices could have led to quite different results.

Indirect costs are also significantly affected by data on the decrease in work capacity by cancer survivors. Recall that although we deduced that the average cancer patient would not work for approximately 20 weeks during the first year past diagnosis and that a significant proportion of cancer patients would not survive to and be working at the beginning of the second year, we also assumed that a survivor who did return to work (or house-keeping tasks) would perform on the job at his prediagnosis level of efficiency. This latter assumption is open to criticism. The effect on indirect costs of changing this assumption can be seen below for the case of a 60-year-

Table 5-26
Sensitivity of Total Indirect Costs of Cancer to the Discount Rate,
Productivity Growth Factor, and Mode of Valuing Household Labor
(Billions of Dollars)

			Rate of Productivity Growth		
			0 Percent	1 Percent	2 Percent
Market-value	Discount rate	2%	21.93	24.53	27.71
approach		6%	15.44	16.73	18.25
		10%	11.98	12.76	13.63
Opportunity-cost	Discount rate	2%	27.93	31.33	35.52
approach		6%	19.48	21.16	23.10
		10%	15.04	16.01	17.14

Note: All costs are in 1975 dollars.

old male localized lung cancer patient. His forgone earnings are computed for three levels of "on-the-job" efficiency upon returning to work: 90, 80, and 50 percent of his prediagnosis level of efficiency.

Relative Efficiency upon Return to Work	Forgone Earnings
100% (original assumption	$32,353
90%	34,338
80%	36,323
50%	42,276

Note that an on-the-job efficiency rate of 50 percent—half that implied in our original assumption—results in an increase in estimated forgone earnings of roughly 30 percent. We judge, however, that a more reasonable possibility might be 90 percent, or perhaps 80 percent at the extreme. In this case, the increase in forgone earnings is no more than 12 percent.

A sensitivity analysis also was performed on the assumption of length of work loss during the first year. Recall that this time varied for the various cancers. We again considered the case of the 60-year-old male localized lung cancer patient. We estimated that he had a loss of 19.9 weeks during the first year. We then consider the two extreme cases: this patient experiences no time off from work, and alternatively, he is out of work for a full year. The results are given below:

Weeks Out of Work First Year	Forgone Earnings
None	$29,021
19.9	32,353
52	36,390

As can be seen, forgone earnings vary from 11 to 12.5 percent of their original value.

Conclusions from the Sensitivity Analysis

We infer from our sensitivity analyses that with the exception of the basic analytical assumptions concerning discount and productivity rates, the most important sources of possible imprecision in our analysis are the assumptions concerning the generation of annual direct-cost components from the TNCS data, the information used to estimate work capacity and return-to-work rates for cancer patients, and the incidence estimates themselves. We have shown that errors in direct costs of up to 5 percent are possible if our assumptions regarding the magnitude and distribution of those costs (as based on the TNCS data) are incorrect. Potential errors in forgone earnings of 12 to 13 percent are possible if the data on return-to-work rates in the first and second years and our assumption regarding patients' work capacity are not exact. In addition, because age-specific incidence rates are not adjusted for possible secular changes between 1970 to 1975, a 3 percent error in both direct and indirect costs is possible.

To refine the analysis reported here it would be important to collect both direct-cost data (including nonhospital data) and work-rate data for at least 3 years past diagnosis (compared with the 2-year period used in the TNCS). Better data on nonhospital costs plus information that provides a more precise picture of how these costs and hospital costs are distributed over the several years past diagnosis would eliminate the need for the "analytical gymnastics" used to estimate annual cost components in this study.

Incidence data disaggregated by stage are critically important in an incidence and economic cost study. As we showed in the mortality section, the stage of the cancer is perhaps a more important predictor of the patient's prognosis, and therefore his costs, than even the cancer site. Proper cost estimation, then, requires incidence data accurately disaggregated by age, sex, cancer site, and *stage*. The SEER Program is continuing to update the incidence data on the TNCS; we would hope that more accurate staging data is also being collected.

In summary, our estimate of $23.1 billion as the total annual cost of cancer in 1975 must be interpreted in light of the possible errors brought out in the sensitivity analysis. In any event, it can be safely concluded that the incidence-based cost of cancer significantly exceeds the cost of all the other conditions considered in this study.

Notes

1. Sidney J. Cutler, Joseph Scotto, Susan S. Devesco, and Roger R. Connelly, Third national cancer survey—An overview of available information, *Journal of the National Cancer Institute* 53(6):1565–1575, 1974.

2. Ibid.

3. Ibid.

4. Howard Birnbaum, *The Cost of Catastrophic Illness* (Lexington, Mass.: Lexington Books, D.C. Heath and Co., 1978), p. 19.

5. Saul A. Rosenberg, Oncology, in Edward Rubenstein and Daniel Federman (eds.), *Scientific American Medicine* (Scientific American, 1979), chap. 12, pp. I-3–4.

6. Ibid., p. I-4.

7. Ibid., p. I-6.

8. Bernard Ferber, Vincent H. Handy, Paul R. Gerhardt, and Murray Solomon, *Cancer in New York State, Exclusive of New York City, 1941–1960* (Bureau of Cancer Control, New York State Department of Health, (1962).

9. Cutler et al., Third national cancer survey.

10. Sidney J. Cutler and John L. Young, eds., *Third National Cancer Survey: Incidence Data*, National Cancer Institute Monograph 41 (U.S. Department of Health, Education and Welfare, Public Health Service, National Institute of Health, Publication No. (NIH) 75-787, 1975), p. 2.

11. Abt Associates, Inc., and Boston University Cancer Research Center, *The Measurement of the Cost of Cancer. Task Two Report. Literature Review and Recommendations for Further Work* (Prepared for the National Cancer Institute, Division of Cancer Control and Rehabilitation, December 1976), p. 61.

12. Interview with Fred Vanderschmidt, Abt Associates, Inc., March 4, 1977.

13. *Current Population Reports: Population Estimates and Projections*, Series P-25, Number 614.

14. This figure reflects a slight underestimation of the number of new lung cancer cases in women.

15. Lillian M. Axtell and Max H. Myers, eds., *Recent Trends in Survival of Cancer Patients 1960–1971* (U.S. Department of Health, Education and Welfare Publication No. NIH 75-767, 1974).

16. Lillian M. Axtell, Sidney J. Cutler, and Max H. Myers, eds. *End Results in Cancer, Report No. 4.* (U.S. Department of Health, Education and Welfare, Public Health Service, National Institute of Health, National Cancer Institute, Publication No. NIH 73-272, 1972).

17. Ibid., p. 5

18. Ibid.

19. See table 5–3.

20. Ibid.

21. Abt Associates and Boston University, *The Measurement of the Cost of Cancer*, p. 48.

22. Joseph Scotto and Leonard Chiazze, Jr., *Third National Cancer Survey: Hospitalizations and Payments to Hospitals. Part A: Summary* (U.S. Department of Health, Education and Welfare Publication No. NIH 76-1094, March 1976).

23. Ibid., pp. 7–9.

24. Ibid., p. 14.

25. Interviews with Dr. Harry Miller, May 16, 1977, and Dr. Allen Korn, April 11, 1977.

26. Abt Associates and Boston University, *The Measurement of the Cost of Cancer*, pp. 56–73.

27. PIB data obtained from Abt Associates and Boston University, *The Measurement of the Cost of Cancer*, table 3.3, pp. 58–59.

28. Scotto and Chiazze, *Third National Cancer Survey*, p. 3; and interviews with Dr. Jerry Cromwell, May 4, 1977, and Dr. Fred Vanderschmidt, March 4, 1977.

29. U.S. Department of Commerce, *Statistical Abstracts of the United States, 1977*, 98th ed. (Washington: U.S. Government Printing Office, 1977), table 135, p. 94.

30. Interviews with Dr. Harry Miller, May 16, 1977; Dr. Allen Korn, April 11, 1977; and Dr. Ernest Weymuller, June 24, 1977.

31. We are grateful to John Young of the National Cancer Institute for making this unpublished data available to us.

32. David Zinman, The war on cancer: Are we winning it? *Newsday* (January 1977):4R.

6   Motor Vehicle Injuries

The motor vehicle is more than representative of our modern technology; it is an integral part of our culture. However, the motor vehicle, like most of our technological advances, is a mixed blessing. Long before attention was focused on motor vehicles in the contexts of energy consumption and environmental pollution, we had come to realize the tremendous economic costs associated with motor vehicle crashes. Although motor vehicles have been around for less than a century, motor vehicle fatalities far outnumber combat deaths suffered by the United States in all its wars. In addition, motor vehicle crashes cause countless injuries, many resulting in severe disability and extensive property damage.

Unlike most chronic diseases, which tend to strike people of middle age and older, motor vehicle crashes are the scourge of youth. According to our estimates, the total incidence of motor vehicle injuries and deaths in 1975 was approximately 4,270,000. More than half these individuals were under the age of 25. Young men between the ages of 15 and 24 experienced the highest incidence rates, suffering close to 25 percent of the total incidence of motor vehicle injuries and approximately 30 percent of the injuries that resulted in either death or severe disability.

Following the criteria of the Federal Highway Administration and the National Center for Health Statistics, a *fatal injury* (*fatality*) is defined as any injury or combination of injuries that results in death within 1 year of the crash.[1] This includes crashes in which the injured person is dead at the scene, dies en route to a hospital, dies during hospitalization, or dies following hospital discharge. We shall consider an injured person who survives at least 1 full year after the crash to have a *nonfatal injury* (*nonfatality*). This person must, moreover, either receive medical care or experience at least 1 full day of restricted activity because of his injury.

Our analysis shall be limited to those injuries suffered in crashes occurring on a public thoroughfare or initiated on a thoroughfare but ending off the road. We omit injuries that involve motor vehicles but do not occur on a public roadway (for example, the case of a person crushed under the weight of an automobile being repaired in a garage or an injury involving an off-the-road recreational or farm vehicle). The incidence of "nonthoroughfare" injuries is small and would be relatively unaffected by improvements in current motor vehicle or highway safety standards (although standards appropriate to recreational or farm vehicles—for example, which would require roll bars on all tractors—could reduce or otherwise affect the injuries they produce).

Throughout the analyses that follow, we examine nonfatalities and fatalities separately, since the incidence data for nonfatalities are considerably less exact than those for fatalities. Data on nonfatalities are usually restricted to statistical estimates based on limited and occasionally biased samples of the population. Data on fatalities, however, represent a virtual census of all occurrences. The overwhelming majority of all fatal motor vehicle injuries are recorded by local and state officials and reported directly to a central federal authority, the National Highway Traffic Safety Administration of the U.S. Department of Transportation. This does not hold for nonfatalities, many of which go unreported by local and state authorities. The problem is such that definitional idiosyncrasies among the reporting agencies have meant that certain cases that qualify as nonfatal injuries in one jurisdiction may not qualify as a reportable injury in another jurisdiction.

Incidence

Fatalities

Among the regional, national, and international studies of motor vehicle fatalities, those of the National Safety Council (1976), U.S. Federal Highway Administration (1975), OECD Road Research Group (1975), and the Metropolitan Life Insurance Company (1973) are representative examples. None, however, exhibits the quality or breadth of analysis found in the Fatal Accident Reporting System (FARS), a computerized data base maintained by the National Highway Traffic Safety Administration (NHTSA).[2] It contains information on fatalities who were occupants of motor vehicles, bicyclists or pedestrians struck by motor vehicles, motorcyclists, and miscellaneous others. Each of the fifty states, as well as the District of Columbia and Puerto Rico, supply fatal crash information to NHTSA. The data sources include police accident reports, medical examiners' records, driver's license files, motor vehicle registration files, and state highway department records.

By convention, FARS restricts its attention to fatalities occurring on public thoroughfares, conforming with our perspective. The FARS data, however, do not mesh perfectly with our incidence parameters. FARS defines a fatality as a death that occurs within 30 days of the crash; we, in contrast, define a fatality as one occurring within 1 year of the crash. According to staff experts at NHTSA, approximately 99 percent of the people who die within 1 year do so during the 30 days immediately following the crash.[3] To conform with our analysis, we have therefore adjusted the

FARS data by increasing each age- and sex-specific estimate of the number of fatalities by a factor of one ninety-ninth, or approximately 1 percent.

A breakdown of fatalities by age and sex based on the adjusted FARS data is presented in table 6–1. As the table indicates, approximately 44,995 individuals died in the United States in 1975 from crash-related injuries. Of this total, approximately 73.5 percent were motor vehicle occupants, 7 percent were motorcyclists, 19 percent were bicyclists or pedestrians struck by motor vehicles, and slightly fewer than 0.5 percent were miscellaneous others.[4] The fatalities occurred in 39,575 crashes, of which roughly 35 percent occurred in urban areas and 65 percent in rural areas.[5] This distribution between urban and rural crashes supports the commonly held belief that a negative correlation exists between crash severity and the population density of the crash site.

Regarding secular trends, the total for fatalities in 1975 represents a clear 15 to 20 percent reduction in the annual totals experienced prior to the countrywide reduction in 1974 of the highway speed limit. The total is representative of the number of fatalities in 1976 and 1977 (approximately 46,000 and 48,000, respectively), although less so of the totals for 1978 and 1979 (approximately 55,000 and 51,000, respectively.[6]

The data in table 6–1 reflect several epidemiological phenomena typical of motor vehicle fatalities:

1. Fatalities are more common among men than women, with approximately 73 percent of all fatalities being men. In fact, the likelihood of a motor-vehicle-related death among males over the age of 15 ranges from a factor of 1.6 to a factor of 3.8 greater than the corresponding likelihood for females of similar age.

2. Fatalities are disproportionately more predominant among the 15 to 24 age group of each sex than among other age groups. Thirty-seven percent of all male fatalities, 29 percent of all female fatalities, and 35 percent of all fatalities are people of this age. This differs from the proportion of 15- to 24-year olds in the 1975 general population, where only 20 percent of all males, 18 percent of all females, and 19 percent of all people were of this age. Whether this trend can be attributed primarily to reckless driving habits among younger people, to their overexposure during more dangerous driving periods, to their immaturity and limited experience, or to a tendency of younger people to drive smaller, less safe vehicles is debatable. What are not in doubt, however, are the societal consequences of this phenomenon. As we will show, the large number of youthful fatalities significantly inflates the forgone productivity losses and thus the total economic costs associated with motor vehicle deaths. Moreover, the inflated economic costs are only a small part of the enormous loss society suffers when thousands of otherwise healthy and vital young people die prematurely.

Table 6-1
Annual Incidence of Motor Vehicle Road Fatalities, by Age and Sex, United States, 1975

	Males			Females			Total Population		
Age Group	Incidence[a]	Percent of All Male Fatalities	Rate[b]	Incidence[a]	Percent of All Female Fatalities	Rate[b]	Incidence[a]	Percent of All Fatalities	Rate[b]
0–14	2,890	8.7	1.1	1,674	14.0	0.6	4,564	10.1	0.9
15–24	12,250	37.1	6.0	3,451	28.8	1.7	15,701	34.9	3.9
25–34	6,017	18.2	3.9	1,604	13.4	1.0	7,621	16.9	2.5
35–44	3,203	9.7	2.9	1,052	8.8	0.9	4,255	9.5	1.9
45–54	2,907	8.8	2.5	1,090	9.1	0.9	3,997	8.9	1.7
55–64	2,368	7.2	2.5	1,083	9.0	1.0	3,451	7.7	1.8
65–74	1,852	5.6	3.1	1,081	9.0	1.4	2,933	6.5	2.1
75+	1,539	4.7	4.9	934	7.8	1.7	2,473	5.5	2.9
Totals	33,026	100.0	3.2	11,969	100.0	1.1	44,995	100.0	2.1

Male fatalities as a percent of total: 73.4%
Female fatalities as a percent of total: 26.6%

[a]U.S. Department of Transportation, National Highway Traffic Safety Administration, *Fatal Accident Reporting System* (FARS). Data current as of May, 1980. (To ensure that the fatality estimates include those individuals dying after 30 days but within 1 year of the crash, the original FARS data have been increased by approximately 1 percent.)

[b]Incidence rate per 10,000. Derived from corresponding incidence data in this table and U.S. population estimates presented in U.S. Bureau of the Census, *Current Population Reports: Population Estimates and Projections*, Series P-25, Number 614, July 1975.

3. For each sex, the fatal incidence rates tend to peak for the 15 to 24 age group and then gradually decrease until age 65. At age 65, the incidence rates again increase. This increase may be explained by two possible factors. First, the rates may reflect the overrepresentation of the elderly, like the very young, among pedestrian crash injuries. On the average, a pedestrian struck by a motor vehicle faces more severe injury and thus a higher likelihood of death than does a motor vehicle occupant. Second, older people are less likely to survive injuries of all varieties, including those resulting from motor vehicle crashes.

Nonfatalities

Data Limitations. In contrast to fatalities, the analysis of nonfatal injuries is less straightforward—we have no single, comprehensive source of incidence data. The existing data are incomplete and none agree on the total of nonfatal injuries. We sought accuracy by pooling information from the competing sources to establish an incidence total for 1975. We break this total down by age and sex based on the reported injury experience of a representative subsample of the fifty states. Using the results of a recent field study of nonfatalities sponsored by NHTSA, the National Crash Severity Study (NCSS), we further disaggregate injury estimates by the severity level of the injury. The result is a distribution of nonfatalities in 1975 by injury-severity level, age, and sex.

Incidence of Nonfatalities. Four sources of information provide data on the total incidence of nonfatalities in 1975. The Federal Highway Administration (FHWA) reports approximately 2,810,000 injury cases, the National Safety Council (NSC) calculates 1,800,000 cases, the Insurance Information Institute of New York estimates 4,987,000 cases, and the National Center for Health Statistics' (NCHS) Health Interview Survey (HIS) estimates approximately 4,225,400 cases.[7] Variations in defining a nonfatal injury and differences in the accuracy of the data collection and sampling procedures contribute to this wide range of estimates for the same statistical parameter.

We feel that the first three data sources contain deficiencies in their methodologies and total incidence estimates. For instance, the estimate reported by the Federal Highway Administration is based exclusively on information gathered from police reports compiled by the individual states and reported to the Department of Transportation. In marked contrast to their accuracy in reporting fatalities, most states traditionally underreport nonfatal crash and injury figures. The FHWA figure, therefore, probably underestimates the actual nationwide total.

For similar reasons, the National Safety Council figure also includes only a subset of total nonfatal cases. The NSC estimate, like the FHWA estimate, is based on incomplete state reports and, moreover, reflects only those injuries that involve permanent impairment or render the person unable to perform regular duties or activities for a full day *beyond* the day of injury. Excluded from the group are those many cases where an injury occurs but results in restricted activity or medical attention only on the day of the crash.

The Insurance Information Institute estimate is debatable for two reasons. First, the injury figure is a projection based on figures submitted by fourteen nonrandom and seemingly nonrepresentative states. Furthermore, the institute assumes that all states in the sample use the same definition of a nonfatal injury—the NSC definition—although this assumption has never been confirmed.

The NCHS Health Interview Survey deserves special consideration. Unlike the other three sources, the NCHS estimate of motor-vehicle-related injuries is derived from a national probability sample (40,000 households containing 116,000 persons in 1975). This statistical procedure is methodologically superior to those employed by the three alternatives. In addition, the NCHS injury definition is more inclusive of minor injuries, for it defines an *injury* as one that is medically attended or causes at lease 1 full day of restricted activity. However, unlike the National Safety Council, NCHS does not require that the full day of restricted activity occur *past* the day of the crash. This recognizes that many injuries result in discomfort and inactivity only on the day of the crash.

The NCHS estimate is, however, imperfect. It is handicapped by an inadequate age and sex breakdown. It is also possible (although not probable) that the estimate includes as injury cases people who were alive at the time of the interview survey but who died within a year of the crash. This creates a potential problem of double counting, for these cases also would be included in our estimate of fatalities. However, according to time-to-death information from the Fatal Accident Reporting System, approximately 86 percent of all fatalities die within 24 hours of the crash, 90 percent die within 48 hours, and fully 97 percent succumb within 15 days.[8] Given this rapidity of death for fatalities, double counting, if it existed, would be insignificant.

These shortcomings of the NCHS survey notwithstanding, we concluded that its figure of 4,225,400 offered the most reasonable and complete estimate of total nonfatal cases. As we will see shortly, the choice of this particular figure over others affects the size of our subsequent estimates of incidence, disaggregated by age, sex, and injury-severity level. In this way, it strongly influences the estimates of total economic costs associated with nonfatal injuries.

Distribution by Age and Sex. Of the fifty states reporting nonfatal injury data in 1975 to the Federal Highway Administration and NHTSA, thirty-two had age and sex breakdowns sufficiently detailed for our analysis. Although virtually all states underrepresent the annual total of nonfatalities, there is little evidence that the age and sex distributions of those cases which are reported display any systematic biases. Furthermore, the thirty-two states supplying information are a representative sample of the country, especially in regard to geographic diversity and their urban/rural population ratios.

Data pooled from the thirty-two states yield a combined sample of approximately 1,883,000 nonfatally injured individuals identified by age and sex. This distribution is then applied against our estimate of total non-fatalities to yield a breakdown of total nonfatalities by age and sex (table 6–2).

Following the trend in fatalities, the majority of nonfatalities for 1975 are men. The overall male/female ratio, however, drops from approximately 3 to 1 in the case of fatalities to approximately 1.3 to 1 in the case of nonfatalities. The 15 to 24 age group again predominates, suffering over 38 percent of all nonfatal injuries with incidence rates 1.5 to 4 times greater than those of other age groups. We estimate that over 1.6 million nonfatal injury cases involve this age group. Broadening the estimate to include everyone under 35, people in the enlarged group account for approximately 3 million cases, or 70 percent of all nonfatal injuries, while representing only 58 percent of the total general population in 1975.

Distribution by Injury-Severity Level. The importance of disaggregating nonfatal injury totals by injury-severity level has been mentioned. The ideal disaggregation would use an injury scale based on cost criteria. Unfortunately, with the exception of some initial research done by Reinfurt et al. (1977) at the University of North Carolina, operational scales of this sort are rare. However, more conventional injury scales do exist, and some have already been tested in empirical studies dealing with trauma cases. Included in this group are the Abbreviated Injury Scale (AIS), the Comprehensive Injury Scale (CIS), the Injury Severity Score (ISS), and the International Classification of Diseases Adapted (ICDA) Code.[9] In addition, there are special injury scales developed by various organizations and a variety of scales and indices for specific trauma, such as burns, head injuries, or shock.

Compared with other scales, the Abbreviated Injury Scale is most useful. First published in 1971 by a joint committee of the American Medical Association, the Society of Automotive Engineers, and the American Association for Automotive Medicine, the AIS provides a consistent scale for collecting, categorizing, and analyzing injury-severity data. Since its introduction, the AIS has gained increasing acceptance in crash-investigation research. It has already been used by NHTSA in its two recent field studies of crash severity and crash-related injuries—the Restraint Systems Evaluation Program (RSEP) conducted during 1974 and 1975 and the National

Table 6–2
Annual Incidence of Motor Vehicle Road Nonfatalities, by Age and Sex, United States, 1975

Age Group	Males			Females			Total Population		
	Incidence[a]	Percent of All Males	Rate[b]	Incidence[a]	Percent of All Females	Rate[b]	Incidence[a]	Percent of All Nonfatalities	Rate[b]
0–14	272,630	11.4	99.6	226,231	12.3	86.1	498,861	11.8	93.0
15–24	985,184	41.3	484.0	654,376	35.5	328.6	1,639,560	38.8	407.1
25–34	486,634	20.4	316.9	341,005	18.5	218.9	827,639	19.6	267.5
35–44	226,397	9.5	203.0	195,097	10.6	167.2	421,494	10.0	184.7
45–54	182,786	7.7	159.1	178,332	9.7	145.2	361,118	8.5	151.9
55–64	125,352	5.3	134.1	130,801	7.1	125.3	256,153	6.0	129.5
65–74	71,494	3.0	118.6	75,349	4.1	96.0	146,843	3.5	105.8
75+	32,649	1.4	103.8	41,083	2.2	76.3	73,732	1.8	86.5
Totals	2,383,126	100.0	228.6	1,842,274	100.0	168.4	4,225,400[c]	100.0	197.8

Male Injuries as a percent of total: 56.4%
Female Injuries as a percent of total: 43.6%

[a]U.S. Department of Transportation, National Highway Safety Administration, National Center for Statistics and Analysis. Motor vehicle injury data reported by 32 states were used to derive age by sex breakdowns for motor vehicle nonfatalities.

[b]Incidence rate per 10,000. Derived from corresponding incidence data in this table and U.S. population estimates presented in U.S. Bureau of the Census, *Current Population Reports: Population Estimates and Projections*, Series P-25, Number 614, 1975.

[c]U.S. Department of Health, Education, and Welfare, National Center for Health Statistics. Current estimates from the health interview survey, United States, 1975. *Vital and Health Statistics* [10] 115, March, 1977.

Crash Severity Study (NCSS) conducted between 1977 and 1979—and is scheduled for use in the forthcoming National Accident Sampling System (NASS). In her analysis of the economic costs associated with motor vehicle injuries, Barbara Faigin (1976) also made exclusive use of this scale.

The AIS is essentially a "threat-to-life" injury scale (although other criteria such as energy dissipation, permanent impairment, and duration of treatment period were considered in its development). It consists of seven numerical codes and asociated injury-severity levels:

AIS Code	Severity Levels
0	No injury
1	Minor
2	Moderate
3	Serious
4	Severe
5	Critical
6	Maximum (currently untreatable and virtually always unsurvivable)

This provides crash investigators and medical personnel with a universal coding system that rates numerically different types of trauma occurring in different body regions.

A selection of various nonfatal injuries occurring in motor vehicle crashes is catalogued by AIS level in table 6–3. Although the examples in the table are restricted to individual injuries, the AIS system also may be used to assign a maximum AIS (MAIS) number. The MAIS number is the highest single AIS code for the person with multiple injuries, and in those cases where only one injury occurs, that AIS code is the MAIS. The MAIS number has special relevance in a motor vehicle setting, where most injured persons, even the less severely impaired, suffer more than one injury. The MAIS coding system has been used in this analysis to classify nonfatalities by injury-severity level.

To implement the MAIS system in our analysis, we used unpublished data from the recent National Crash Severity Study (NCSS). The NCSS provides the best currently available data base on the statistical inter-relationships between crash conditions and occupant injury severity, focusing on passenger vehicles involved in tow-away crashes. (Passenger vehicles include passenger cars, light trucks, vans, and multipurpose vehicles, such as jeeps.) Data from the NCSS constitute a "purposive" sample of passenger vehicle tow-away crashes occurring in seven geographic areas of the United States.[10] By *purposive* we mean that the NCSS areas were predetermined rather than random. The areas, however, comprise a variety of geographic locales (at least one NCSS area was located in each of the nation's four demographic regions) and collectively display a distribution of central-city,

Table 6–3
Representative Nonfatal Motor Vehicle Injuries by
Abbreviated Injury Scale (AIS) Level

AIS Code[a]	Injury-Severity Level	Representative Injuries
0	No injury	—
1	Minor injury	Superficial abrasion or laceration of skin; digit sprain; first-degree burn; head trauma with headache or dizziness (no other neurological signs).
2	Moderate injury	Major abrasion or laceration of skin; cerebral concussion (unconscious less than 15 minutes); finger or toe crush/amputation; closed pelvic fracture with or without dislocation.
3	Serious injury	Major nerve laceration; multiple rib fracture (but without flail chest); abdominal organ contusion; hand, foot, or arm crush/amputation.
4	Severe injury	Spleen rupture; leg crush; chest-wall perforation; cerebral concussion with other neurological signs (unconscious less than 24 hours).
5	Critical injury	Spinal cord injury (with cord transection); extensive/deep laceration of kidney or liver; extensive second- or third-degree burns; cerebral concussion with severe neurological signs (unconscious more than 24 hours).
6	Maximum (currently untreatable, immediately fatal)	Decapitation; torso transection; massively crushed chest.

Source: Information presented in *The Abbreviated Injury Scale (AIS)*, the American Association for Automotive Medicine, 1980 revision.

[a]In this analysis, motor vehicle injuries coded AIS 1 through AIS 5 include only persons with nonfatal injuries who survive at least 1 full year following the crash. In coding individuals with multiple injuries use has been made of the maximum AIS (MAIS).

suburban, small-town, and rural populations that closely resembles that of the nation. This is important because crash severity has a high negative correlation with population density, thereby making the urban/rural mix of the NCSS areas a critical factor in evaluating the study's representativeness. Moreover, although the areas themselves were not selected by a probability-sampling procedure, crashes and motor vehicle occupants within each area were chosen by strict adherence to a stratified probability-sampling scheme.

The May 1980 NCSS file, from which data for the incidence analysis are drawn, contains a weighted sample of 111,563 occupants of towed passenger vehicles. Of this number, 39,243 suffered nonfatal injuries, and within the nonfatal sample, 23,900 were identified by MAIS level (and by age and sex).

Although it was not possible to identify the MAIS level of the remaining 15,343 injuried occupants, NCSS investigators felt that most of these individuals, like occupants in the identified group, sustained MAIS 1 injuries. The distribution of the identified group by MAIS level and sex is presented in table 6–4.

Although more damage and destruction is associated with towaway crashes than with non-tow-away crashes, about 90 percent of the injured cases in the preceding sample were minor or moderate (MAIS 1 or 2 injuries), and only 2.8 percent of the sample suffered injuries that were life-threatening (MAIS 4 or 5 injuries). Despite the small percentage of MAIS 4 and 5 injuries recorded in the NCSS sample, one can still argue that vehicular occupants in tow-away crashes suffer a greater proportion of severe, life-threatening injuries than their counterparts in non-tow-away crashes. Therefore, as an indicator of injuries suffered by *occupants* in *all* crashes, the NCSS figures may be biased in the direction of greater severity. This does not necessarily invalidate their use when we think in terms of *all* motor-vehicle-related nonfatalities, for the NCSS surveyed only vehicular occupants and overlooked injuries to nonoccupants (for example, pedestrians, bicyclists, motorcyclists). The average nonoccupant, relatively unprotected, has a higher likelihood of serious injury even when compared with an occupant in a tow-away crash. As a result, the bias toward greater severity introduced by tow-away crashes is partially counterbalanced by the exclusion of nonoccupants from the sample.

To what degree the biases offset each other depends on a number of factors about which we have little or no empirical information. What is suggested, however, is that we can rank the nonfatally injured by increasing overall severity if we consider the source of their injury. The rank ordering is (1) occupants injured in non-tow-away crashes, (2) occupants injured in tow-away crashes, and (3) injured nonoccupants. Based on this assumption, we

Table 6–4
MAIS Level Distribution of Identified Nonfatal Injuries in NCSS May 1980 File

	Number Injured			Percent of Total Injured		
MAIS Level	Male	Female	Both Sexes	Male	Female	Both Sexes
1	8,679	8,553	17,232	70.6%	73.7%	72.1%
2	2,082	1,943	4,025	16.9	16.7	16.8
3	1,105	889	1,994	9.0	7.7	8.3
4	317	175	492	2.6	1.5	2.1
5	109	48	157	0.9	0.4	0.7
Total nonfatal	12,292	11,608	23,900	100.0	100.0	100.0

have taken the injury distribution by MAIS level of tow-away occupants from the NCSS sample as a first-order estimate of the corresponding distribution for all nonfatalities in 1975. Percentage breakdowns by MAIS level and sex have been developed for nonfatalities in seven age groups: 0 to 14, 15 to 24, 25 to 34, 35 to 44, 45 to 54, 55 to 64, and 65 years of age and older. These have been combined in table 6–5 with the estimates of the number of nonfatalities by age and sex presented in table 6–2 to yield an overall breakdown by MAIS level, age, and sex. The minor or moderate injuries, MAIS 1 or MAIS 2, account for the preponderance of injury cases: approximately 3,053,035 MAIS 1 injuries (72.3 percent of the total) and 702,923 MAIS 2 injuries (16.6 percent of the total). In contrast, there are only an estimated 87,262 MAIS 4 and 28,611 MAIS 5 injuries who survive the first year. This means that less than 2.8 percent of the nonfatalities in 1975 suffered severe or critical injuries.

Spinal Cord Injuries. Within the category of MAIS 5 injuries, spinal cord injuries (SCI) stand out as being both devastating to the patient and costly to society (Smart and Sanders, 1976). A spinal cord injury is presently an irreversible injury characterized by an acute, traumatic lesion of the spinal cord that results in varying degrees of paralysis and/or sensory loss below the level of the lesion. Its other ramifications include extensive medical and rehabilitative treatment immediately following the injury, follow-on care for the remainder of the individual's life, and increased physical and emotional dependency that may threaten the patient's career, marriage, family, and social relationships.

The cost estimates in Smart and Sanders and others are significantly more precise than those of other injury subtypes in the MAIS 5 category. The costs associated with diagnostic subcategories of spinal cord injury provide a reasonable basis for estimating the corresponding costs associated with the remainder of MAIS 5 injuries. We thus analyze spinal cord injuries as a separate class within the general MAIS 5 grouping.

Following the example of Smart and Sanders and others, we subdivide spinal cord injuries into four impairment subcategories: quadriplegic–complete lesion (quad complete), quadriplegic–incomplete lesion (quad incomplete), paraplegic–complete lesion (para complete), and paraplegic–incomplete lesion (para incomplete). This partition of the SCI population separates patients according to the two major levels of injury, quadriplegic (injury to the cervical or upper portion of the spinal cord) and paraplegic (injury to the thoracic/lumbar or lower portion of the spinal cord), and the two major extents of injury, complete lesion (complete physiological transection of the cord) and incomplete lesion (incomplete or partial physiological transection of the cord).

Smart and Sanders developed incidence rates by age, sex, and

Table 6–5
Annual Incidence of Motor Vehicle Road Nonfatalities, by Maximum Abbreviated Injury Scale (MAIS) Level, Age, and Sex, United States, 1975

Sex/Age	MAIS 1		MAIS 2		MAIS 3		MAIS 4		MAIS 5		Total Nonfatalities	
	Incidence	Rate[a]	Incidence	Rate[a]	Incidence	Rate[a]	Incidence	Rate[a]	Incidence	Rate[a]	Incidence	Rate[a]
Males												
0–14	213,442	78.0	33,670	12.3	20,338	7.4	2,590	0.9	2,590	0.9	272,630	99.6
15–24	695,244	341.5	171,422	84.2	82,460	40.5	25,812	12.7	10,246	5.0	985,184	484.0
25–34	348,562	227.0	80,789	52.6	40,054	26.1	15,039	9.8	2,190	1.4	486,634	316.9
35–44	158,365	142.0	34,435	30.9	25,107	22.5	6,067	5.4	2,422	2.2	226,397	203.0
45–54	126,081	109.7	32,758	28.5	18,390	16.0	4,223	3.7	1,334	1.2	182,786	159.1
55–64	84,237	90.1	22,024	23.6	14,503	15.5	3,121	3.3	1,467	1.6	125,352	134.1
65–74	46,104	76.5	14,915	24.7	8,259	13.7	1,601	2.7	615	1.0	71,494	118.6
75+	21,055	66.9	6,811	21.7	3,771	12.0	731	2.3	281	0.9	32,649	103.8
Subtotal	1,693,091	162.4	396,824	38.1	212,882	20.4	59,184	5.7	21,145	2.0	2,383,126	228.6
Females												
0–14	187,003	71.1	27,148	10.3	8,212	3.1	3,190	1.2	679	0.3	226,231	86.1
15–24	488,508	245.3	114,832	57.7	39,520	19.8	8,440	4.2	3,076	1.5	654,376	328.6
25–34	262,234	168.3	51,321	32.9	20,801	13.4	5,217	3.3	1,432	0.9	341,005	218.9
35–44	139,748	119.7	33,147	28.4	18,242	15.6	2,848	2.4	1,112	1.0	195,097	167.2
45–54	123,585	100.6	35,238	28.7	15,354	12.5	3,620	2.9	535	0.4	178,332	145.2
55–64	89,664	85.9	21,922	21.0	16,939	16.2	1,818	1.7	458	0.4	130,801	125.3
65–74	44,784	57.1	14,555	18.6	13,991	17.8	1,906	2.4	113	0.1	75,349	96.0
75+	24,418	45.4	7,936	14.7	7,628	14.2	1,039	1.9	62	0.1	41,083	76.3
Subtotal	1,359,944	124.3	306,099	28.0	140,687	12.9	28,078	2.6	7,466	1.0	1,842,274	168.4
Total	3,053,035	142.9	702,923	32.9	353,569	16.6	87,262	4.1	28,611	1.3	4,225,400	197.8

Source: Data presented in table 6–2 and unpublised data on MAIS levels obtained from the *National Crash Severity Study*, National Highway Traffic Safety Administration. U.S. Department of Transportation (data as current as of May 1980).
[a]Incidence rate per 10,000.

impairment subcategory for nonfatal, permanently impaired SCI suffered in motor vehicle crashes in 1974. We combine these rates with U.S. population estimates by age and sex for 1975 to establish the incidence of nonfatal SCI in crashes during 1975 (table 6–6). Nonfatal SCI cases total approximately 2700, or slightly less than 10 percent of all MAIS 5 cases in 1975. As in the general category of MAIS 5 injuries, males predominate over females. The 15 to 24 age group again dominates, accounting for 47 percent of all SCI cases—the same proportion, as for all MAIS 5 cases.

Mortality and Life Expectancy

Approaches to the Data

For most trauma victims, the increased risk of death is short-term and normally manifests itself only during the first few days, weeks, or months following the injury. Since all nonfatalities in our study, by definition, survive at least 1 year after the crash, it is reasonable to assume that cases in the three least severe injury subcategories (MAIS 1, 2, and 3) *do not* experience any significant increase in their risk of death relative to their uninjured peers in the general population. This assumption simplifies the mortality analysis, for over 97 percent of the nonfatalities in the 1975 incidence group fall into these three categories.

Determining if the more severely injured nonfatalities, the MAIS 4 and 5 cases, experience any sustained increase in their risk of death is complex and, at this time, not amenable to a purely rational deductive analysis. One approach that has substantial heuristic appeal is to construct a frequency distribution of injuries by anatomic site for each of the higher injury-severity groups. We could then combine this with data on the intermediate and long-term increases in the risk of death produced by traumas at these anatomic sites to project the increased relative mortality for cases within a particular severity group. We define the *relative mortality rate (RMR)* as the ratio of the actual mortality experience of individuals suffering a particular injury or class of injuries to the expected mortality of individuals of the same age (and normally, the same sex) in the general population.

This approach would require an averaging procedure in which the relative mortality rate for each type of injury would be weighted by the proportion of injuries of that type and the results summed over the different types of injuries within the severity group. This would yield an overall or average relative mortality rate applicable to the "average" cases within the severity group.

Although implementing this approach should be straightforward, several factors limit its applicability. First, the only data currently available to construct the required injury distributions would come from either the

Table 6–6

Annual Incidence of Nonfatal Motor-Vehicle-Related SCI, by Age, Sex, and Impairment Category, United States, 1975[a]

Sex/Age Category	Quad Complete	Quad Incomplete	Para Complete	Para Incomplete	Total SCI
Males					
0–14	5	8	14	14	41
15–24	132	206	313	287	938
25–34	75	117	101	94	387
35–44	41	64	52	48	205
45–54	46	70	39	36	191
55–64	40	61	19	17	137
65–74	15	24	10	9	58
75+	8	12	5	5	30
Subtotal	362	562	553	510	1987
Females					
0–14	8	13	26	24	71
15–24	36	56	121	112	325
25–34	8	12	47	44	111
35–44	4	7	29	26	66
45–54	10	16	20	17	63
55–64	13	20	6	6	45
65–74	2	5	6	5	18
75+	2	3	4	4	13
Subtotal	83	132	259	238	712
Total	445	694	812	748	2699

Source: C.N. Smart and C.R. Sanders, *The Costs of Motor Vehicle Related Spinal Cord Injuries* (Insurance Institute for Highway Safety, 1976), tables 5 and 6, pp. 26 and 29; and U.S. Bureau of the Census, *Current Population Reports: Population Estimates and Projections*, Series P-25, Number 614, 1975. U.S. population estimates for 1975 by age and sex.

[a]Incidence figures represent estimates of the number of permanently impaired SCI patients who survive their initial hospitalization period. This is a good approximation of the number of permanently impaired patients surviving 1 year or more past injury.

National Crash Severity Study (NCSS) or the Restraint Systems Evaluation Program (RSEP). Although the more recent NCSS data are more accurate than the RSEP information, these data have their limitations. For example, the data on injury location and severity are keyed primarily to the individual injury and not to the injury case. The listing of injuries suffered by nonfatal MAIS 5 cases thus includes all AIS 5 injuries but none of the less-severe injuries—for instance, AIS 3 or 4 injuries—that may have occurred to multiply injured MAIS 5 individuals. Although many of these other injuries may not, by themselves, be life-threatening, they may nevertheless increase an individual's risk of death when occurring in a multiple-injury setting (see Baker et al., 1974). Another factor to consider is that the data available on relative mortality rates for trauma victims are sparse, limited both in scope and in depth. This further constrains the implementation of the approach just described.

Our methodology to measure the increased risk of death for motor vehicle nonfatalities is, of necessity, ad hoc. Despite the problems with available NCSS and RSEP data, we develop frequency distributions of injuries by anatomic site based on those data. We assume that these distributions are indicative, although not entirely representative, of the actual frequency distributions 1 year after the crash. If one recognizes their innate limitations, the distributions provide valuable insights regarding the parts of the body most frequently injured in MAIS 4 and 5 cases and the impact of these injuries on mortality and life expectancy.

Distribution of AIS 4 and 5 Injuries by Anatomic Site

The operational problem with the NCSS data relative to the listing of multiple injuries has been discussed. Despite this difficulty, the sample sizes for AIS 4 and 5 injuries (occurring to MAIS 4 and MAIS 5 cases, respectively) surveyed in the NCSS are relatively large. For AIS 4, the sample size N is 1333 weighted injuries; for AIS 5, N is 418 weighted injuries.[11] This indicates that the general injury profile implied by these data may be more representative than expected.

The RSEP survey did not benefit from the large sample sizes observed in the NCSS effort. In fact, the sample sizes are quite small—for AIS 4, N is 50 injuries, and for AIS 5, N is 22 injuries.[12] This factor plus structural problems in the data base limits the representativeness of the RSEP data and recommends their use exclusively as a rough point of comparison with the NCSS results.

In figures 6–1 and 6–2, distributions of AIS 4 and 5 injuries disaggregated both by body region and by system or organ injured are presented for the NCSS sample; in figure 6–3, corresponding distributions disaggregated by body region alone are presented for the RSEP sample. (Lack of sufficient data prevented further disaggregation of the RSEP injuries by system or organ injured.) In the NCSS, head and face injuries account for 31 percent and abdominal injuries account for 16 percent of all AIS 4 injuries. The RSEP data tend to support this, showing that 28 percent of the AIS injuries are sustained in the head/face region but 32 percent occur in the abdominal area. Of the AIS 4 head/face injuries in the NCSS, fully 67 percent occur without concurrent injury to the brain or other parts of the nervous system. This is important, since information presented in the next section shows that patients with head injuries who experience little or no damage to the nervous system do not show increases in mortality rates or reductions in average life expectancy.

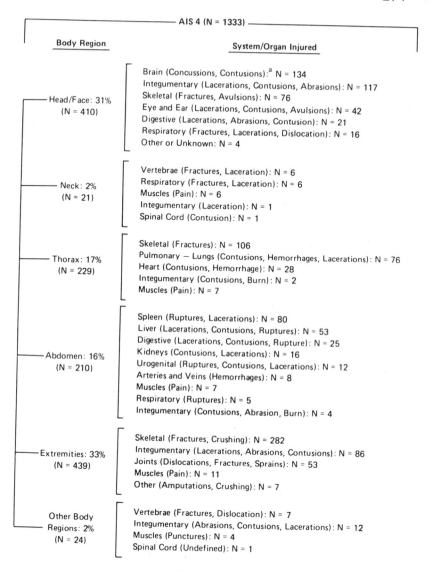

AIS 4 (N = 1333)

Body Region   **System/Organ Injured**

Head/Face: 31%
(N = 410)
- Brain (Concussions, Contusions):[a] N = 134
- Integumentary (Lacerations, Contusions, Abrasions): N = 117
- Skeletal (Fractures, Avulsions): N = 76
- Eye and Ear (Lacerations, Contusions, Avulsions): N = 42
- Digestive (Lacerations, Abrasions, Contusion): N = 21
- Respiratory (Fractures, Lacerations, Dislocation): N = 16
- Other or Unknown: N = 4

Neck: 2%
(N = 21)
- Vertebrae (Fractures, Laceration): N = 6
- Respiratory (Fractures, Laceration): N = 6
- Muscles (Pain): N = 6
- Integumentary (Laceration): N = 1
- Spinal Cord (Contusion): N = 1

Thorax: 17%
(N = 229)
- Skeletal (Fractures): N = 106
- Pulmonary — Lungs (Contusions, Hemorrhages, Lacerations): N = 76
- Heart (Contusions, Hemorrhage): N = 28
- Integumentary (Contusions, Burn): N = 2
- Muscles (Pain): N = 7

Abdomen: 16%
(N = 210)
- Spleen (Ruptures, Lacerations): N = 80
- Liver (Lacerations, Contusions, Ruptures): N = 53
- Digestive (Lacerations, Contusions, Rupture): N = 25
- Kidneys (Contusions, Lacerations): N = 16
- Urogenital (Ruptures, Contusions, Lacerations): N = 12
- Arteries and Veins (Hemorrhages): N = 8
- Muscles (Pain): N = 7
- Respiratory (Ruptures): N = 5
- Integumentary (Contusions, Abrasion, Burn): N = 4

Extremities: 33%
(N = 439)
- Skeletal (Fractures, Crushing): N = 282
- Integumentary (Lacerations, Abrasions, Contusions): N = 86
- Joints (Dislocations, Fractures, Sprains): N = 53
- Muscles (Pain): N = 11
- Other (Amputations, Crushing): N = 7

Other Body Regions: 2%
(N = 24)
- Vertebrae (Fractures, Dislocation): N = 7
- Integumentary (Abrasions, Contusions, Lacerations): N = 12
- Muscles (Punctures): N = 4
- Spinal Cord (Undefined): N = 1

Source: Data on injury location and severity were derived from the NCSS file of May 1980.
[a]Items in parentheses represent the types of injury lesions listed in order of frequency.

Figure 6–1. Frequency Distribution of AIS 4 Injuries by Body Region and System/Organ Injured, Based on NCSS Data

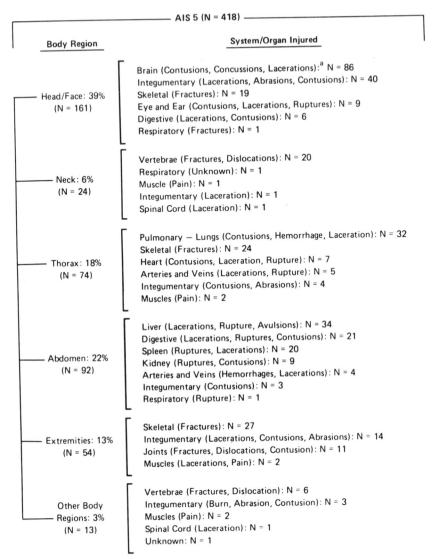

AIS 5 (N = 418)

| Body Region | System/Organ Injured |

Head/Face: 39% (N = 161)
- Brain (Contusions, Concussions, Lacerations):[a] N = 86
- Integumentary (Lacerations, Abrasions, Contusions): N = 40
- Skeletal (Fractures): N = 19
- Eye and Ear (Contusions, Lacerations, Ruptures): N = 9
- Digestive (Lacerations, Contusions): N = 6
- Respiratory (Fractures): N = 1

Neck: 6% (N = 24)
- Vertebrae (Fractures, Dislocations): N = 20
- Respiratory (Unknown): N = 1
- Muscle (Pain): N = 1
- Integumentary (Laceration): N = 1
- Spinal Cord (Laceration): N = 1

Thorax: 18% (N = 74)
- Pulmonary — Lungs (Contusions, Hemorrhage, Laceration): N = 32
- Skeletal (Fractures): N = 24
- Heart (Contusions, Laceration, Rupture): N = 7
- Arteries and Veins (Lacerations, Rupture): N = 5
- Integumentary (Contusions, Abrasions): N = 4
- Muscles (Pain): N = 2

Abdomen: 22% (N = 92)
- Liver (Lacerations, Rupture, Avulsions): N = 34
- Digestive (Lacerations, Ruptures, Contusions): N = 21
- Spleen (Ruptures, Lacerations): N = 20
- Kidney (Ruptures, Contusions): N = 9
- Arteries and Veins (Hemorrhages, Lacerations): N = 4
- Integumentary (Contusions): N = 3
- Respiratory (Rupture): N = 1

Extremities: 13% (N = 54)
- Skeletal (Fractures): N = 27
- Integumentary (Lacerations, Contusions, Abrasions): N = 14
- Joints (Fractures, Dislocations, Contusion): N = 11
- Muscles (Lacerations, Pain): N = 2

Other Body Regions: 3% (N = 13)
- Vertebrae (Fractures, Dislocation): N = 6
- Integumentary (Burn, Abrasion, Contusion): N = 3
- Muscles (Pain): N = 2
- Spinal Cord (Laceration): N = 1
- Unknown: N = 1

Source: Data on injury location and severity were derived from the NCSS file of May 1980.

[a]Items in parentheses represent the types of injury lesions listed in order of frequency.

Figure 6–2. Frequency Distribution of AIS 5 Injuries by Body Region and System/Organ Injured, Based on NCSS Data

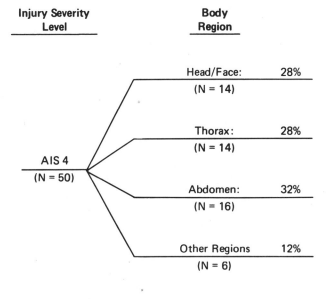

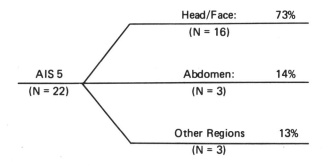

Source: Unpublished data on unweighted injuries in the RSEP study sample, National Highway Traffic Safety Administration, USDOT.

Figure 6–3. Frequency Distributions of AIS 4 and AIS 5 Injuries by Body Region, Based on RSEP Data

The NCSS data also indicate that a significant proportion of the AIS 4 injuries occur in the extremities (at least 33 percent) and in the thorax (at least 17 percent). Of these injuries, approximately 83 percent are either skeletal fractures, integumentary problems (that is, burns, lacerations, abrasions, or contusions affecting the body's skin), or other injuries that involve little or no disturbance to internal cardiovascular, circulatory, digestive, or nervous system organs. In fact, of the 1333 AIS 4 injuries, close to 65 percent represented trauma without any apparent damage to an internal organ.

The NCSS data on AIS 5 injuries indicate that a plurality of these injuries (39 percent) are to the head/face region, with more than half of those injuries involving damage to the brain. Compared with AIS 4 injuries in the NCSS sample, the proportion of all AIS 5 injuries that involve the brain is twice as great (21 versus 10 percent), and on average, these injuries are potentially far more harmful, since they include lacerations and other serious injuries to the brain itself. The proportion of AIS 5 injuries to the abdomen is larger than for AIS 4 injuries (22 versus 16 percent); the proportion of injuries to the thorax, approximately the same (18 and 17 percent, respectively); and the proportion to the extremities, far less (13 versus 33 percent). The RSEP data also show a plurality of the AIS 5 injuries in the head/face region, but in this case, the plurality turns out to be a staggering majority, approximately 73 percent of the total.

In general, the NCSS data show that while the AIS 4 injuries are characterized by serious skeletal fractures to the head, thorax, and extremities, together with integumentary problems and abdominal injuries, the AIS 5 injuries are primarily critical brain injuries together with ruptures and lacerations of the abdomen and thorax and their contents. The dramatic fact stands out that the majority of all AIS 5 head injuries have resulted in extensive nervous system/brain damage, in contrast to the AIS 4 head injuries, most of which have not; these injuries also comprise a significant proportion of all AIS 5 injuries. This does not bode well for the "average" MAIS 5 case compared with the "average" MAIS 4 case, for patients with head injuries involving substantial nervous system trauma are, as we shall see, subject to serious complications. They are at a greater risk of death both in the short and long run than their uninjured peers in the general population.

Mortality Rates for Different Injuries

Spinal Cord Injuries (SCI). In their analysis of survival data for motor-vehicle-related SCI, Smart and Sanders (1976) found that SCI patients as a group have higher mortality rates than individuals of similar age and sex in the general population: they are more susceptible to medical complications (for example, urinary tract infections and decubitus ulcers) that lead to infection and death.

Smart and Sanders summarized the changes in SCI mortality rates observed over the last 50 to 60 years and reviewed the major research efforts on SCI. They determined that the most important empirical research correlating the level and extent of spinal cord injury to patient mortality was performed by Jousse et al. (1968) using a sample of 965 patients in Toronto, Canada. All of the patients in this group had passed through a period of initial hospitalization and rehabilitation, and all suffered permanent neurological impairment. Geisler et al. (1977) updated and extended this research. For each of the four major impairment categories considered in the studies— paraplegic (complete and incomplete) and quadriplegic (complete and incomplete)—both Jousse and Geisler compared the actual mortality experience of the discharged SCI patients with the expected mortality of individuals of the same age in the Canadian general population. Geisler's updated results, based on a sample of 1501 patients, are documented in table 6–7.

The results in the third column of table 6–7 can be interpreted as the relative mortaity rates (RMR) for patients in each of the four impairment categories. On this basis, paraplegic incompletes have a mortality rate approximately twice as great as their peers in the general population, while quadriplegic completes suffer mortality rates that are almost a factor of 12 greater than normal. Although the RMR for an impairment group as a whole does not necessarily apply to every patient in that group, it is reasonable to assume that the rate does apply to the "average" patients within the group. For instance, one might assume that the annual mortality rate for an "average" incomplete quadriplegic of a certain age is roughly equivalent to the annual mortality rate for a person of the same age (and sex) in the general population multiplied by a factor of 2.23.

Table 6–7
Mortality Rates of Spinal Cord Injury (SCI) Patients Following Hospital Discharge Compared with Rates of the General Population

SCI Impairment Category	Patient Sample (N = 1501)	SCI Mortality Rate Divided by General Population Rate
Para incomplete	450	1.81
Quad incomplete	353	2.23
Para complete	484	4.64
Quad complete	214	11.63
All SCI	1501	4.22

Source: Data abstracted from W.O. Geisler, A.T. Jousse, and Megan Wynne-Jones, Survival in traumatic transverse myelitis, *Paraplegia* 14: 263 (Table I), 1977. Reprinted with permission.

Other Injuries. The literature on mortality rates for trauma victims is limited in both scope and depth. For AIS 4 and non-SCI AIS 5 injuries, useful information is available for five conditions:

1. Aortic aneurysm owing to aortic laceration or rupture
2. Hypertension resulting from renal injury (that is, trauma to the kidney)
3. Cerebral concussion or contusion or depressed skull fracture with neurological signs owing to serious head injuries
4. Resection of the spleen resulting from blunt abdominal trauma
5. Resection of the pancreas, liver, or gall bladder resulting from blunt abdominal trauma

Aortic Aneurysm. A chronic aortic aneurysm (a permanent abnormal dilation of the aorta) may result from an aortic injury. Bennett and Cherry (1967) report that the frequency of aneurysm formation following aortic ruptures is approximately 5 percent. To complicate matters, an aneurysm may remain asymptomatic and undetected for months or years and then may break at any time.

Although elective surgery to repair aneurysms has become relatively safe, the best survival information is available for a series of unoperated aneurysm patients. Data in Joyce (1964) indicates that the relative mortality rate for unoperated aneurysm patients over a 10-year period following injury is approximately 3.12. We expect that a relative mortality rate based on the unoperated patients' experience would be higher than that for a more heterogeneous group of patients including individuals who successfully underwent surgery. Moreover, this rate applies at most to the 5 percent of the population that actually develops an aneurysm after aortic injury; for the other 95 percent, we assume an RMR of 1.00. An upper bound for the overall RMR of people suffering and surviving an aortic laceration may thus be obtained by computing a weighted average. This RMR equals approximately 1.11 (that is, $0.95 \times 1.00 + 0.05 \times 3.12$), a value close to the expected mortality experience of the general population.

Hypertension from Renal Injury. A review article by Grant et al. (1971) summarizing several other sources presents data that indicate the rate of hypertension (elevated blood pressure) development following renal injury is about 11 percent. Grant also found that the average time interval between injury and discovery of hypertension is slightly less than 3 years. Furthermore, nephrectomy (removal of a damaged kidney) or partial nephrectomy lowers the blood pressure to normal levels in approximately 75 percent of the cases.

For simplicity, we assume that 11 percent of the renal injuries suffered by MAIS 4 and MAIS 5 cases become hypertensive upon injury, that these cases are operated on an average of 3 years following the injury, and that 75 percent of the operated cases become normal and thus have an RMR of 1.0 while 25 percent continue at the increased RMR of hypertensives. Kannel (1974) has reported the annual mortality experience by age and sex for normotensives and hypertensives participating in the Framingham Heart Study. His data suggest the following relative mortality rates for hypertensives:

Age Interval	Relative Mortality Rate (RMR)	
	Male	Female
35–44	5.31	3.92
45–54	2.16	2.05
55–64	2.10	1.05
65–74	2.05	2.38
All ages ≥ 35	2.17	1.99

For our disease paradigm, the preceding RMR values apply to only 11 percent of the renal-injured cases for an average of 3 years after injury, with the other 89 percent experiencing an RMR of 1.0. At the 3-year juncture, all members of the hypertensive group who receive appropriate follow-on treatment would have a nephrectomy or partial nephrectomy, which would return approximately 75 percent of the previously hypertensive cases to an RMR of 1.0. Under our assumptions, therefore, only 2 to 3 percent of all renal injury cases will experience any significant increase in their relative mortality rates 3 years or more after the injury, and for these cases, the relative mortality rates will lie, on average, between 1.99 and 2.17.

Serious Head Injuries. The most detailed follow-up study of serious head injuries was performed by Walker et al. (1971). Walker and his collegues examined a sample of male German war veterans who sustained head injuries in World War I and a control group of uninjured veterans. Members of the injured group had sustained both penetrating and nonpenetrating wounds. Although the war veterans incurred their injuries considerably earlier in the history of medicine than those currently injured in crashes and thus may have been at a disadvantage medically compared with their present-day counterparts, they presented a unique study opportunity. The German war veteran sample was one of the few head-injured groups that had been tracked over a sufficiently long enough period to indicate the long-term increase in the risk of death faced by patients with this general type of injury. In the World War I study, Walker provided survival rates from ages 35 to 85 for men in the German general population, all members of the head-injured veterans' sample, and those within the sample who both experienced nervous system/brain damage and developed posttrauma epilepsy. The survival rates for the head-injured sample were calculated under alternative assumptions: (1) that those not located during the follow-up survey were dead, and (2) that they were alive. Rates based on the former assumption are used here.

Studies of head-injured veterans of World War II and the Korean conflict also have been performed by Walker and various other researchers (Caveness et al., 1962; Walker et al., 1959; and Walker, 1957). Walker's 1957 study of a sample of World War II veterans is representative of this research. He found that during the 10-year period immediately following injury, the risk of death increased by a factor of 2 to 3 for those patients experiencing brain damage and posttrauma epilepsy.

Since our analysis focuses on head injuries suffered in motor vehicle crashes and most of these injuries are (unlike war wounds) non-missile-related, a relevant piece of research for our purposes is Jennett's 1975 study, *Epilepsy after Non-Missile Head Injuries*. Jennett examines the increased risk of death experienced by head injury patients and presents evidence that brain damage and ensuing posttrauma epilepsy are critical factors in determining whether the head injury will be fatal or not. He argues that patients experiencing early epilepsy—an initial epileptic seizure within 1 week of injury—are at a significantly higher risk of death than those who do not. Furthermore, patients with severe head injuries (that is, those involving brain damage) are at risk of epilepsy and its consequences for the remainder of their lives, with some individuals having initial seizures 30 to 40 years after the date of original injury.

Caveness et al. (1979) found a clear correlation between the severity of head injuries and the onset of epileptic seizures. One of their major conclusions is that the likelihood of seizures developing in an injured patient is determined by the location and extent of brain damage. Their incidence data for seizures following head injury are essentially the same as for individuals injured in World War I.

For our mortality analysis, we assume that members of Walker's World War I head-injured sample correspond to MAIS 4 patients and that those within the sample with substantive brain damage and posttrauma epilepsy (that is, those with more critical aftereffects) correspond approximately to MAIS 5 patients. To obtain rough estimates of the relative mortality rates for these two injured groups, we compute the conditional probability of surviving to age 60 given survival to age 35 for all German men and for members of the two groups. Subtracting these probabilities from 1 in each case yield conditional mortality rates for estimating the RMR for each group. The RMR is expressed algebraically as

$$RMR_{\text{Injured group}} = \left(\frac{1 - \text{conditional probability of survival, injured group}}{1 - \text{conditional probability of survival, general population}} \right)$$

For the entire head-injured sample, the computed RMR is slightly less than 1.0. This suggests that MAIS 4 head-injured patients, the vast majority of which have not experienced serious trauma to the nervous system, suffer little or no change in their probability of survival. The RMR for the epileptic subgroup, used in our analysis as surrogates for MAIS 5 head-injury patients, is approximately 1.35. This is only slightly higher than the expected mortality experience for the general population. However, this RMR value applies to epilepsy patients who received their injuries at an average age of 20 and had already survived to age 35. Clearly, patients of this sort who had already survived 15 years should have a lower RMR than similar patients who had been tracked immediately from time of injury or from a point in time only 1 year after injury. Despite the advances in the medical treatment of epilepsy that have occurred since the German sample was injured, we feel confident in arguing that the RMR for those individuals who were known to have survived 15 years past injury should serve as a *lower* bound for the expected RMR of today's head-injured patients who, to date, are known to have survived only 1 year after injury—our MAIS 5 head-injured nonfatalities.

Resection of Abdominal Organs. With one exception, resection (the surgical removal of part of an organ or structure) of selected abdominal organs as a result of blunt trauma has little or no negative impact on survival. At least two studies, Eraklis et al. (1967) and Haller and Jones (1966), show no increased tendency toward infection or death in children after removal of the spleen; the RMR for rupture of the spleen, predominantly an MAIS 4 injury, is tentatively assumed to be 1.00 based on this evidence. Quattlebaum (1953) indicates that removing even a relatively large section of the liver, as might be necessary after serious trauma, would not impair its function, and Donovan et al. (1972) states that after an operation for the most common pancreatic injury—rupture of the body of the pancreas—there is little or no persistent endocrine insufficiency. A RMR of 1.00 for these injuries thus seems reasonable.

Ironically, the one organ that seems to produce a limited increase in mortality following surgical removal is often considered insignificant—the gallbladder. A study reported in the *Statistical Bulletin of the Metropolitan Life Insurance Company* (1966) estimates that the expected mortality after gall bladder removal is approximately 35 percent above normal during the first 2 years following the operation. If the patient survives 5 years after surgery, however, his mortality rate reverts, more or less, to that for the general population. In addition, since the sample included patients with both disease-induced and injury-induced gallbladder conditions, it is difficult to determine if the short-term increase in mortality experienced by the whole sample would still manifest itself if the injury cases were analyzed alone.

When all the available evidence is considered, patients with injured gallbladders, especially those surviving 1 year or more past injury and operation, probably experience little change in their relative mortality rates. This makes them similar to the other abdominal injury cases described earlier. As a group, the abdominal cases seem to suffer little increased mortality despite the apparent severity of their injuries.

Relative Mortality Rates for MAIS 4 and 5 Injury Cases

Using the information on mortality rates summarized in table 6–8, we estimate an average relative mortality rate for cases in each of the two serious injury-severity groups. These estimates are judgmental, but make use of the relative mortality rates for each type of injury given in the table and the frequency distributions of injuries found in figures 6–1 through 6–3.

MAIS 4 Cases. Figure 6–1 indicates that roughly one-half of the AIS 4 injuries sampled in the NCSS are to the head/face and abdominal regions, while another third are to the extremities. The NCSS data also indicate that the AIS 4 head injuries were confined in most instances to trauma that did not involve significant nervous system damage. Based on Walker's (1971) analysis of head-injured World War I veterans and the more recent studies by Jennett (1975) and Caveness et al. (1979), it appears that head injuries relatively free of neurological complications produce little or no change in the expected mortality rates and life expectancies of the injured individuals. We assume, therefore, a relative mortality rate of 1.00 for people experiencing these "less serious" head injuries. Likewise, injuries to the abdomen, even those requiring surgery, usually do not place the victim at any greater risk of death in the long run. Because of the predominance among injuries to the extremities of skeletal fractures and integumentary problems not involving burns, those injuries are also assumed not to be life-threatening on a long-term basis. Both these classes of injuries, like head injuries, are thought to have an RMR of 1.00.

A good argument can be made that 80 percent of the AIS 4 injuries should produce relative mortality rates of approximately 1.00. (Mortality information on the remaining 20 percent was either not available or inconclusive.) However, all nonfatalities analyzed in our present study are assumed to have survived at least 1 year past injury. Therefore, virtually all cases with AIS 4 injuries have successfully passed through the most critical periods following their injuries. For this reason, and from the existing evidence, we conclude that it is reasonable to assign a relative mortality rate of 1.00 to all AIS 4 injuries and MAIS 4 cases. We feel that any error in the RMR value is small and compatible with our general analysis.

Table 6–8
Relative Mortality Rates Associated with Trauma at Selected Anatomic Sites

Anatomic Site/Condition	Estimated Relative Mortality Rate
I. Spinal cord injuries	
Paraplegic incomplete	1.81
Quadriplegic incomplete	2.23
Paraplegic complete	4.64
Quadriplegic complete	11.63
II. Head injuries	
Few (if any) neurological complications	1.00
Posttrauma epilepsy	≥1.35
III. Renal (kidney) damage	
No hypertension	1.00
Hypertensive complications	2.11
IV. Blunt trauma and resection of abdominal organs	
Spleen	1.00
Pancreas	1.00
Liver	1.00
Gallbladder	1.00 to 1.35
V. Trauma to cardiovascular system[a]	
Aortic rupture, no aneurysm	1.00
Aortic aneurysm	3.2

Source: Information in text.

[a]This table deals with survivors only. The percentage of all aortic ruptures that are not fatal is quite small.

MAIS 5 Cases. For MAIS 5 cases, it is easier to estimate relative mortality rates for the SCI patients than to develop a RMR for the remaining non-SCI cases. Geisler et al. indicate relative mortality rates ranging from 1.81 to 11.63 for spinal cord patients. As tables 6–7 and 6–8 show, the value of the RMR depends on the level and extent of the spinal cord lesion, with paraplegic incompletes having the lowest RMR (1.81) and quadriplegic completes the highest (11.63).

The RMR estimate for non-SCI MAIS 5 cases is developed more circuitously, incorporating information and opinions from a variety of sources. The approach is similar to that used earlier for MAIS 4 cases. From the NCSS data presented in figure 6–2, we observe that a plurality of the AIS 5 injuries involve trauma to the head/face region. There is further evidence that most of these head injuries involve significant neurological damage resulting from injury to the brain. The RSEP data in figure 6–3 confirm the large incidence of head injuries. Within the RSEP sample of twenty-two AIS 5 injuries, 73 percent of the cases involved head/face trauma.

We assume that head-injured patients with concurrent brain damage are likely to experience debilitating neurological complications. Their complications will rival and, in some cases, exceed those of the brain-injured patients in Walker's World War I study who developed posttrauma epilepsy. We recall that the epileptic group had a long-term relative mortality rate of 1.35. We expect that the RMR of the brain-injured MAIS 5 cases is at least as great as this value and perhaps greater, because Walker's result is based on a sample of patients who had already successfully survived 15 years past injury, while the MAIS 5 patients are only known to have survived 1 year past injury. If the RMR value is greater, the question becomes: How much greater? Here the data wear thin. Some guidance may be obtained from considering the RMRs for the less pernicious spinal cord injuries, the paraplegic incompletes (RMR = 1.81) and quadriplegic incompletes (RMR = 2.23). Walker's 1957 study of head-injured World War II veterans found that the short-term RMR for head-injured patients developing post-trauma epilepsy was approximately 2.0 to 3.0. As an upper bound, we might also consider the RMR for MAIS 5 patients experiencing an aortic rupture with aneurysm complications (RMR = 3.12).

We decided to err on the conservative side by assigning a RMR of 1.81 to the head-injured MAIS 5 cases. This essentially associates these cases for mortality and life-expectancy purposes with the least severely injured SCI patients. In addition, this RMR value is midway between that of Walker's World War I epileptic group (RMR = 1.35) and that of his corresponding World War II group (RMR = 2.0 to 3.0). Because of the predominance of head-injured cases among the AIS 5 injuries in the RSEP and NCSS samples (and also because of the critical nature of all AIS 5 injuries), we assume that this RMR value applies to the MAIS 5 group in general.

To summarize our results, we assume that the relative mortality rate for MAIS 4 cases, like the relative mortality rates for MAIS 1 through MAIS 3 cases, is approximately 1.00. Patients in those severity groups who survive 1 year experience no significant increases in mortality rates or reductions in life expectancies compared with individuals in the general population. The MAIS 5 cases are disaggregated into two major subgroups—the SCI patients and the non-SCI patients (the plurality of whom suffer from head and brain injuries). For the non-SCI patients, we initially assign a RMR of 1.81, and for the SCI patients, a RMR value commensurate with the level and extent of the spinal cord injury. The RMR values for SCI patients range from 1.81 to 11.63. In the next section we examine the effect of relative mortality rates greater than 1.00 on survival probabilities and average life expectancies.

Survival Probabilities and Life Expectancies for
MAIS 5 Cases

Survival Probabilities. From the relative mortality rates just developed and the annual mortality rates for the general population derived from the 1977

U.S. Life Tables, we estimate survival probabilities for MAIS 5 patients of different ages and sex. The procedure was discussed in chapter 2 and replicates that used by Smart and Sanders (1976) in their analysis of the survival patterns of spinal cord injury patients. Standard life-table techniques are used for the calculations. The mathematical relationship between key variables entering the calculations is expressed by the probability formula

$$P^i_{l+1,s}(n) = \prod_{t=l+2}^{t=n-1} [1 - \alpha_i t i\, Q_s t)] \qquad \text{for } n = l + 1;\ P^i_{l+1,s}(n) = 1 \\ \text{by assumption}$$

where $Q_s(t)$ = probability of a person of sex s in the general population dying during the year following his tth birthday, given that he survives to age t

α_i = relative mortality rate for patients with injury type i

$P^i_{l+1,s}(n)$ = probability of a patient of sex s with injury type i surviving to age n, conditional on being injured at age l and surviving at least 1 year past injury

(Note: All nonfatalities injured at age l are assumed to have survived at least 1 year after injury. Therefore, it follows for MAIS 5 cases that their probability of surviving to age $l + 1$, expressed by $P^i_{l+1}(l + 1)$ is equal to 1.)

The probability formula illustrates the relationship assumed between the average annual mortality rate for an MAIS 5 case, the relative mortality rate for that type of case, and the corresponding mortality rate for a member of the general population of similar age and sex:

MAIS 5 mortality rate = relative mortality rate
                      $\times$ general population mortality rate

Because of the scarcity of data, we are forced to assume that the value of the relative mortality rate depends only on injury type, that injury types are differentiated for mortality purposes at a very aggregate level (that is, SCI versus non-SCI patients), and that the age or the sex of the person at injury, as well as the time past onset of injury, has little or no variable effect on the relative mortality rate. (The effects on survival patterns and thus on economic costs of changing these assumptions are examined later in the section on sensitivity analysis.)

Sets of survival probabilities have been computed for patients in each of the eight age groups and for both sexes. Examples of the stream of survival probabilities applicable to 20-year-old male and female MAIS 5 cases are presented in tables 6–9 and 6–10. Survival probabilities are presented in

Table 6–9
A Comparison of Survival Probabilities between 20-Year-Old Males in the MAIS 5 and General Populations

		Probability of Surviving to Subsequent Age for 20-Year-Old Male				
			Member of MAIS 5 Population[a]			
	Member of		Paraplegic		Quadriplegic	
Subsequent Age	General Population	Non-SCI Patient	Incomplete	Complete	Incomplete	Complete
21	1.0000	1.0000	1.0000	1.0000	1.0000	1.0000
22	0.9978	0.9960	0.9960	0.9897	0.9950	0.9741
23	0.9955	0.9918	0.9918	0.9792	0.9900	0.9482
24	0.9932	0.9877	0.9877	0.9688	0.9849	0.9229
25	0.9910	0.9838	0.9838	0.9587	0.9800	0.8990
26	0.9889	0.9799	0.9799	0.9492	0.9753	0.8765
27	0.9868	0.9762	0.9762	0.9400	0.9708	0.8553
28	0.9848	0.9726	0.9726	0.9311	0.9664	0.8350
29	0.9828	0.9691	0.9691	0.9223	0.9620	0.8153
30	0.9808	0.9655	0.9655	0.9136	0.9576	0.7959
31	0.9787	0.9618	0.9618	0.9048	0.9532	0.7766
32	0.9767	0.9581	0.9581	0.8958	0.9486	0.7574
33	0.9745	0.9543	0.9543	0.8867	0.9440	0.7381
34	0.9723	0.9503	0.9503	0.8772	0.9392	0.7184
35	0.9699	0.9461	0.9461	0.8673	0.9340	0.6979
36	0.9674	0.9417	0.9417	0.8568	0.9286	0.6767
37	0.9646	0.9369	0.9369	0.8456	0.9227	0.6545
38	0.9617	0.9317	0.9317	0.8337	0.9165	0.6315
39	0.9586	0.9262	0.9262	0.8211	0.9099	0.6076
40	0.9552	0.9204	0.9204	0.8078	0.9028	0.5828
.	.	.	.	.	.	.
.	.	.	.	.	.	.
.	.	.	.	.	.	.
.	.	.	.	.	.	.
65	0.6803	0.4956	0.4956	0.1580	0.4198	0.0070
66	0.6577	0.4658	0.4658	0.1336	0.3887	0.0043
67	0.6343	0.4357	0.4357	0.1115	0.3578	0.0025
68	0.6099	0.4054	0.4054	0.0916	0.3271	0.0014
69	0.5845	0.3749	0.3749	0.0739	0.2968	0.0007
70	0.5582	0.3443	0.3443	0.0585	0.2670	0.0003
71	0.5310	0.3139	0.3139	0.0453	0.2379	0.0001
72	0.5030	0.2840	0.2840	0.0342	0.2100	0.0001
73	0.4743	0.2546	0.2546	0.0251	0.1832	0.0000
74	0.4449	0.2261	0.2261	0.0179	0.1579	
75	0.4150	0.1986	0.1986	0.0123	0.1343	
76	0.3848	0.1724	0.1724	0.0082	0.1125	
77	0.3544	0.1478	0.1478	0.0052	0.0927	
78	0.3242	0.1250	0.1250	0.0031	0.0750	
79	0.2943	0.1041	0.1041	0.0018	0.0596	
80	0.2652	0.0855	0.0855	0.0010	0.0465	
81	0.2371	0.0691	0.0691	0.0005	0.0355	
82	0.2104	0.0550	0.0550	0.0002	0.0266	
83	0.1854	0.0432	0.0432	0.0001	0.0195	
84	0.1625	0.0335	0.0335	0.0000	0.0141	
85	0.1420	0.0259	0.0259		0.0102	
.	.	.	.	.		.

Source: Derived from data in USDHEW, NCHS, Life tables, *Vital Statistics of the United States, 1977*; and W.O. Geisler et al., Survival in traumatic transverse myelitis, *Paraplegia* 14: 262–275, 1977.

Table 6-10

A Comparison of Survival Probabilities between 20-Year-Old Females in the MAIS 5 and General Populations

Probability of Surviving to Subsequent Age for 20-Year-Old Female

| | | Member of MAIS 5 Population[a] | | | | |
| | Member of | | Paraplegic | | Quadriplegic | |
Subsequent Age	General Population	Non-SCI Patient	Incomplete	Complete	Incomplete	Complete
21	1.0000	1.0000	1.0000	1.0000	1.0000	1.0000
22	0.9993	0.9987	0.9987	0.9967	0.9984	0.9918
23	0.9986	0.9974	0.9974	0.9933	0.9968	0.9834
24	0.9978	0.9961	0.9961	0.9899	0.9952	0.9749
25	0.9971	0.9947	0.9947	0.9865	0.9935	0.9665
26	0.9963	0.9934	0.9934	0.9831	0.9918	0.9580
27	0.9956	0.9920	0.9920	0.9795	0.9901	0.9494
28	0.9948	0.9906	0.9906	0.9759	0.9884	0.9406
29	0.9939	0.9891	0.9891	0.9721	0.9865	0.9315
30	0.9931	0.9875	0.9875	0.9681	0.9846	0.9219
31	0.9921	0.9858	0.9858	0.9639	0.9825	0.9118
32	0.9911	0.9840	0.9840	0.9594	0.9803	0.9010
33	0.9900	0.9820	0.9820	0.9546	0.9779	0.8897
34	0.9889	0.9799	0.9799	0.9493	0.9753	0.8774
35	0.9876	0.9777	0.9777	0.9437	0.9725	0.8643
36	0.9862	0.9752	0.9752	0.9375	0.9695	0.8501
37	0.9847	0.9724	0.9724	0.9308	0.9662	0.8349
38	0.9830	0.9695	0.9695	0.9235	0.9625	0.8186
39	0.9812	0.9663	0.9663	0.9157	0.9586	0.8011
40	0.9793	0.9628	0.9628	0.9072	0.9543	0.7825
:	:	:	:	:	:	:
65	0.8249	0.7050	0.7050	0.4039	0.6496	0.0960
66	0.8119	0.6849	0.6849	0.3743	0.6268	0.0784
67	0.7981	0.6638	0.6638	0.3448	0.6030	0.0629
68	0.7833	0.6415	0.6415	0.3151	0.5780	0.0493
69	0.7673	0.6178	0.6178	0.2852	0.5517	0.0376
70	0.7499	0.5924	0.5924	0.2552	0.5238	0.0277
71	0.7310	0.5655	0.5655	0.2254	0.4944	0.0196
72	0.7108	0.5371	0.5371	0.1964	0.4639	0.0133
73	0.6889	0.5072	0.5072	0.1684	0.4320	0.0085
74	0.6653	0.4757	0.4757	0.1416	0.3990	0.0051
75	0.6398	0.4427	0.4427	0.1164	0.3649	0.0028
76	0.6124	0.4084	0.4084	0.0933	0.3301	0.0014
77	0.5834	0.3734	0.3734	0.0728	0.2952	0.0006
78	0.5528	0.3380	0.3380	0.0551	0.2607	0.0003
79	0.5211	0.3029	0.3029	0.0404	0.2273	0.0001
80	0.4884	0.2685	0.2685	0.0286	0.1955	0.0000
81	0.4550	0.2352	0.2352	0.0196	0.1657	
82	0.4212	0.2036	0.2036	0.0128	0.1383	
83	0.3872	0.1739	0.1739	0.0080	0.1134	
84	0.3534	0.1464	0.1464	0.0048	0.0913	
85	0.3199	0.1213	0.1213	0.0027	0.0720	
:	:	:	:	:	:	:

Source: Same as for table 6-9.

[a]In formulating the survival probabilities for a 20-year-old MAIS 5 female, there is the implicit assumption that the individual survived at least 1 year following her injury. Thus the probability of surviving to age 21 is 1.0000.

these tables for MAIS 5 patients in different injury subgroups, as well as for members of the general population. As one might expect, the data show that the probability of surviving to each subsequent age is greatest for members of the general population and lowest for people suffering the most severe form of spinal cord injury, quadriplegia complete.

Life Expectancies. To illustrate the excess mortality caused by an injury, we compare the estimated life expectancies of patients suffering MAIS 5 injuries and those of age- and sex-matched peers in the general population. This comparison is shown in table 6–11. For people in the general population and patients in each injury subgroup, the life expectancies are derived by summing the stream of survival probabilities applicable to individuals of that age and sex in that group. Like the survival probabilities, the values in the life-expectancy table reflect the difference in mortality rates observed between males and females and assumed between patients in different injury

Table 6–11
Life Expectancies of MAIS 5 Patients, by Age, Sex, and Injury Type

			SCI Patients			
Age at Injury	Member of General Population	Non-SCI Patient[a]	Paraplegic Incomplete[b]	Paraplegic Complete[c]	Quadriplegic Incomplete[d]	Quadriplegic Complete[e]
Male Life Expectancy (Years)						
0–14	60.2	53.2	53.2	41.4	50.6	30.0
15–24	48.9	42.3	42.3	31.5	39.8	21.5
25–34	39.8	33.7	33.7	24.2	31.5	16.2
35–44	30.8	25.2	25.2	16.8	23.2	10.3
45–54	22.4	17.5	17.5	10.6	15.9	5.9
55–64	15.2	11.4	11.4	6.2	10.1	3.0
65–74	9.3	6.8	6.8	3.4	6.0	1.6
75+	4.0	3.3	3.3	1.8	3.0	1.0
Female Life Expectancy (Years)						
0–14	66.6	61.0	61.0	50.3	58.8	39.2
15–24	54.9	49.6	49.6	39.3	47.4	29.2
25–34	45.3	40.2	40.2	30.6	38.2	21.5
35–44	35.9	31.2	31.2	22.4	29.3	14.5
45–54	27.0	22.8	22.8	15.4	21.2	9.2
55–64	18.7	15.5	15.5	9.7	14.2	5.4
65–74	11.1	9.0	9.0	5.3	8.2	2.6
75+	4.3	3.7	3.7	2.5	3.5	1.1

Source: Same as for table 6–9.
[a]RMR = 1.81.
[b]RMR = 1.81.
[c]RMR = 4.64.
[d]RMR = 2.23.
[e]RMR = 11.63.

subgroups. Certain general patterns appear that we can summarize roughly: uninjured people life longer than injured people; females live longer than males; and regardless of sex and injury status, life expectancy is a decreasing function of age at time of injury.

Among spinal cord patients, those who have less severe forms of spinal impairment—the paraplegic incompletes—tend to live longer than their counterparts who suffer from more debilitating forms of impairment, for instance, the quadriplegic completes. In addition, the life expectancies of non-SCI MAIS 5 patients are equal to the life expectancies of paraplegic incompletes of the same age and sex (we recall that the relative mortality rate for non-SCI patients was assumed equal to the relative mortality rate for paraplegic incompletes).

Direct Costs of Motor Vehicle Injuries

As in our analysis of incidence, we shall examine separately the direct costs for fatalities and for nonfatalities. This division is important because direct costs for most fatalities are small and, on average, accrue for no more than a day or so after the crash. Direct costs for seriously injured nonfatalities, in contrast, tend to be large and often continue for years.

The resources necessary to care for a fatality depend on the length of time that he or she survives after the crash. The magnitude of the costs of this care vary depending on the case, but the cost components will normally be limited to emergency services, inpatient hospital services, physician and surgeon services rendered on an inpatient basis, and insurance administration expenses. Unlike Faigin's (1976) analysis of the costs of motor vehicle injuries, we make no attempt to evaluate the more esoteric direct costs associated with fatalities. Examples of these costs include coroner or medical examiner services rendered in lieu of emergency medical services and costs developing from the difference in present value of funeral expenses now versus similar expenses accruing at the end of a normal lifespan. Like Faigin, however, we do estimate litigation and court costs associated with fatal (and nonfatal) injuries.

For nonfatalities, the cost components we evaluate include all the preceding costs plus the costs of outpatient care and, for chronically injured patients requiring long-term care, the following additional costs:

Structural alterations to one's home

Rehabilitation services following hospital discharge

Institutional or home attendant care

Medical equipment and appliances

Drugs and medical supplies

Rehospitalization

Miscellaneous supplies and services

We emphasize that since many years may be required to determine the ultimate consequences of a chronic injury, the long-term medical effects and costs of these injuries are more difficult to estimate than the immediate effects and costs. Since to the best of our knowledge neither the Department of Transportation nor any other public or private agency has surveyed systematically the costs of long-term care of nonfatalities, our estimates are approximate. We again rely on Smart and Sanders (1976), extrapolating from their results on SCI costs to develop estimates of similar costs for all catastrophically injured nonfatalities.

Figure 6–4 presents a schematic overview of the treatment and direct-cost model for motor vehicle injuries. It highlights the differences in treatment procedures and medical needs between fatalities and nonfatalities and, among nonfatalities, the differences in the level of resource utilization between those injuries which are initially life-threatening and those which are not. For each class of patients, it outlines the factors involved in initial treatment and follow-on care.

Fatalities

Treatment Subcategories. We identified three categories of deaths within the overall fatality group: (1) those who die at the crash scene or are dead on arrival at an emergency medical facility (DOAs), (2) those who die during treatment in the emergency facility but prior to admission to the hospital and (3) those who die during hospitalization. (We assume implicitly that the severity of a fatal injury requires hospitalized treatment or other comparable institutional care until death for all fatalities who survive past emergency treatment.) The average fatality in each patient category generates distinctly different costs because of the difference in medical resources consumed. DOAs typically require police and fire services, as well as those of the emergency medical facility, but only perfunctory medical care at the medical facility. Those who die after arrival at the emergency room require all the preceding services plus significant emergency medical treatment. Those who die following hospital admission receive, in addition, medical, surgical, and ancillary services that span both intensive and routine hospital care.

Although we lack definitive information on the proportion of fatalities falling into each of the three patient categories, we have data on times to death following the crash for fatalities in the Fatal Accident Reporting

System (FARS) sample. Using these data, we construct frequency-based distributions of times to death for all fatalities (adjusted to take account of those deaths not appearing in the FARS sample and occurring more than 30 days after the crash). The results, disaggregated by age and sex, are presented in table 6–12.

Information on time to death may be used with other data to estimate the proportion of fatalities in each patient category. If we assume that fatalities dying prior to a specified period of time after the crash never reach the emergency medical facility alive, they effectively constitute the group of DOAs. Similarly, fatalities dying after that time but before the lapse of another time period may be assumed to have died while in the emergency room. Finally, for those remaining fatalities dying after the second time interval, we may assume that death occurred after emergency room treatment and hospital admission.

Table 6–12
Distribution of Times to Death Following Crash for Motor Vehicle Fatalities, by Age and Sex, United States, 1975

	Proportions of Fatalities Dying during Following Time Intervals after Crash		
Age and Sex Group	$T \le 1$ hour	1 hour $< T \le 3$ hours	3 hours $< T \le 1$ year
Males			
0–14	57.8	14.0	28.2
15–24	61.6	15.4	23.0
25–34	65.1	14.4	20.5
35–44	64.6	14.9	20.5
45–54	65.5	12.7	21.8
55–64	63.7	13.7	22.6
65–74	53.5	13.8	32.7
75+	44.7	12.6	42.7
All males	61.4	14.5	24.1
Females			
0–14	58.9	15.6	25.5
15–24	61.4	15.1	23.5
25–34	58.9	16.7	24.4
35–44	63.4	15.1	21.5
45–54	62.9	15.3	21.8
55–64	60.9	14.0	25.1
65–74	52.7	14.3	33.0
75+	42.4	15.1	42.5
All females	58.7	15.2	26.1
Total fatalities	60.7	14.7	24.6

Source: U.S. Department of Transportation, National Highway Traffic Safety Administration Fatal Accident Reporting system. FARS data adjusted to reflect estimated 1.05 percent of fatalities dying after 30 days.

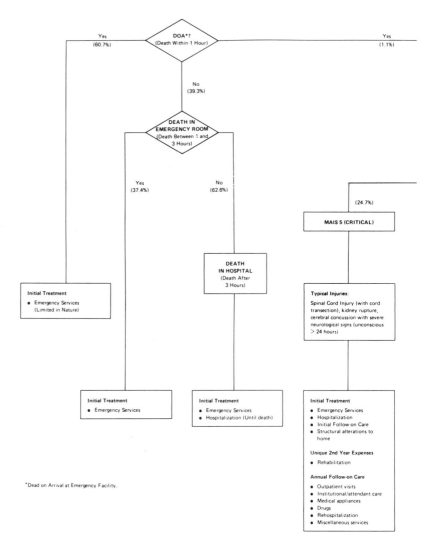

Figure 6–4. Treatment and Direct-Cost Model for Motor Vehicle Injuries

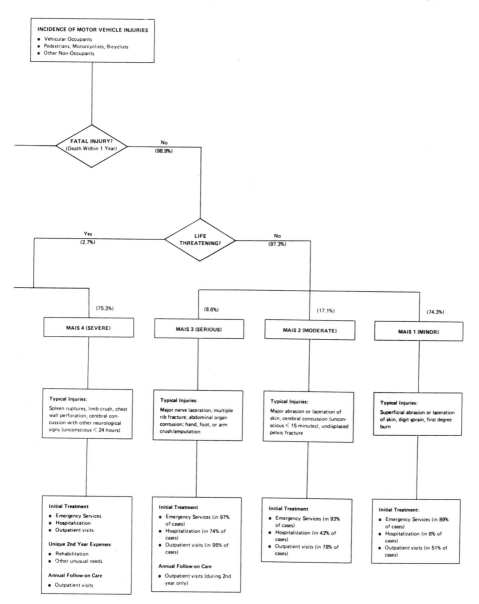

INCIDENCE OF MOTOR VEHICLE INJURIES
- Vehicular Occupants
- Pedestrians, Motorcyclists, Bicyclists
- Other Non-Occupants

FATAL INJURY?
(Death Within 1 Year)

No
(98.9%)

Yes
(2.7%)

LIFE THREATENING?

No
(97.3%)

(75.3%)

(8.6%)

(17.1%)

(74.3%)

MAIS 4 (SEVERE)

MAIS 3 (SERIOUS)

MAIS 2 (MODERATE)

MAIS 1 (MINOR)

Typical Injuries:
Spleen ruptures, limb crush, chest wall perforation, cerebral concussion with other neurological signs (unconscious < 24 hours)

Typical Injuries:
Major nerve laceration; multiple rib fracture; abdominal organ contusion; hand, foot, or arm crush/amputation

Typical Injuries:
Major abrasion or laceration of skin, cerebral concussion (unconscious < 15 minutes), undisplaced pelvic fracture

Typical Injuries:
Superficial abrasion or laceration of skin, digit sprain, first degree burn

Initial Treatment
- Emergency Services
- Hospitalization
- Outpatient visits

Unique 2nd Year Expenses
- Rehabilitation
- Other unusual needs

Annual Follow-on Care
- Outpatient visits

Initial Treatment
- Emergency Services (in 97% of cases)
- Hospitalization (in 74% of cases)
- Outpatient visits (in 95% of cases)

Annual Follow-on Care
- Outpatient visits (during 2nd year only)

Initial Treatment
- Emergency Services (in 93% of cases)
- Hospitalization (in 42% of cases)
- Outpatient visits (in 78% of cases)

Initial Treatment:
- Emergency Services (in 89% of cases)
- Hospitalization (in 6% of cases)
- Outpatient visits (in 51% of cases)

While we must estimate the values for the inclusive time periods as precisely as possible, true or actual values for these time periods may vary depending on the crash location (rural or urban), on the working procedures and idiosyncrasies of personnel at the emergency facility, and on other factors. As an example, the rural or urban crash location may affect the elapsed time from crash occurrence to the patient's arrival at the nearest emergency medical facility. The cutoff time for classification as a DOA thus may differ for urban and rural crashes. The skill of the emergency room staff can affect the average time a patient spends in the emergency room and the proportion of fatalities who survive to be admitted to the hospital.

From interviews with ambulance personnel, doctors, and nurses experienced in emergency treatment, we estimate *upper bounds* for the time it takes to transfer a critically injured patient from the crash scene to an emergency medical facility and the time required there to stabilize the patient before admitting him to the hospital. Our estimates of these values are 1 hour and 2 hours, respectively.[13] According to the sequence just described, DOAs thus include all fatalities who die within 1 hour of the crash (essentially those fatalities who die prior to arrival at the emergency facility); fatalities succumbing between 1 and 3 hours after the crash constitute the group dying in the emergency room; and those fatalities dying after 3 hours comprise the deaths following hospital admission.

This model and the data in table 6–12 on times to death for fatalities suggest that 60.7 percent of all fatalities in 1975 were DOAs, 14.7 percent were deaths in the emergency room, and the remaining 24.6 percent were deaths following hospital admission. These proportions vary little by sex. The proportions do, however, differ by age: fatalities over 65 years of age have fewer DOAs and more inhospital deaths than younger fatalities. Since we have attempted to estimate upper bounds rather than lower bounds for the time intervals, we expect that the proportion of fatalities that are DOAs implied by the times-to-death data is a generous estimate, while the proportion of fatalities dying inhospital is more conservative. Since a DOA requires fewer medical resources than an inhospital death, we feel that the estimates of average direct costs per fatality and total direct costs of all fatalities calculated in later sections should, *ceteris paribus*, be conservative.

Costs of Emergency Services. Except for the few fatalities who survive 3 or more hours following the crash, most will not require inpatient hospital treatment. All, however, will require emergency services at the scene of the crash, at an emergency medical facility, or at both. These include the cost of police and fire assistance at the scene of the crash, the cost of first aid at the scene and transportation to an emergency medical facility, and the cost of emergency treatment upon arrival at the medical facility.

When a vehicle crash occurs involving a serious or fatal injury, police and fire personnel are normally called to the scene. The police aid crash victims, direct traffic, and investigate the circumstances of the crash. Firefighters prevent fires from gasoline leakage, extricate occupants from damaged vehicles, and provide first aid.

In a national study sponsored by the Federal Highway Administration, Wuerdemann and Joksch (1973) estimated the opportunity costs of police assistance at motor vehicle crashes in 1969. These costs represented the value of time for the duties of police officers at the crash scene and for routine investigation following the crash, as well as a fractional share of expenditures for agency supervision and other support activities. For fatalities, average police assistance costs per crash in 1969 dollars were $65 nationally;[14] in 1975 dollars this becomes $105. Since the number of fatal crashes in 1975 is estimated at 39,575 and the number of fatalities occurring in those crashes is 44,995, the cost per fatality in 1975 is approximately $90 [that is, (39,575/ 44,995) × $105]. Smart and Sanders (1976) estimated the costs of fire-fighters' time at serious crashes (in 1974), assuming the equivalent of 1.5 hours of a firefighter's time and approximately 0.75 to 1.5 hours of supervisory time per crash. Adjusted to 1975 levels, this cost becomes $34 per crash and $30 per fatality. From these figures, a first-order estimate of the average cost per fatality of police and fire assistance nationally is $120.

Ground ambulance is the most common form of emergency transporta-tion used to convey motor vehicle crash victims from the crash site to an emergency medical facility. Since we assume that all fatalities receive care at an emergency facility (even if it is only a medical confirmation of death), we also assume that each requires ground ambulance transportation to the facility.[15] (Because helicopter transfer of patients from the crash scene is rare, we do not include it as a transportation alternative.)

Costs of ground ambulance services vary by state and region. Costs of the most widely used local or public ambulance services are difficult to assess since their funding is buried in municipal budgets. Private ambulance services, then, represent the best measure of actual emergency transportation costs. Private ambulance charges depend on a base rate plus mileage costs for the distance traveled to and from the scene of the crash. A survey of ambulance companies serving metropolitan and rural areas in the Northeast revealed that the 1977 base rate for ambulance service ranged from $35 to $60 per trip and the mileage rate ranged from $.75 to $2 per mile.[16] From these data, we estimate that $40 is a reasonable value to assign for the average base rate and $1 a reasonable value for the mileage rate in 1975 dollars. The average base rate corresponds well with the 1975 Massachusetts Medicaid reimbursement rate for ambulance service of $41.

Federal Highway Administration statistics for 1975 indicate that 61 percent of all motor vehicle fatalities occurred in rural areas and only 39 percent in urban areas.[17] This implies that the majority of motor vehicle fatalities were transported a relatively long distance to the nearest medical facility (approximately 10 to 20 miles one way) and the remainder were transported a much shorter distance (less than 5 to 10 miles one way). If we take the average base rate of $40 and add mileage charges of $25 (25 miles round trip $\times$ $1 per mile) for rural ambulance service and $10 (10 miles round trip $\times$ $1 per mile) for urban service, the total ambulance costs amount to an average of $65 for a rural ambulance run and $50 for an urban ambulance run. Weighting these costs by the percentage of fatalities occurring in rural and urban areas, we arrive at $60 as an estimate of the average cost per fatality of emergency transportation ($65 $\times$ 0.61 + $50 $\times$ 0.39 = $60).

The first truly substantive costs of medical treatment for motor vehicle fatalities are generated in the emergency room, since physicians or nurses are rarely sent to the crash scene and the costs of ambulance personnel (most often emergency medical technicians) are included in the cost of ambulance service. The extent of emergency treatment for a fatality depends on his condition upon arrival at the medical facility. If the patient is dead on arrival (DOA) at the hospital with no obvious hope of resuscitation, the treatment provided is usually limited. Based on the rates at a major Boston municipal hospital, adjusted to national levels, the costs for this care often do not exceed $36.[18] These include a minimal charge for basic emergency room services, a small fee for physician's services, and an estimate of the marginal cost of certain hospital administrative functions (issuing certificate of death, informing family, and occasionally arranging for autopsy).

For those fatalities who are alive upon arrival at the medical facility, the level of resources provided in the emergency room increases substantially, regardless of whether the patient dies there or survives to hospital admission. The increased care includes longer physician time, more ancillary services (laboratory tests, x-rays, medication, medical and surgical supplies), and more frequent use of costly resuscitation and life-support equipment. A survey of several acute-care hospitals in Massachusetts suggests that the costs of this care, again expressed in 1975 dollars adjusted to national levels, usually ranges from $200 to $325 per patient and in some cases may go as high as $400 or $500.[19] We used a rough midpoint estimate of $265.

Totaling the estimated expenses for police and fire assistance, ambulance service, and emergency room treatment, the overall cost for emergency service averages approximately $215 for a DOA and $445 for a fatality who survives the crash but dies either in the emergency room or following admission to the hospital. For a DOA or a fatality dying in the emergency room, this cost constitutes the extent of his direct expenses resulting from injury. This cost, however, is only a small portion of the overall direct expenses for the average fatality requiring hospitalization.

Costs of Hospitalization and Physician/Surgeon Services. We estimate that 24.6 percent of all fatalities survive more than 3 hours after the crash, successfully pass through emergency room care, and are admitted to a hospital. Because of their severe injuries, fatalities in this category generate significant inpatient costs. We lack comprehensive information on the many different types of fatal injuries that occur, as well as on the hospitalization costs associated with those injuries. A more general (albeit less exact) approach, however, is available to develop estimates of the average hospitalization costs per fatality. As in the analysis of coronary heart disease, one may express average hospitalization costs as the product of the average length of stay and the average per-diem cost.

Because of the critical nature of fatal injuries, we assume that all fatalities that initially require inpatient treatment will continue to require this level of care until death. Under this assumption, an estimate of the average length of stay for hospitalized fatalities is obtained by computing their average time to death. For convenience, we divide hospitalized fatalities into two subgroups: those who survive more than 3 hours but less than 30 days after the crash, and those who survive more than 30 days but less than 1 year after the crash. According to unpublished Fatal Accident Reporting System (FARS) data for 1975, fatalities in the first subgroup have an average time to death following the crash of approximately 4.2 days. This ranges from a low of 2.5 days for girls under 15 years of age to a high of 6.3 days for men aged 65 to 74. For fatalities in the second subgroup, there are no good data on times to death. We assume that their times to death follow a triangular probability distribution extending over a range from 30 to 365 days, reflecting our belief that proportionally more of these people will die during the first 6 months than during the second 6 months after the crash. This distribution implies an average time to death for fatalities in the second subgroup of approximately 140 days, assumed uniform for different ages and sexes.[20]

To obtain an overall average applicable to all *hospitalized* fatalities, we multiply the average time to death of fatalities in each subgroup by the proportion of fatalities in that subgroup and sum the results over the two subgroups. We recall that 24.6 percent of *all* fatalities in 1975 were hospitalized. Of these, approximately 23.6 percent died between 3 hours and 30 days after the crash (the first subgroup of hospitalized fatalities) and 1 percent died 30 days or more after the crash (the second subgroup). Considering only hospitalized fatalities, we estimate that 95.9 percent (that is, 23.6/24.6 × 100%) died within 30 days of the crash and 4.1 percent (that is, 1.0/24.6 × 100%) died 30 days or more following the crash. Taking a weighted average of times to death, we conclude that the average time to death for all hospitalized cases is 10 days (that is, 0.959 × 4.2 days + 0.041 × 140 days). If it is true (as we assume) that time to death and length of stay are roughly equivalent for a hospitalized fatality, then this result also serves as our best estimate of the average length of stay for those individuals.

Estimates of average length of stay for hospitalized fatalities of different ages and sex are presented in table 6–13. These estimates extend from 8.1 days for girls under the age of 15 to 11.9 days for men aged 55 to 64. The differences in the estimates reflect differences among the age and sex cohorts in the proportion of fatalities surviving less than 30 days and the average time to death for these cases.

Table 6–13 also presents estimates of average hospitalization costs. As we mentioned earlier, these costs are estimated by multiplying average length of stay by the average cost per day of medical care. We assume that fatalities receive inpatient care in a short-term acute-care hospital. We used the American Hospital Association's estimate of $136 for the average cost per day of regular inpatient care in 1975 and Cretin's (1977) estimate of $325 for the cost per day of treatment in an intensive care (or coronary care) unit

Table 6–13
Length of Stay, Hospitalization Costs per Capita, and Physician and Surgeon Costs per Capita for Hospitalized Fatalities, by Age and Sex, United States, 1975

Age and Sex Group	Average Length of Stay (in Days)		Hospital Per-Diem Charge		Hospital Costs per Fatality	Professional Charges per Fatality[a]
Males						
0–14	8.5	×	$250	=	$2125	$680
15–24	9.8		250		2450	784
25–34	10.9		250		2725	872
35–44	11.3		250		2825	904
45–54	11.8		250		2950	944
55–64	11.9		250		2975	952
65–74	10.5		250		2625	840
75+	8.8		250		2200	704
All males	10.2		250		2550	816
Females						
0–14	8.1	×	250	=	2025	648
15–24	9.4		250		2350	752
25–34	9.9		250		2475	792
35–44	11.0		250		2750	880
45–54	11.0		250		2750	880
55–64	10.7		250		2675	856
65–74	9.5		250		2375	760
75+	8.7		250		2175	696
All females	9.6		250		2400	768
All hospitalitized fatalities	10.0		250		2500	800

[a]0.318 of hospital costs.

during the same year. Using data from Boyd's (1972) analysis of the clinical needs of nonsurviving trauma victims, we weighted these values by our estimate of the proportion of days spent under routine and intensive care—40 and 60 percent, respectively[21]—yielding a composite per diem of $250. Hospitalization costs based on this per-diem charge and the length-of-stay data range from $2025 to $2975 per fatality, and average $2500. They include the standard hospital costs of room and board, basic nursing services, and ancillary services, plus the additional costs of life-supporting procedures provided in intensive care.

The amount of time required of internists, neurologists, neurosurgeons and general surgeons, and orthopedic specialists can be significant and the opportunity costs of their time substantial. However, the data on professional charges for hospitalized fatalities are extremely limited. Both DeLorean (1975) and Struble (1975) have done some initial research in this area, and their work laid the basis for Faigin's (1976) estimates of physician and surgeon fees. Data from Faigin's analysis suggest that, on average, the costs of professional services utilized in treating hospitalized fatalities are approximately 32 percent of the costs of all other inhospital services.[22] From table 6–13, we may thus obtain estimates of physician and surgeon costs ranging from $648 to $952, depending on the age and sex of the patient, and averaging $800.

Treatment Costs per Fatality. To summarize the cost-component analysis, we have tabulated the cost of care rendered to fatalities as (1) emergency services, including police and fire assistance, emergency transportation, and emergency room treatment; (2) inhospital services other than physician- and surgeon-related services; and (3) physician and surgeon services rendered on an inpatient basis. Cost estimates have been computed for fatalities in each of the three *time-to-death-dependent* patient categories (that is, DOA, death in the emergency room, and death following hospital admission) as well as overall averages for all fatalities. The results are presented in table 6–14.

As one might anticipate, the treatment costs generated by a hospitalized fatality ($3745) dramatically exceed analogous costs for either a DOA ($215) or a fatality succumbing in the emergency room ($445). However, since fatalities requiring hospitalization represent less than 25 percent of the total, the estimate of average treatment costs applicable to *all* fatalities ($1121) is much closer to the per-capita averages for nonhospitalized fatalities than to the corresponding average for hospitalized cases.

To provide a further perspective on how our data and modeling assumptions have caused age- and sex-specific differences in the treatment-cost estimates, we have computed average per-capita costs by age and sex for DOAs, deaths in the emergency room, deaths following hospital admission, and all fatalities. The results are presented in table 6–5. As the table shows,

Table 6–14
Average Treatment Costs per Fatality
(Dollars)

Patient Category	Emergency Services	Hospitalization	Professional Services	Total Per Capita
DOA	215	0	0	215
Death in emergency room	445	0	0	445
Death following hospital admission	445	2500	800	3745
Total fatalities[a]	307	616	198	1121

[a]Derived by taking a weighted average of costs of fatalities in each of three patient categories. Weights correspond to proportion of fatalities in each category and are for DOAs, 60.7 percent; for deaths in the emergency room, 14.7 percent; and for deaths following hospital admission, 24.6 percent.

estimates of average treatment costs of a DOA or a death in the emergency room are, by assumption, the same for all ages and both sexes. The costs associated with the treatment of hospitalized fatalities, however, vary by age and sex as the average length of stay (table 6–13) estimated for these fatalities varies. The differences in direct costs for all fatalities among the various age and sex groups is explained by concomitant differences among the groups in the costs for hospitalized fatalities and in the distribution of fatalities among the three patient categories.

Total Direct Costs of Fatalities. The cost estimates in the last column of table 6–15 are multiplied by 1.045 to account for insurance administration costs; the results are presented in the third column of table 6–16. These figures, which represent average direct costs per fatality, are then multiplied by the corresponding number of fatalities in each incidence category to obtain the total direct costs generated by fatalities in each category. We then sum these costs—presented in the fourth column of table 6–16—over the various incidence categories to find the total direct costs sustained by all fatalities in the incidence population.

In table 6–16 we see that estimated total direct costs associated with the incidence of motor vehicle fatalities in 1975 are approximately $52.7 million, with an overall average cost per fatality of about $1171 (this does not include legal and court costs, which are calculated in a later section). Males generate significantly more direct costs than females—73 percent of the total versus 27 percent—but this is to be expected since males constitute approximately 73 percent of total incidence. Younger fatalities between the

Table 6–15
Treatment Costs per Fatality for Dead on Arrivals (DOAs), Deaths in the Emergency Room, Deaths Inhospital, and All Fatalities, by Age and Sex, United States, 1975
(Dollars)

Age and Sex Group		Average Treatment Costs per Fatality		
	DOA	Death in Emergency Room	Death Inhospital	All Fatalities[a]
Males				
0–14	215	445	3250	1098
15–24	215	445	3679	1046
25–34	215	445	4042	1035
35–44	215	445	4174	1061
45–54	215	445	4339	1146
55–64	215	445	4372	1184
65–74	215	445	3910	1458
75+	215	445	3349	1577
All males	215	445	3811	1117
Females				
0–14	215	445	3118	996
15–24	215	445	3547	1034
25–34	215	445	3712	1103
35–44	215	445	4075	1082
45–54	215	445	4075	1092
55–64	215	445	3976	1193
65–74	215	445	3580	1356
75+	215	445	3316	1570
All females	215	445	3613	1133
Total fatalities	215	445	3745	1121

[a]Derived by taking a weighted average of costs of fatalities in each of three patient categories— DOA, death in emergency room, and death inhospital. Weights correspond to proportion of fatalities in each category.

ages of 15 and 24 account for nearly 33 percent of direct costs, but this is not unusual, given their disproportionately large representation in the incidence population (35 percent of total incidence).

Our estimates of the average cost of fatalities differ substantially from those of Faigin (1976), who focused on the same incidence year, 1975. Faigin contends that the cost of emergency assistance, hospitalization, and physician services averages approximately $515 per fatality, less than half our estimate of $1171.[23] Faigin underestimates the proportion of fatalities who are hospitalized (5.9 percent versus our 24.6 percent) and does not fully acknowledge the large fraction of hospital care for fatalities in the more costly

Table 6–16
Total Direct Costs of Motor Vehicle Fatalities, by Age and Sex, United States, 1975

Age and Sex Group	Incidence	Average Cost Per Capita	Total Direct Cost
Males			
0–14	2,890	$ 1,147	$ 3,314,830
15–24	12,250	1,093	13,389,250
25–34	6,017	1,082	6,510,394
35–44	3,203	1,109	3,552,127
45–54	2,907	1,198	3,482,586
55–64	2,368	1,237	2,929,216
65–74	1,852	1,524	2,822,448
75+	1,539	1,648	2,536,272
All males	33,026	1,167	38,537,123
Females			
0–14	1,674	1,041	1,742,634
15–24	3,452	1,081	3,731,612
25–34	1,604	1,153	1,849,412
35–44	1,052	1,131	1,189,812
45–54	1,090	1,141	1,243,690
55–64	1,082	1,247	1,349,254
65–74	1,081	1,417	1,531,777
75+	934	1,641	1,532,694
All females	11,969	1,184	14,170,885
Total fatalities	44,995	1,171	52,708,008

Note: All costs are in 1975 dollars.

intensive care setting (approximately 60 percent of the hospitalized care of fatalities).[24] Both factors make Faigin's estimates of hospitalization and physician costs lower than ours. She also does not include a component for insurance administration expenses. At the same time, however, Faigin includes as direct costs the expenditures for coroner/medical examiner services ($130) and the differences in present value of funeral expenses now versus those occurring at the end of a normal lifespan ($925), whereas we do not.[25] If these two costs are added to the total for "core" direct costs, Faigin's average cost per capita becomes $1570. The situation is then interestingly reversed: our estimate is now lower, but the percentage difference between the two estimates, now 25 percent, is not as extreme as before. Faigin's per-capita cost implies a bill of $70.6 million in direct expenditures for fatalities compared with our total of $52.7 million, a difference of approximately $17.9 million.

Nonfatalities

The analysis of the direct costs of fatalities did not require an examination of medical costs accruing in future years. This is not always the case for nonfatalities. Although most minor and moderate injuries will require medical treatment only during the year of incidence, this is not true for more serious, chronic conditions. For example, spinal cord injuries, extensive second- or third-degree burn cases, or cases of cerebral trauma with severe residual neuroogical deficits all require long-term treatment resulting in significant future costs.

Data Limitations. The data to formulate direct-cost estimates for nonfatalities combine both limited objective data and judgmental assessments derived from a number of sources. As noted earlier, we have few national data bases that include information on the treatment experience of nonfatal motor vehicle injuries. Of these, the two field studies of crash severity and crash-related injuries completed by NHTSA, the Restraint Systems Evaluation Program (RSEP) conducted during 1974 and 1975, and the more recent National Crash Severity Study (NCSS) conducted between 1977 and 1979 are the most useful. Because they cover similar ground and the data from the NCSS effort are considered to be more statistically representative, we used the NCSS information.

Even the NCSS data, however, have shortcomings. As we mentioned before, the NCSS data were derived entirely from the experience of motor vehicle occupants injured in tow-away crashes. The tow-away crash, with its increased public visibility, may have encouraged the treatment of minor injuries that would otherwise have gone untreated in a non-tow-away setting. The NCSS data on the frequency of treatment of minor injury cases (essentially MAIS 1 cases) thus should be viewed critically, for they may be overestimates. In addition, the observation period for injury cases followed in the study was normally restricted to the first 45 days or, at most, the first year following the crash. The short observation period reduced substantially data collection on the long-term medical effects and costs of chronic injuries. Finally, the NCSS focused on "cost-related" variables (for example, proportion of injury cases hospitalized, length of hospital stay per patient, number of outpatient visits per patient) rather than on the actual dollar costs of medical treatment. While this information is important, it does not provide a complete basis from which to develop economic estimates. These problems prevent the study from serving as an exhaustive, sole source of information on direct costs.

We supplemented the NCSS data with additional information from

Professional Activities Survey (PAS) hospitals, the American Hospital Association, the Federal Highway Administration, DeLorean's (1975) analysis of physician/surgeon costs generated in motor vehicle cases, Smart and Sanders' (1976) analysis of spinal cord injuries, and other sources. In addition, assessments based on informal surveys of institutions and medical personel experienced in the emergency care of motor vehicle trauma as well as our own estimates contributed to the somewhat eclectic data base. Where possible, we checked our values for consistency against those of Faigin (1976) and the recent All-Industry Research Advisory Committee (AIRAC) study of auto insurance claims and injury expense reimbursement, *Automobile Injuries and Their Compensation in the United States (1979)*.

Direct-Cost Model. Following the general guidelines of chapter 2, we use a four-step approach to model and analyze the direct costs of nonfatalities:

Step 1: Model the average direct costs per nonfatality.
Step 2: Estimate values for patients in each of the five injury severity groups (MAIS 1 through 5).
Step 3: Compute the present value of the per-patient direct costs for the different age, sex, and injury-severity categories.
Step 4: Multiply the per-patient costs by the corresponding nonfatal incidence estimate and sum the results over all incidence categories to find total direct costs.

For a nonfatality whose age l, sex s, and injury-severity type i are specified, the present value of averge direct costs may be expressed as

$$PVC = F_l^i + \frac{S^i}{(1 + r)} + \sum_{n=l+1}^{99} \frac{P_{l+1,s}^i(n) \times AFOC_l^i}{(1 + r)^{n-l}}$$

or equivalently,

$$PVC = F_l^i + \frac{S^i}{(1 + r)} + AFOC_l^i \times \sum_{n=l+1}^{99} \left[\frac{P_{l+1,s}^i(n)}{(1 + r)^{n-l}} \right]$$

where $PVC =$ present value of average direct costs accruing over a nonfatality's lifetime

$r =$ average direct costs generated during the first year past injury

$S^i =$ average costs of unique and unusual services delivered during the second year past injury (these may include the costs of physical and vocational rehabilitation services and other unusual clinical needs)

$AFOC_l^i$ = average annual follow-on costs generated during any subsequent year past the first (these may include the costs of outpatient medical/surgical care, medical appliances, drugs, institutional and attendant care, rehospitalization, and miscellaneous services and supplies)

$P_{l+1,s}^i(n)$ = probability of a person of injury-severity type i and sex s surviving to age n, given injury occurrence at age l and survival at least 1 year past injury

The term F_l^i, which encompasses all injury-related expenses generated during the first year, may be further defined as

$$F_l^i = ES_l^i + IH_l^i + MD_l^i + HM^i + AFOC_l^i(1)$$

where ES_l^i = average cost per patient of emergency services

IH_l^i = average initial hospitalization costs

MD_l^i = average cost of physician and surgeon services rendered on an inpatient basis

HM^i = average cost of structural modifications to a person's home

$AFOC_l^i(1)$ = average cost of follow-on care during the first year

The terms ES_l^i, IH_l^i, and MD_l^i, in turn, may be modeled as

$$ES_l^i = PF^i + \alpha_l^i (ET^i + ER^i)$$

$$IH_l^i = \beta_l^i \times LOS_l^i \times [\delta_{ICU}^i \times C_{ICU} + (1 - \delta_{ICU}^i) \times C_R]$$

$$MD_l^i = \gamma^i \times IH_l^i$$

where PF^i = average cost per patient of police and fire assistance

ET^i = average cost of ambulance service for a patient using emergency transportation following the crash

ER^i = average cost of emergency room treatment for a patient receiving emergency care following the crash

α_l^i = proportion of patients receiving emergency room treatment following the crash (the proportion using emergency transportation is also assumed equal to this value)

$\beta_I^i =$ proportion of patients requiring hospitalization following the crash

$LOS_I^i =$ average length of stay for a *hospitalized* patient

$\delta_{ICU}^i =$ proportion of inhospital time spent in intensive care by a *hospitalized* patient

$C_R =$ per-diem cost in 1975 of regular inpatient care in a short-term, acute-care hospital ($136)

$C_{ICU} =$ per-diem cost in 1975 of intensive hospitalized care ($325)

$\gamma^i =$ the ratio of average costs of inpatient physician and surgeon services to average hospitalization costs.

The preceding model illustrates the analytical techniques we use to evaluate direct costs and the technical relationships existing between cost components and other variables. It contains many of the same relationships found in the more descriptive model of the direct costs of fatalities. The analysis of fatalities, however, considers only four cost components— emergency services, initial hospitalization, inpatient physician and surgeon services, and insurance administration expenses associated with the reimbursement of other health-related costs. All costs end within the first year following injury and do not require discounting. For nonfatalities, the number of cost components examined during the first year is expanded to include charges for follow-on care after hospital discharge and structural modifications to a patient's home if necessitated by his medical condition. The time perspective also includes the costs of such services as rehabilitation delivered during the second year following injury and the costs of follow-on care that may continue over the lifetime of the patient. Follow-on care could include expenditures for outpatient medical/surgical care, medical appliances, drugs, institutional and attendant care, rehospitalization, and miscellaneous supplies and services. All expected future costs are discounted to the present, which here is taken to be the year of occurrence of the injury (1975). As for fatalities, we account for insurance administration expenses by multiplying all other direct costs by a factor of 1.045.

Despite the model's precision, its form remains general. It in no way attempts to incorporate all the variations in treatment protocols and costs that are possible when the multitude of individual injury cases is scrutinized. The model seeks rather to reflect the "average" treatment experience and associated costs of patients in each of eight age cohorts, two sex categories, and nine injury-severity groups—a formidable task given the relatively limited data base.

To reconcile the model with existing data, we made six main simplifying assumptions:

1. *The direct costs of MAIS 1 and MAIS 2 patients are limited to charges that accrue only during the first year past injury.* Depending on the case, these charges may include expenditures for emergency services, initial hospitalization, inpatient physician and surgeon services, and outpatient follow-on care. We restricted these costs to the first year because these injuries have limited severity (for example, abrasion or laceration of the skin, digit sprain, minor cerebral concussion). This also accords with a similar assumption made by Faigin (1976) in her analysis of the direct costs of MAIS 1 and MAIS 2 patients.

2. *MAIS 3 patients generate the same types of first-year costs as MAIS 1 and 2 patients and, in addition, limited costs for outpatient care in the second year.* While MAIS 3 injuries (for example, multiple rib fracture, abdominal organ contusion, nerve laceration) are considered more severe than MAIS 1 or 2 injuries, they are not life-threatening and, in general, do not require the types of continuing follow-on care characteristic of chronic injuries. Treatment for patients with MAIS 3 injuries is therefore assumed to conclude not later than during the second year.

3. *MAIS 4 patients generate (a) the types of first-year costs common to MAIS 1, 2, and 3 patients, (b) second-year costs for unusual clinical care (for example, rehabilitation), and (c) moderate outpatient costs for the rest of their lives.* Many MAIS 4 injuries are severe, often producing chronic sequelae (for example, leg crush), and hence are likely to require continuing costs.

4. *MAIS 5 injuries (for example, serious head injury with concurrent brain damage, and spinal cord injury), the most critical and debilitating of all nonfatal injuries, generate substantial direct costs.* First-year costs may include not only charges for emergency services, initial hospitalization, and physician and surgeon services rendered on an inpatient basis, but also charges for various forms of follow-on care and structural modifications to the patient's home. We assume that second-year rehabilitation services are necessary and that their cost is significant. Given the normally chronic, catastrophic nature of these injuries, annual follow-on care is expected to be extensive, to continue for the remainder of the patient's (now reduced) lifespan, and to produce large annual costs.

5. *The costs of unique and unusual clinical services rendered to many MAIS 4 and MAIS 5 patients reflect their need for specialized vocational and/or physical rehabilitation programs after hospital discharge, beginning in the second year following injury.* This assumption is based on Smart and Sanders' (1976) analysis of the rehabilitative needs of spinal cord

patients. Although some programs require formal education, continued counseling, or extensive physical retraining that may extend beyond the end of the second year, the average duration of a program is normally short enough that assigning all rehabilitation costs to that year does not significantly alter their true present value. (In the case of those programs which actually start in the first year after injury and extend into the second, the difference between the estimated and true present value of program costs caused by assigning all such costs to the second year is also expected to be small.)

6. *The costs of rehabilitation services and future follow-on care estimated for the least severely injured spinal cord patients, the incomplete paraplegics, provide an adequate basis for similar cost estimates for the non-SCI MAIS 5 patients.* This is consistent with our decision to group the non-SCI MAIS 5 cases with the incomplete paraplegics to examine their mortality and life expectancy. It was an expedient measure we adopted in view of the paucity of data on the long-term medical needs and costs of chronic, catastrophic injuries (except for selected studies on the lifetime care and costs of spinal cord injuries).

First-Year Costs. We examine in the next subsections the different types of direct costs that may accrue to a nonfatality during the first year past injury: costs of emergency services, hospitalization charges, physician and surgeon fees, charges for follow-on medical care, and home modification expenses.

Emergency Services. We have assumed that police and fire assistance costs vary directly with crash and injury severity. MAIS 5 nonfatalities are believed to generate the same costs of police-related activities as fatalities—$90 per injury case—and less seriously injured patients, progressively lower costs.[26] The costs of fire personnel ($30 per injury case) are included only for patients in the MAIS 4 and MAIS 5 severity groups.

Our analysis of the average costs for ground ambulance service for nonfatalities is similar to that used in the section on fatalities. Assuming that the distribution of cases between rural and urban areas is similar for critically injured nonfatalities and fatalities, the average cost of an ambulance run for a fatality ($60) is a good estimate of the same cost for an MAIS 5 patient. Federal Highway Administration statistics indicate that approximately 33 percent of all motor vehicle nonfatalities in 1975 occurred in rural areas and 67 percent in urban areas.[27] A weighted average of rural and urban ambulance charges yields an average cost of $55 (that is $60 $\times$ 0.33 + $50 $\times$ 0.67) for all MAIS 1, 2, 3, and 4 cases requiring emergency transportation.

Emergency room treatment normally includes physician services, ancillary services, and basic emergency medical services (those functions whose costs are included in the floor charge or base rate). In general, the costs of these services vary directly with injury severity ranging, for example, from small costs for limited drugs and medical and surgical supplies for MAIS 1 patients to more extensive costs for blood studies, urinalysis, x-rays, intravenous fluids, catheterization, and life-support equipment for MAIS 5 spinal cord patients. Estimates of emergency room costs for spinal cord cases are taken from Smart and Sanders' (1976) estimates of the costs of their care in 1974, updated to 1975.[28] We surveyed emergency medical-care procedures and charges in selected Massachusetts hospitals (adjusted to national levels) to obtain cost estimates for injured persons in other severity groups.[29] These costs range from $30 for a MAIS 1 patient up to $310 for a spinal cord patient.

We can reasonably assume that *all* nonfatalities with MAIS 4 or 5 injuries and a high proportion of less severely injured persons receive emergency room treatment. If we include as emergency-care recipients (1) those patients recorded as having been transported from the crash scene to the hospital in an emergency (or police) vehicle and then released prior to admission, thus yielding overestimates for MAIS 1 injuries, as well as (2) those patients who are eventually admitted to the hospital, the proportion receiving emergency care in the NCSS is 89 percent or more for each severity group.

We further assumed that each nonfatality receiving emergency room treatment requires emergency transportation. This links the proportion requiring transportation with the proportion receiving emergency medical care. Combining the values for the different emergency-service parameters, we obtain estimates of the average costs of emergency services that range from approximately $100 for an MAIS 1 patient to $490 for a spinal cord patient.

Hospitalization. We assume that all nonfatalities in the MAIS 4 and 5 groups require and receive inpatient care. The 1979 NCSS data and Faigin (1976) support this. If, for each severity group, we weight the proportion hospitalized by the proportion of the incidence population in that group and sum the results over the various groups, the result shows that roughly 19 percent of all nonfatalities were hospitalized. This agrees with the All-Industry Research Advisory Committee (AIRAC, 1979) insurance study of motor vehicle injury cases where reparation data indicate that slightly fewer than 20 percent were hospitalized.[30]

Average length of hospital stay has been calculated using data in Smart and Sanders (1976) and a 26,100-case sample pooled from NCSS and Professional Activities Survey (PAS) injury cases identified by MAIS level and age.[31] As we might expect, length of stay is an increasing function of injury-severity status. Estimates range from a low (yet significant) value of

5.2 days for MAIS 1 cases who are hospitalized up to 235 days for the most severely injured spinal cord patients.

Following Smart and Sanders' (1976) estimates of per-diem costs for initial care at SCI treatment centers and adjusting to 1975 price levels, we find per-diem estimates ranging from $172 to $189 for *all* inpatient services for an SCI patient.[32] For other nonfatalities, we have used values that reflect the costs per day in 1975 of regular inpatient care ($136) and intensive care ($325) at short-term, acute-care hospitals. As in the case of fatalities, we fully expect that a seriously injured patient will spend a certain proportion of his hospital stay in intensive care. For non-SCI MAIS 5 patients, this proportion is assumed the same as that of hospitalized fatalities, 60 percent; for MAIS 4 patients, the proportion drops to 30 percent. Only about 10 percent of MAIS 3 cases need intensive care, and MAIS 1 and MAIS 2 patients require none.

If we combine the parameter values representing proportion hospitalized, average length of stay for hospitalized cases, costs per day of inpatient care, and the percentage division between different types of inpatient care, we obtain estimates of average hospitalization costs for patients in each of the injury-severity groups. These costs vary substantially among groups. MAIS 1 patients, with no or short hospitalization, have average costs of only $44. The costs, however, escalate rapidly with increasing injury severity. MAIS 2 patients generate average costs of $561 per case; MAIS 3 patients, $1300 per case; MAIS 4 patients, $3257 per case; and non-SCI MAIS 5 patients, $6459 per case. Because of their long average lengths of stay, SCI patients produce by far the highest average costs: from $17,930 to $44,300 per case depending on the individual's impairment.

Physician and Surgeon Services. Although the per-diem charges for SCI patients include the costs of inpatient care by physicians and surgeons, this is not true of the per-diem charges estimated for other nonfatalities. To estimate physician and surgeon costs for these other groups, we rely on the initial research done on this subject by DeLorean (1975). DeLorean utilized physician cost data taken from a variety of automobile insurance and workmen's compensation sources to estimate that average physician and surgeon charges equal to approximately 40 percent of average hospitalization costs were not inconsistent with the available data. Refining these down to the level of the individual injury-severity groups, DeLorean found that the following percentage ratios apply: MAIS 1, 27 percent; MAIS 2, 36 percent; MAIS 3, 38 percent; MAIS 4, 40 percent; and non-SCI MAIS 5, 40 percent.[33] Multiplying these percentages by the corresponding estimates of average hospitalization costs yields estimates of physician and surgeon costs. Like similar costs estimated for fatalities, they approximate the economic value of professional medical service rendered during inpatient care.

Follow-On Medical Care. We assume that most follow-on care for nonfatalities with MAIS 1, 2, 3, and 4 injuries is provided on an outpatient basis after hospital discharge. Estimates of the average costs of outpatient care are derived from NCSS data on outpatient visits and physician-charge data in *Medical Economics.* The NCSS data indicate that, on average, in the first year: MAIS 1 patients make 1.2 outpatient visits, MAIS 2 patients make 2.4 visits, MAIS 3 patients make 4.3 visits, and MAIS 4 patients make 6.5 visits. We assume that all outpatient visits are made to an internist or other medical specialist charging similar fees. From *Medical Economics,* the average charges for internists in 1975 were approximately $20.60 for the initial visit and $12.30 for each subsequent visit.[34] Under this set of assumptions, the average cost of outpatient care during the first year following injury will be between $23 and $88, depending on the patient's severity group.

Because of the chronic, catastrophic nature of MAIS 5 injuries, annual follow-on care in these cases is expected to transcend the simple requirements of outpatient care. In fact, Smart and Sanders (1976) determined that follow-on care for a surviving spinal cord patient will be extensive and perpetual. This care includes special drugs and medical supplies; medical equipment and appliances; home attendant care or, in more extreme cases, institutional care in nursing homes and chronic-care hospitals; periodic rehospitalization for treatment of complications; and other miscellaneous supplies and services. Following the lead of Smart and Sanders, we assume that SCI patients received initial hospitalization and rehabilitation training at a specialized SCI treatment center and, consequently, require less in the way of extensive institutional and rehospitalization care than patients who have not had the benefit of SCI center care. Even so, annual follow-on care is expensive and average costs extend from $2905 for an incomplete paraplegic to $14,080 for a complete quadriplegic.[35]

We recognize that during the period immediately following injury, SCI patients are hospitalized continuously and thus do not generate costs for follow-on care. Therefore, to obtain a more realistic estimate of these costs accruing during the first year after injury, we prorated the cost for a full year to take account of the initial long hospitalization period. In the case of incomplete paraplegics, this means that the average cost of follow-on care in the first year is approximately $2905 \times 0.72 = 2075, where 0.72 represents the fraction of that year when the patient *is not* hospitalized continuously. [To obtain the value of 0.72, we evaluated the following fraction: $(365 - LOS^i)/365$. For incomplete paraplegics, this equals $(365 - 104)/365 = 261/365 = 0.72$.] Similar "first-year" costs were developed for patients in the three other spinal cord impairment categories.

The dearth of data, except for spinal cord injuries, on the costs of lifelong care for catastrophic injuries hinders the analysis of the costs of follow-on care for non-SCI MAIS 5 patients and, indeed, of the costs of any services provided to this group after initial hospitalization. One major assumption we made is that such costs for the least severely injured SCI patients, the incomplete paraplegics, provide a reasonable basis from which to develop estimates for other catastrophically injured patients. We have further assumed that the average cost of follow-on care, home modifications, or rehabilitation services for a non-SCI MAIS 5 patient is proportional to the corresponding cost for an incomplete paraplegic (the same proportion that exists between these two classes of patients for costs prior to hospital discharge).

The average cost of initial treatment prior to discharge is $9423 for a non-SCI MAIS 5 case and $18,420 for an incomplete paraplegic. The ratio of these costs is approximately 0.512. Under our cost-proportionality assumption, the multiple of this ratio and the cost of first-year follow-on care for an incomplete paraplegic provides a working estimate of the average follow-on costs during the first year for a non-SCI MAIS 5 patient. This value, which is incorporated in our analysis, is $1062 (that is, $2075 × 0.512). We emphasize that this cost-estimation procedure is an expediency. It does not imply that follow-on care for non-SCI patients is necessarily similar to that for spinal cord cases. It suggests, rather, that substantial follow-on care is necessary for other catastrophically injured nonfatalities and that the *costs* of this care can be approximated as a fractional multiple of similar costs for spinal cord patients.

Home Modifications. We assume that structural modifications to an individual's home are necessary for catastrophically injured nonfatalities. SCI patients who are not institutionalized certainly require them, and by association, we expect that most other MAIS 5 cases who return to a home setting need them. Smart and Sanders estimated the costs of alterations on a typical two-story house for a paraplegic and quadriplegic. These costs, adjusted to 1975 levels and corrected for the proportion of SCI patients who are expected to receive institutional care, average $3000 and $6025, respectively.[36] (The large cost differential between paraplegics and quadriplegics results from the quadriplegics' need for more extensive modifications.) Home modification costs for a non-SCI MAIS 5 case, like the costs of first-year follow-on care, are estimated by taking the analogous expenditures for an incomplete paraplegic and multiplying by the ratio of initial treatment costs (0.512) to obtain $1536 as a rough estimate of those costs. Except in rare instances, we assume that structural modifications are not required for MAIS 1 through 4 patients.

Totaling the average costs of emergency services, initial hospitalization, physician and surgeon services rendered on an inpatient basis, follow-on care during the first year, and home modifications yields an estimate of average injury-related expenditures during the first year after injury occurrence. These expenditures are $179 for a MAIS 1, $957 for a MAIS 2, $2049 for a MAIS 3, $4963 for a MAIS 4, $12,021 for a non-SCI MAIS 5, and between $23,495 and $55,830 for spinal cord patients.

Unique Second-Year Costs. In general, the costs of unique clinical services for MAIS 4 and MAIS 5 patients reflect their need for specialized vocational and physical rehabiliation programs. Based on Smart and Sanders' analysis of the rehabilitative needs of spinal cord patients following hospital discharge, we assume that these costs accrue primarily during the second year of injury. Since SCI patients receiving care in a specialized spinal cord treatment center normally undergo extensive physical retraining prior to discharge, most of their postdischarge rehabilitation emphasizes vocational counseling, adjustment, and educational programs. Smart and Sanders assumed that the percentage of SCI patients electing a vocational rehabilitation program would equal the percentage of those patients who are eventually reemployed—conservatively, 63 percent of all paraplegics and 48 percent of all quadriplegics. (Smart and Sanders define *reemployed* individuals to include those who return directly to competitive employment, the self-employed, homemakers, and those enrolling in formal education and training programs leading to future employment possibilities.) With this caveat and using data from several SCI center programs, they projected average vocational rehabilitation costs (adjusted to 1975 levels) of $1545 for paraplegics and $1905 for quadriplegics.[37] These estimates are used in our analysis.

For the non-SCI MAIS 5 patients, rehabilitative efforts following hospital discharge are expected to include both physical and vocational rehabilitation programs. Again, to obtain a ball-park estimate of their costs, we have taken the rehabilitation costs estimated for incomplete paraplegics ($1545) and multiplied by 0.512, yielding an average cost of $790 per case. For MAIS 4 patients, some rehabilitation services are probably necessary, although on a reduced scale. Accordingly, we assigned an average cost of $300 to cover the expenses of rehabilitation and other unusual services for MAIS 4 cases. Neither vocational nor physical rehabilitation is considered a substantive factor in the care of MAIS 1, 2, or 3 patients.

Annual Follow-On Care. The cost per year of follow-on care for surviving SCI patients was discussed earlier. To estimate the corresponding cost for non-SCI MAIS 5 patients, we once again use the average cost for an incomplete paraplegic ($2905) as a benchmark. Multiplying this value by 0.512 gives $1485, our estimate of the average annual cost of follow-on care for the remaining MAIS 5 cases.

Because these injuries frequently are chronic, we believe that MAIS 4 patients, as a group, require moderate levels of outpatient care over their remaining lifetimes. During each year that a patient lives, we assume that he requires an amount of outpatient care that corresponds approximately with the number of outpatient visits necessary during the first year after injury (an average of 6.5 visits per person). If this care is priced at the cost of a subsequent outpatient visit ($12.30 per visit), the average cost is $80 per case.

Although the outpatient care of MAIS 1 and 2 patients is not believed to extend beyond the end of the first year after injury, we concede that MAIS 3 patients may require care that spills over into the second year. To be consistent with the approach taken for MAIS 4 patients, we assume that the number of outpatient visits during that year is, on average, the same as the number during the first year (4.3 visits per case) and the appropriate cost to apply is that of a subsequent outpatient visit. This provides for an average cost of $53 for outpatient care during the second year. For our analysis, we assume that the injury-related treatment of a MAIS 3 patient is brought to a successful conclusion by the end of that year.

Cost Components by Injury-Severity Level. Table 6–17 displays the values of key parameters used in our direct-cost model to estimate annual cost components; Table 6–18 summarizes the cost components obtained. As table 6–17 shows, a separate value of each parameter has been estimated for each of the nine injury-severity groups. When the data also permitted subclassification by age (that is, under 65 years of age and 65 years of age and older), this is indicated in the table and incorporated in the final results. We found that further disaggregation by sex was either unnecessary or statistically infeasible.

Table 6–18 groups the annual cost components into three categories: costs in the first year after injury, unique costs for second-year care, and costs of annual follow-on care past the first year.

Average Direct Costs per Nonfatality. The direct-cost component values in table 6–18 coupled with the age- and sex-specific survival probabilities permit us to estimate the present value of the average direct costs (PVC) for nonfatalities in each incidence category. As a demonstration of the model, the cost calculations for a male spinal cord injury victim who suffers incomplete paraplegia at age 20 are outlined in subsequent paragraphs.

An incomplete paraplegic generates direct costs during the year of injury and in subsequent years. The costs of annual follow-on care ($AFOC$) are substantial and accrue as long as the individual survives. Under these circumstances, the model of direct costs per capita (using a 6 percent discount rate) can be expressed as

$$PVC = F^i + \frac{S^i}{(1.06)} + \sum_{n=21}^{99} \frac{P^i_{21,s}(n) \cdot AFOC^i}{(1.06)^{n-20}}$$

or equivalently,

$$PVC = F^i + \frac{S^i}{(1.06)} + AFOC^i \cdot \left[\sum_{n=21}^{99} \frac{P^i_{21,s}(n)}{(1.06)^{n-20}} \right]$$

where i = incomplete paraplegic

s = male sex

and all other terms are as defined earlier in our direct-cost model. Since

$$F^i = ES^i + IH^i + MD^i + HM^i + AFOC^i(1)$$

(indicating the sum of the average costs of emergency services, initial hospitalization, physician and surgeon services, home modifications, and follow-on care during the first year, respectively) and, for an incomplete paraplegic,

$$ES^i = \$490$$

$$IH^i + MD^i = \$17,930$$

$$HM^i = \$3000$$

$$AFOC^i(1) = \$2075$$

we have

$$F^i = (\$490 + \$17,930 + \$3000 + \$2075) = \$23,495$$

In addition, the following relationships hold:

$$S^i = \$1545$$

$$AFOC^i = \$2905$$

and

$$\sum_{n=21}^{99} \frac{P^i_{21,s}(n)}{(1.06)^{n-20}} = 14.684$$

Table 6–17
Values of Selected Direct-Cost Parameters for Nonfatalities, by Injury-Severity Group

| | | | | | *Injury-Severity Groups* | | MAIS 5 | | |
Direct-Cost Parameter	MAIS 1	MAIS 2	MAIS 3	MAIS 4	Non-SCI Patient	Para Incomplete	Para Complete	Quad Incomplete	Quad Complete
Emergency Services:									
Police and fire cost ($): PF^i	25	35	50	100	120	120	120	120	120
Emergency transport cost ($): ET^i	55	55	55	55	60	60	60	60	60
Emergency room care cost ($): ER^i	30	75	100	160	200	310	310	310	310
Proportion receiving E.R. care (%): α^i_j	88.8[a]	92.5[a]	96.7[a]	100.0	100.0	100.0	100.0	100.0	100.0
Initial Hospitalization:									
Proportion hospitalized (%): β^i_j	6.2[a]	41.9[a]	74.1[a]	100.0	100.0	100.0	100.0	100.0	100.0
ALOS in days per hospitalized case: LOS^i_j	5.2[a]	9.9[a]	11.3[a]	16.9	25.9	104.0	127.0	174.0	235.0

Proportion of inhospital time in ICU (%): δ_{ICU}	0	0	10.0	30.0	60.0	NA[b]	NA	NA	NA
Per-diem cost, regular inpatient care ($): C_R	136.	136.	136.	136.	136.	172.	172.	189.	189.
Per-diem cost, intensive care ($): C_{ICU}	—	—	325.	325.	325.	NA	NA	NA	NA
Physician and surgeon services: Ratio, physician and surgeon costs to hospitalization costs: γ	0.270	0.360	0.380	0.400	0.400	NA	NA	NA	NA

[a]Separate estimates exist for this variable for persons under 65 and those 65 years of age and older. Age-specific estimates are incorporated in direct-cost results presented in tables 6–19 and 6–20.
[b]NA = Not available or not applicable.

Table 6-18
Average Direct Costs per Patient: A Summary of Component Costs of MVI Nonfatalities, by Injury-Severity Group
(Dollars)

| | | | | | | Injury-Severity Groups | | | | |
| | | | | | | | MAIS 5 | | | |
Direct Cost Category	MAIS 1	MAIS 2	MAIS 3	MAIS 4	Non-SCI Patient	Para Incomplete	Para Complete	Quad Incomplete	Quad Complete
First-year costs:									
Emergency services[a]	$ 101	$ 155	$ 200	$ 315	$ 380	$ 490	$ 490	$ 490	$ 490
Initial hospitalization[a]	44	562	1,300	3,257	6,459	17,930	21,895	32,805	44,300
Inpatient physician and surgeon services[a]	12	202	488	1,303	2,584	—[b]	—[b]	—[b]	—[b]
Follow-on care during first year	22	38	61	88	1,062[d]	2,075	2,950	4,200	5,015
Home modifications	0	0	0	0	1,536[d]	3,000	3,000	6,025	6,025
Subtotal[a]	179	957	2,049	4,963	12,021	23,495	28,335	43,520	55,830
Unique services in second year	0	0	0	300	790[d]	1,545	1,545	1,905	1,905
Annual follow-on care (past first year)	0	0	53[c]	80	1,485[d]	2,905	4,525	8,025	14,080

Note: All costs are in 1975 dollars.

[a]For patients in MAIS 1, 2, and 3 injury-severity groups, separate estimates exist for this cost component for persons under 65 and those 65 years of age and older. Age-specific estimates are incorporated in direct-cost results presented in tables 6–19 and 6–20.

[b]For SCI patients, physician and surgeon fees are already included in initial hospitalization costs.

[c]No follow-on care is assumed necessary for MAIS 3 patients past the end of the second year.

[d]These costs for a MAIS 5 non-SCI patient are obtained by multiplying corresponding costs for para incompletes by 0.512.

Therefore, it follows that

$$PVC = \$23,495 + \frac{\$1545}{1.06} + \$2905 \cdot 14.684 = \$67,609$$

Multiplying this figure by 1.045 to incorporate insurance administration expenses yields $70,651, the present value (at time of injury) of the lifelong directs costs of a 20-year-old male incomplete paraplegic. This estimate will apply for each MAIS 5 nonfatality in the incidence category defined to include male incomplete paraplegics between the ages of 15 and 24.

Similar estimates have been calculated for patients in each of the other nonfatal incidence categories. The results are shown in table 6–19. Several trends are evident from the values in the tables:

1. The difference in per-capita costs incurred by people suffering minor injuries and people suffering chronic, catastrophic injuries is enormous. MAIS 1 patients have average costs of only $192, while MAIS 5 patients have average costs that range from $34,293 to $184,407, depending on the injury-severity group. This implies that MAIS 5 per-capita costs can be greater than corresponding MAIS 1 costs by a factor of 180 to 960.

2. Based on incidence figures, over 72 percent of all nonfatalities have average direct costs per capita under $195 (MAIS 1 cases), about 89 percent have costs per capita of $1000 or less (MAIS 1 and 2 cases), and only 0.7 percent have costs per capita that exceed $34,000 (MAIS 5 cases). This results in average direct costs per capita of approximately $910 for all nonfatalities.

3. Patients in the MAIS 1, 2, and 3 injury-severity groups, for whom disaggregation of the cost-component data by age was possible, show average costs that are significantly higher for individuals 65 years of age and older. In fact, within these severity groups, the costs of people 65 and over are approximately twice those of people under 65. This phenomenon is best explained by the traditionally higher frequency at which the elderly demand medical care if injured and the relatively larger amounts of medical resources necessary to care for them.

4. For patients in the MAIS 4 and 5 severity groups, average costs show a different dependency on age. In these groups, costs per capita are a monotonically decreasing, rather than increasing, function of age. In the most extreme instance (female quad completes), the present-value costs of children under 14 are a factor of 2.2 greater than those of middle-aged adults 55 to 64 years of age and a factor of 3.5 greater than those of the elderly over 75. This trend prevails because chronically injured patients, such as those in the MAIS 4 and 5 groups, generate much of their costs in the form of annual

Table 6-19
Present Value of Direct Costs per Nonfatality, by Age, Sex, and Injury-Severity Group, United States, 1975
(Dollars)

Age and Sex Group	MAIS 1	MAIS 2	MAIS 3	MAIS 4	MAIS 5 Subgroups				
					Non-SCI Patient	Para Incomplete	Para Complete	Quad Incomplete	Quad Complete
Males									
0–14	187	948	2,073	6,809	37,371	73,085	99,701	175,767	250,014
15–24	187	948	2,073	6,760	36,127	70,651	93,680	168,275	222,588
25–34	187	948	2,073	6,702	34,744	67,945	88,124	160,218	204,187
35–44	187	948	2,073	6,601	32,335	63,232	78,235	146,154	168,690
45–54	187	948	2,073	6,457	29,089	56,883	66,303	127,617	131,238
55–64	187	948	2,073	6,279	25,390	49,646	54,782	107,186	101,320
65–74	298	1,791	3,323	6,084	21,771	42,566	45,704	88,034	83,080
75+	298	1,791	3,323	5,906	18,858	36,868	39,470	73,235	58,342
All males	191	994	2,144	6,655	33,915	67,022	86,741	147,034	178,632
Females									
0–14	187	948	2,073	6,834	38,087	74,484	103,731	180,215	271,395
15–24	187	948	2,073	6,801	37,236	72,819	99,523	175,072	251,730
25–34	187	948	2,073	6,755	36,065	70,530	94,079	168,081	228,477
35–44	187	948	2,073	6,678	34,192	66,864	85,728	156,983	194,523
45–54	187	948	2,073	6,567	31,601	61,796	75,423	141,973	158,328
55–64	187	948	2,073	6,413	28,281	55,302	64,036	123,291	124,898
65–74	298	1,791	3,323	6,213	24,259	47,433	52,291	101,336	97,418
75+	298	1,791	3,323	6,000	20,434	39,951	42,756	81,212	77,591
All females	193	1,010	2,265	6,659	35,366	69,598	92,759	157,200	209,594
All nonfatalities	192	1,001	2,192	6,657	34,293	67,841	88,660	148,968	184,407

Note: All costs are in 1975 dollars, discounted at 6 percent.

follow-on care in future years, while patients in the MAIS 1, 2, and 3 groups generate few if any charges beyond the first year after injury. Since the total for follow-on charges depends heavily on patient age and life expectancy—with older people generating smaller charges—total direct costs for a chronically injured patient will be inversely proportional to the person's age at injury. (It was impossible to disaggregate the input cost data by age for MAIS 4 and 5 patients and, therefore, impossible to measure whether *component costs* were greater for older people, as they were in the case of MAIS 1, 2, and 3 patients. Even if this were the case, however, we do not believe that this factor alone would reverse the general trend of lower direct costs for progressively older patients.)

Total Direct Costs of Nonfatalities. Multiplying the cost estimates in table 6–19 by the corresponding number of patients in each incidence category yields estimates of total direct costs for patients in each category. Summing these costs over the various categories gives an estimate of the present value of total direct costs for all nonfatalities in the incidence population (table 6–20). (Litigation and court costs associated with motor vehicle injuries are considered separately in the next section.)

Because of the large number of minor and moderate injuries that occur in any given year (89 percent of total nonfatal incidence in 1975), MAIS 1 and MAIS 2 cases account for a substantial portion of total direct costs. In 1975 they contributed $1.290 billion, or 34 percent, of a $3.843 billion total, despite the comparatively low values determined for per-capita costs in those groups. MAIS 3 patients accounted for $0.775 billion of total costs (20 percent); MAIS 4 patients, $0.581 billion (15 percent); and MAIS 5 patients, who constitute only 0.7 percent of the incidence population but generate extremely large per-capita costs, an astounding $1.197 billion (31 percent). Within the MAIS 5 group, spinal cord injuries had a disproportionate influence on costs. Of the $1.197 billion in direct costs generated, SCI patients accounted for 26 percent of this figure while comprising slightly less than 10 percent of the MAIS 5 incidence population.

The age- and sex-related split of total direct costs is also revealing. The distribution of costs accords broadly with the incidence distribution. The 15 to 24 age group again predominates, contributing over 40 percent of total costs (and 39 percent of total incidence). Men supersede women both in their incidence of injury and in their generation of costs, accounting for 64 percent of total costs and 56 percent of total incidence. People 65 years of age and older account for approximatly 8 percent of total direct costs while constituting only 5 percent of the nonfatal incidence population. This disproportion is not surprising, given the significantly higher per-capita costs estimated for elderly patients in the MAIS 1, 2, and 3 groups.

At 4.5 percent of all other treatment-related direct costs, insurance

Table 6-20
Present Value of Total Direct Costs of Motor Vehicle Nonfatalities, by Age, Sex, and Injury-Severity Group, United States, 1975
(Thousands of Dollars)

Age and Sex Group	MAIS 1	MAIS 2	MAIS 3	MAIS 4	MAIS 5 Non-SCI Patients	MAIS 5 SCI Patients	Total Direct Costs
Males							
0–14	39,925	31,913	42,166	17,635	95,259	5,075	231,973
15–24	130,049	162,476	170,963	174,499	336,271	113,646	1,087,904
25–34	65,200	76,573	83,043	100,794	62,643	49,347	437,600
35–44	29,623	32,638	52,054	40,048	71,686	23,373	249,422
45–54	23,584	31,049	38,128	27,268	33,249	19,604	172,882
55–64	15,757	20,875	30,069	19,596	33,769	12,476	132,542
65–74	13,731	26,715	27,448	9,740	12,126	4,199	93,959
75+	6,271	12,199	12,533	4,318	4,733	1,727	41,781
Subtotal	324,140	394,438	456,404	393,898	649,736	229,447	2,448,063
Females							
0–14	34,980	25,731	17,026	21,802	23,157	8,999	131,695
15–24	91,378	108,839	81,936	57,404	102,435	39,064	481,056
25–34	49,052	48,643	43,126	35,239	47,642	11,370	235,072
35–44	26,141	31,417	37,820	19,020	35,764	6,101	156,263
45–54	23,117	33,399	31,833	23,772	14,915	6,414	133,450
55–64	16,772	20,778	35,119	11,660	11,680	4,806	100,815
65–74	13,338	26,070	46,498	11,842	2,305	1,253	101,306
75+	7,272	14,214	25,351	6,235	1,001	730	54,803
Subtotal	262,050	309,091	318,709	186,974	238,899	78,737	1,394,460
Total nonfatalities	586,190	703,529	775,113	580,872	888,635	308,184	3,842,523

Note: All costs are in 1975 dollars, discounted at 6 percent.

administration expenses are estimated at $165.5 million of a $3.843 billion total for nonfatal injuries in 1975.

Faigin (1976) estimates average direct costs per patient by injury-severity group.[38] Although her methodology and data sources differ in several respects from our own, her results are of interest, especially since they imply differences in the estimate of total direct costs. The following chart compares her estimates with ours:

Injury-Severity Group	Average Direct Costs per Capita	
	Faigin (1976)	*Present Analysis*
MAIS 1	$ 128	$ 192
MAIS 2	650	1,001
MAIS 3	1,665	2,192
MAIS 4	7,520	6,657
MAIS 5	17,425	41,829

With the exception of the MAIS 4 severity group, Faigin's values in each instance are lower than ours. This highlights what we feel is a significant underestimation on Faigin's part of follow-on care costs for MAIS 5 patients, of hospitalization and professional costs during the first year for MAIS 2 patients, and of hospitalization and outpatient costs for MAIS 3 patients. As for fatalities, no component was included in her analysis to account for insurance administration expenses. Faigin's values together with our nonfatal incidence estimates produce $2.591 billion in direct expenditures for non-fatalities, $1.252 billion lower than our total estimate of $3.843 billion.

Legal and Court Costs

In addition to health resources necessary to care for fatal and nonfatal injuries, motor vehicle crashes may result in the consumption of valuable legal resources. Legal action owing to crash sequelae causes the diversion of resources that could be channeled into resolving other problems. The economic loss equals the opportunity cost of the time and materials devoted to the legal proceedings. In order to assess this cost, we must (1) identify the legal resources that crashes consume, (2) determine how best to measure them, (3) estimate the proportion of crashes that actually involve legal action, and (4) combine the results in order to estimate both average costs per case and total economic costs owing to legal action. Our focus is the legal costs related to motor vehicle injuries—not legal costs owing to motor vehicle property damage or non-injury-related traffic offenses—and then, only those costs not already included in health insurance administration charges.

A motor vehicle crash may result in either criminal or civil action, or both. The costs of civil action are determined by the stage of the legal process at which the case is terminated, ranging from retention of counsel with no suit filed to settlement in court. The resources consist of the time and services of the lawyers, judges, and legal and court personnel who process the case. A portion of the variable court overhead expenditures also must be included as resource costs. For civil cases, one must include the costs of plaintiff and defense attorneys and their support staffs; for criminal cases, the costs of prosecutors, defense attorneys, and their associated staffs apply. All criminal and some civil cases incur court costs.

To assess the legal and court costs of motor-vehicle-related litigation in 1975, one would ideally need to know the number of crashes or, equivalently, the number of injuries that result in civil and criminal cases and the average cost of processing such cases. Several studies have assessed different elements of legal and court costs. The U.S. Department of Transportation 1970) assessed the legal and court costs of civil cases involving serious injuries and fatalities to be $831.8 million in 1968. This total includes $470 million for plaintiff attorneys' fees and expenses, $230 million for defense attorneys, and $131.8 million for state and federal court costs.[39] Wuerdemann and Joksch (1973) estimated that criminal court costs in state and local courts during 1969 amounted to $100 million to $150 million, with an additional $2 million to $7 million for prosecutors' fees.[40] Unfortunately, they made no estimates for defense attorneys.

We have distinguished between legal costs for cases involving less severe injuries (MAIS 1, 2, and 3 cases) and those involving more severe injuries (MAIS 4 and 5 cases and fatalities). We have assumed that, in general, civil and criminal cases involving progressively more serious injuries are more time- and resource-consuming and therefore more costly. Although the time spent processing a case also may be influenced by factors unconnected with the severity of the injury, we assume that they have minimal effect on the average legal resources and, hence, average legal costs required per case.

The positive correlation assumed between injury severity and legal resources consumed is supported by several sources. The AIRAC Study (1979), which combined data collected cooperatively by twenty-nine major automobile insurance companies in the United States and a consumer survey of 60,000 households, found that insurance claimants with larger financial losses (and presumably, more severe injuries) were more likely to require the services of legal counsel than were those with smaller losses. The study found that only 16 percent of bodily injury claimants with financial losses less than $100 were represented by counsel, while 85 percent of the claimants with losses over $10,000 were similarly represented.[41] Practicing attorneys surveyed during the course of our study confirmed that in civil cases, suits for larger sums of money are normally made for the more severe injuries. The lawyers also felt that the financial size of the suit (and hence, the severity of the injury) and the time spent on pleading, interrogation, depositions, and investigatory work were positively related.

To help ascertain the average legal and court costs of a motor vehicle injury case, we developed a simple, yet complete, model of the legal process distinguishing between civil and criminal actions. In the case of civil action, an individual injured in a motor vehicle crash may or may not initiate legal action. If he chooses to do nothing, no legal costs are generated. However, if he chooses to enter into litigation, we assume that legal counsel will be necessary. The crash victim and his attorney then have three alternatives: (1) do not file suit, (2) file suit but settle out of court, or (3) file suit and settle in court. If the first alternative is chosen, the legal costs are the basic attorney's fee, which we estimate to be $300 in 1975.[42] In the second case, legal counsel adopts the plaintiff attorney's role and charges, on average, $750 to $8045 depending on the severity of the injury.[43] Additional fees for a defense attorney to defend the individual being sued will average $815 for a MAIS 1, 2, or 3 nonfatality and $1485 for a more severe motor vehicle injury.[44] The final scenario, where the case is settled in court, adds extensive court costs ranging from $2415 for a MAIS 1, 2, or 3 up to $4830 for a fatality or MAIS 4 or 5.

When criminal charges are filed, the full legal process is intitated. The defendant, who normally is a driver of one of the motor vehicles involved in the crash (and occasionally one of the injured parties as well), must retain legal counsel. We estimated the cost of defense counsel in criminal action to be approximately $100 in cases relating to MAIS 1, 2, or 3 injuries and $500 in cases relating to MAIS 4 or 5 injuries or fatalities. Based on Wuerdemann and Joksch, the cost of prosecutors' time was estimated to be $65 for cases involving a MAIS 1, 2, or 3 nonfatality and up to $140 for cases involving more severe injuries.[46] Court costs in criminal cases were $45 for a MAIS 1, 2, or 3 nonfatality and $100 for a fatality or a MAIS 4 or 5 nonfatality.[47] Although we feel the estimates of Wuerdemann and Joksch concerning the costs of criminal litigation are unusually conservative, we used them to help minimize double counting. (According to the U.S. Departments of Justice and Commerce, in *Expenditure and Employment Data for the Criminal Justice System, 1975*, court costs are usually impossible to segregate by classification as "civil" or "criminal." Some double counting is thus inevitable.)

Table 6–21 summarizes the legal and court costs per case for motor vehicle injuries that result in civil or criminal action. These costs, however, are conditioned on the injury case leading to a particular form of legal action. To extrapolate to all injury cases, we must first ascertain the proportion of those cases actually involved in legal action. Data from Faigin (1976) and the Department of Transportation (1970) allowed us to estimate the proportion of the motor vehicle injured who retained counsel in civil actions. By

Table 6–21
Legal and Court Costs per Case for Motor Vehicle Injuries Involving Legal Action
(Dollars)

Injury-Severity Group	Civil Action				Criminal Action		
	Cost of Legal Counsel (No suit filed)	Cost of Plaintiff Attorney[a] (Suit filed)	Cost of Defense Attorney (Suit filed)	Court Costs (Suit Filed and In-Court settlement)	Cost of Prosecutor's Time	Cost of Defense Attorney	Court Costs
MAIS 1	300	740	815	2415	65	100	45
MAIS 2	300	1080	815	2415	65	100	45
MAIS 3	300	2380	815	2415	65	100	45
MAIS 4	300	2400	1485	4830	140	500	100
MAIS 5	300	5260	1485	4830	140	500	100
Fatality	300	8045	1485	4830	140	500	100

Note: All costs are in 1975 dollars. Costs for each service (plaintiff attorney, defense attorney, court costs, and so forth) are conditioned on the service being required and utilized; for example, court costs in civil actions apply only to cases in which a suit is settled in court.
[a] Abstracted from data in Faigin (1976, p. 20, Table 42).

injury-severity group, those proportions are MAIS 1 and 2, 4.8 percent; MAIS 3, 19.2 percent; MAIS 4 and 5, 26.5 percent; and fatalities, 34.5 percent.[48] From this information and additional results in Faigin's study, we computed the proportion of MVI cases who retained legal counsel but did not file suit, the proportion who retained counsel and filed suit but settled out of court, and the proportion who retained counsel, filed suit, and settled in court:[49]

| | Percentage Retaining Counsel | | |
Injury-Severity Group	But Not Filing Suit	Filing Suit but Settling Out of Court	Filing Suit and Settling in Court
MAIS 1 and 2	1.4	3.0	0.4
MAIS 3	5.1	12.3	1.8
MAIS 4 and 5	7.0	17.0	2.5
Fatality	9.1	22.1	3.3

The AIRAC (1979) Study estimated that 20 percent of bodily injury liability claims involved an attorney and 1.5 percent of these claims went to trial to reach settlement.[50] Depending on the injury-severity group, we estimate that from 4.8 to 34.5 percent of the people suffering motor vehicle injuries in 1975 retained attorneys pending civil action and from 0.4 to 3.3 percent required an in-court settlement of their civil suits. If we compute a weighted average of these results, however, we find that only 7 percent of the entire incidence population retained legal counsel and only 0.6 percent processed civil suits that required a trial or other in-court settlement. The apparent discrepancies between our percentages and those of the AIRAC Study may lie in the fact that MAIS 1 and 2 injury cases, which have a small likelihood of retaining counsel, constitute a substantial portion of the overall incidence population (approximately 90 percent) but may comprise only a small portion of the bodily injury claims surveyed in the AIRAC Study. If we exclude the MAIS 1 and 2 cases from our global sample, our results are consistent with those of the AIRAC investigators. We then find that approximately 22 percent of the fatalities and remaining nonfatalities retain legal counsel and 2 percent require in-court settlement of their suits.

In civil action, an injured person either retains legal counsel, in which case costs are generated at one of three possible stages in the legal process, or does not retain counsel and hence has no legal or court costs. As an example, we estimate that 73.5 percent of the MAIS 5 incidence group did not retain counsel and therefore, did not produce legal and court costs related to civil proceedings. For the 26.5 percent that took legal action, we expect that 7 percent retained counsel but did not file suit (stage 1), 17 percent filed suit and settled out of court (stage 2), and only 2.5 percent filed suit and required an in-court settlement (stage 3). Multiplying each percentage by the average legal and court costs for that stage (see table 6–21) and summing the products gives $1460 [that is, $0.7 \times \$300 + 0.17 \times (\$5260 + \$1485) + 0.025 \times (\$5260 + \$1485 + \$4830)$] as the average legal and court costs related to civil proceedings for a MAIS 5 injury case. Similar calculations for the other injury-severity groups are displayed below:

Injury-Severity Group	Average Cost for Civil Action per Injury Case
MAIS 1	$ 70
MAIS 2	80
MAIS 3	510
MAIS 4	900
MAIS 5	1460
Fatality	2600

Average costs of criminal action were calculated similarly. It was assumed that all three cost elements (the opportunity costs of prosecutors' time, the cost of defense attorneys, and court costs) would apply to each case involving legal action, since by law any person charged with a criminal offense has a right to counsel and, usually, the right to in-court adjudication of his alleged offense. We estimated that the average costs of criminal legal action were $210 for MAIS 1, 2, and 3 nonfatalities and $740 for MAIS 4 and 5 nonfatalities and fatalities (table 6–21). Multiplying these by the percentage of cases leading to criminal action (approximately 17.7 percent for MAIS 1, 2, and 3 nonfatalities and 21.8 percent for MAIS 4 and 5 nonfatalities and fatalities) yields an average cost per injury case of $40 and $160 for these two groups.[51]

Table 6–22
Legal and Court Costs Associated with Motor Vehicle Injuries, United States, 1975

Injury-Severity Group	Cost per Injury Case			Total Incidence	Total Costs (Thousands of Dollars)
	Civil Action	Criminal Action	Total Legal and Court		
MAIS 1	$ 70	$ 40	$ 110	3,053,035	$335,834
MAIS 2	80	40	120	702,923	84,351
MAIS 3	510	40	550	353,569	194,463
MAIS 4	900	160	1,060	87,262	92,498
MAIS 5	1,460	160	1,620	28,611	46,350
Fatality	2,600	160	2,760	44,995	124,186
All injury cases	160	45	205	4,270,395	877,682

Note: All costs are in 1975 dollars.

Combining the average litigation costs per case for civil and criminal action gives us the average legal and court costs associated with motor vehicle fatalities and nonfatalities in 1975. These costs are summarized by injury-severity group in column 4 of table 6–22. Multiplying the per-case costs by the aggregate incidence data in column 5 and summing across injury groups yields total legal and court costs. We estimate that in 1975 approximately $877.7 million was expended to settle legal action resulting from injuries occurring in motor vehicle crashes. (We implicitly assume for our analysis that all legal and court costs occur in the first year after injury and thus do not require discounting.) Although they account for only 1 percent of total incidence, fatalities contributed $124.2 million, or 14 percent of all legal and court costs. Of the $753.5 million in legal costs owing to nonfatalities, over 50 percent was generated by MAIS 1 cases.

Indirect Costs of Motor Vehicle Injuries

Fatalities

As for the three diseases we discuss in this book, the largest portion of total economic costs for motor vehicle injuries is the lost productivity owing to premature death or injury-related disability. For motor vehicle fatalities, the enormity of this productivity loss—measured in terms of forgone earnings— vastly overshadows their direct costs. It serves as an unambiguous example of the relative importance of indirect costs in the economic evaluation of the consequences of health impairments.

Because fatalities have no earnings expectations after injury, their forgone earnings are equivalent to the expected earnings of demographically matched, but uninjured persons in the general population. (In this respect, the per-person earnings loss of a motor vehicle fatality is no different than the corresponding loss of an age- and sex-matched sudden death or fatal myocardial infarction (MI) owing to coronary heart disease.) Estimates of forgone earnings per fatality broken down by age and sex are presented in the third column of table 6–23. Multiplying these values by the corresponding fatal incidence figures in the second column and summing over incidence categories, we obtain a staggering $7.052 billion as the estimate of total forgone earnings resulting from motor vehicle fatalities in 1975. This indicates an average loss of approximately $156,700 for each of the 44,995 fatalities in that year.

It is clear from the table that men suffer greater forgone earnings per person than women of the same age, reflecting the significant discrepancies in wage levels between the sexes. This factor coupled with the disproportionate representation of men in the incidence population (73.5 percent of all

Table 6–23
Present Value of Total Forgone Earnings of Motor Vehicle Fatalities,
by Age and Sex, United States, 1975

Age and Sex Group	Incidence	Average Forgone Earnings per Fatality (Dollars)	Total Forgone Earnings (Millions of Dollars)
Males			
0–14	2,890	130,863	378.2
15–24	12,250	225,992	2,768.4
25–34	6,017	247,881	1,491.5
35–44	3,203	205,687	658.8
45–54	2,907	135,972	395.3
55–64	2,368	52,199	123.6
65–74	1,852	5,754	10.7
75+	1,539	533	0.8
All males	33,026	176,445	5,827.3
Females			
0–14	1,674	92,241	154.4
15–24	3,451	156,059	538.7
25–34	1,604	153,131	245.6
35–44	1,052	126,642	133.2
45–54	1,090	87,150	95.0
55–64	1,083	39,950	43.2
65–74	1,081	11,682	12.6
75+	934	2,556	2.4
All females	11,969	102,366	1,225.1
Total fatalities	44,995	156,739	7,052.4

Note: Forgone earnings are expressed in 1975 dollars, discounted at 6 percent.

fatalities) makes them account for 83 percent of total earnings. Moreover, men between the ages of 15 and 24 generate close to 40 percent of all forgone earnings, and men between 15 and 44 account for fully 70 percent of the total. This underscores the high loss per capita experienced by adolescents and young men in these age groups and the comparatively high motor vehicle fatality rates that they suffered.

Nonfatalities

The lost productivity of motor vehicle nonfatalities may take either of two general forms. The first derives from absence from work or homemaking activities owing to *temporary* disability caused by the injury. As we explained in chapter 2, this loss normally is measured in terms of the number of days during which an individual's activity is sufficiently restricted (because of hospitalization, other medical attention, bed rest, or general lassitude) so that he is unable to perform his primary vocational role. This form of disability is limited and usually concludes well before the end of the first year following injury. We feel that patients in MAIS 1 through 4 groups experience varying levels of temporary disability and account for commensurate amounts of lost productivity.

The second form of lost productivity is more typical of MAIS 5 patients. It is characterized by *permanent* disability that prevents individuals from performing most or all of their work-related functions. In most critical trauma cases, lost productivity resulting from permanent disability is expected to accrue for several years after injury and, in the absence of sufficient vocational and physical rehabilitation, for the remainder of the individual's life. Even if the individual returns to work or homemaking tasks, some loss in productivity may still occur because of (1) reduced performance levels while on the job and (2) reductions in life expectancy induced by injury-related complications. As in the case of fatalities, both forms of forgone productivity are measured in terms of forgone earnings.

Forgone Earnings per Person of MAIS 1 through 4 Cases. As we mentioned in chapter 2, the most general classification of temporary disability employed by the National Center for Health Statistics is the *day of restricted activity*. This is defined as a day on which a person substantially reduces his or her amount of normal activity because of a specific disease or injury. Although complete inactivity is not always presumed, a person experiencing a day of restricted activity is normally incapable of carrying out his or her role as a worker or homemaker. Therefore, if we multiply the average number of days of restricted activity experienced by an injured person by the average value of each of those days (measured as forgone earnings), we obtain a rough estimate of the average loss in earnings and productivity owing to that temporary disability.

We assume that nonfatalities in the MAIS 1, 2, 3, and 4 severity groups experience days of restricted activity during the first year. (We implicitly assume that no days of restricted activity will be experienced by MAIS 3 and 4 patients during the second of subsequent years after the injury, despite the outpatient care and rehabilitation services they may demand. We feel that the scheduling of clinical services will be sufficiently well integrated into a patient's daily routine at that time that no reduction in productive activities will occur.) From NCSS data on (1) the number of days spent in the hospital, (2) the number of days of bed rest (outside the hospital), and (3) the number of days of "other restricted activity" (period when the use of cast, crutches, braces, or walker are required), we can estimate the number of days of restricted activity during the first year for MAIS 1 through 4 injury groups. Averages derived from these data are presented in table 6–24. Because of the

Table 6-24
Average Number of Days of Restricted Activity per Case, by Injury-Severity Group and Age

Injury-Severity Group	Hospital Days per Case		Bed-Rest Days per Case		Days of Other Restricted Activity per Case		Total Days of Restricted Activity per Case[a]	
	<65 Years	≥65 Years	<65 Years	≥65 Years	<65 Years	≥65 Years	<65 Years	≥65 Years
MAIS 1	0.2	0.8	0.8	1.1	1.1	0.8	1.9	2.5
MAIS 2	2.4	7.3	2.4	11.9	9.9	16.3	12.7	32.2
MAIS 3	10.0	13.0	6.9	16.4	32.7	41.6	43.1	62.7
MAIS 4	19.6	32.0	21.5	21.5	84.3	109.5	108.5	141.1

Source: Derived from data in the NCSS file of May 1980.

[a]Derived by summing hospital days, bed-rest days, and (0.8 × days of other restricted activity).

manner in which the latter two pieces of data were collected, double counting may exist. We compensate for this by assuming that 20 percent of the days of "other restricted activity" are also days of nonhospitalized bed rest. With this proviso, the actual number of days of restricted activity per case may be estimated using the formula

Number of days of = Number of hospital days + number of bed-rest days
restricted activity   + 0.8 × number of days of other restricted activity

We estimated the value of a day of restricted activity (VDR) as

$$VDR = \frac{Y_s(n) \cdot E_s(n)}{365}$$

where $Y_s(n)$ = mean average earnings of employed people and homemakers in the general population of age n and sex s measured at incidence-year 1975 levels

$E_s(n)$ = proportion of the general population of age n and sex s employed in the labor force or engaged in housekeeping tasks

Estimates of the value of a day of restricted activity by age and sex were presented in chapter 2. There we saw that, as in the case of fatalities, men have a higher value placed on their productive activity than women of the same age because of the current wage differentials existing between the sexes. In addition, for each sex, people aged 25 to 54 have the greatest value per day. For men in that age group, the average value of a day of restricted activity in 1975 is estimated between $37 and $44; for women, the average value of a day is $25 to $26.

To determine the average individual's forgone earnings, we simply multiply the estimate of the average number of days of restricted activity by the value of a day of restricted activity. Estimates of average forgone earnings for patients in severity groups MAIS 1 through MAIS 4 are presented in table 6–25. As we might anticipate, the amount of forgone earnings varies directly with injury severity. Within severity groups, men aged 25 to 54 have the highest average forgone earnings because of the higher value placed on a day of restricted activity for these men compared with per-diem values for individuals in other age and sex groups.

Forgone Earnings per Person of MAIS 5 Cases. Estimating the present value of forgone earnings for MAIS 5 patients is more complex. Unlike the less severely injured patients, the period of disability, and hence of forgone earnings, frequently lasts beyond the first year after injury. In contrast to

Table 6–25
Forgone Earnings per Person, by Age and Sex, for MAIS 1 through 4
Injury-Severity Groups, United States, 1975
(Dollars)

Age and Sex Group	Injury-Severity Group			
	MAIS 1	*MAIS 2*	*MAIS 3*	*MAIS 4*
Males				
0–14	0	0	0	0
15–24	26	173	588	1481
25–34	70	465	1578	3972
35–44	83	554	1879	4731
45–54	79	528	1793	4513
55–64	57	383	1298	3268
65–74	16	207	402	905
75+	2	23	45	102
All males	42	291	1006	2660
Females				
0–14	0	0	0	0
15–24	23	155	526	1324
25–34	49	324	1100	2770
35–44	49	326	1107	2786
45–54	47	311	1056	2660
55–64	32	213	724	1821
65–74	17	223	435	979
75+	5	66	128	287
All females	30	211	706	1733
All nonfatalities	36	256	887	2362

Note: Forgone earnings expressed in 1975 dollars.

fatalities, however, MAIS 5 patients may return to a paid job or homemaking role and thus recoup earnings that might otherwise be lost. To manage these complicating aspects, we have separated the MAIS 5 group into spinal-cord-injured and non-spinal-cord-injured patients. As for the analysis of direct costs, we show how our estimate of lost productivity for SCI patients may be extended to apply to non-SCI patients.

To estimate the forgone earnings of spinal cord patients, we make direct use of the methodology of Smart and Sanders (1976). Their approach involves the estimation of the expected earnings of an SCI patient following injury. This, in turn, requires an estimation of the reemployment rates for patients with different types of spinal cord impairments.

Smart and Sanders estimated the likelihood of an SCI patient returning to a paid job or homemaking role from data on the postdischarge status of patients treated at foreign and domestic spinal cord treatment centers. The values represent the percentage of persons in each SCI impairment category who return to work, to homemaking roles, or to educational and training programs presumably leading to employment. Smart and Sanders estimated "employment" rates following discharge and rehabilitation for each of the four major impairment categories: incomplete paraplegics, 66 percent; complete paraplegics, 61 percent; incomplete quadriplegics, 55 percent; and complete quadriplegics, 33 percent.[52] We used these rates to calculate the expected postmorbid earnings of an SCI patient. Subtracting these earnings from the earnings expectation had there been no injury (which corresponds to the average forgone earnings for fatalities of similar age and sex in table 6–3) gives the average forgone earnings per person resulting from injury.

This postmorbid earnings model assumes that

1. SCI patients who return to employment, school, or housekeeping tasks do so approximately 2 years after injury.
2. A patient's *future* employment rate (or likelihood of remaining employed in future years) is constant over time and equal to his original chance of returning to employment, school, or homemaking tasks following injury. (The only exception is when the employment rate for people of the same age and sex in the general population is less than that proposed for the patient; in this case, the employment rate is lowered to conform with the rate applicable to the general population.)
3. The mean earnings of employed SCI patients are roughly equal to the mean earnings of their counterparts in the general population of similar age and sex.

Each of these assumptions is a first approximation of the actual employment situation facing SCI patients. The second and third assumptions are optimistic, but permit us to set an upper limit to postmorbid earnings and thus to estimate conservatively forgone earnings.

The present value of the expected postmorbid earnings of an SCI patient surviving at least 1 year past injury (*PVPM*) is now modeled as

$$PVPM = \sum_{n=l+2}^{85} P_{l+1,s}^i(n) \cdot Y_s(n) \cdot E^i \left(\frac{1+\gamma}{1+r}\right)^{n-l}$$

where $P_{l+1,s}^i(n)$ = probability of a MAIS 5 SCI patient of impairment type i and sex s surviving to age n given injury occurrence at age l and survival for at least 1 year past injury

E^i = proportion of the SCI population with impairment type i that is employed, in school, or engaged in housekeeping tasks and all other parameters are as defined in chapter 2. Unlike analogous parameters in earnings models for cancer, heart disease, and stroke, the value of parameter E^i does not reflect an employment rate relative to that of an injury-free population but rather an absolute employment rate specific to the SCI-impaired group. (The consequences of using the value of this parameter as an approximation of the relative employment rate are considered later in the sensitivity analysis.) In line with the other models, the future earnings of SCI patients are expected to accrue over a significantly reduced lifespan.

The average forgone earnings owing to injury are summarized in table 6–26 by age, sex, and impairment category. The table shows that incomplete paraplegics, because of their higher likelihood of reemployment and smaller reductions in life expectancy, experience the smallest amount of forgone earnings. For males, the range is approximately $325 to $94,600; for females, it is about $1485 to $60,690. Complete quadriplegics, however, experience forgone earnings that approach the large losses of fatalities. These extend from approximatly $575 to $194,700 for males and from $2600 to $116,120 for females. Except for people 65 and older, men forgo more earnings than women. For both sexes, individuals injured between the ages of 15 and 44 sustain greater losses than people of other ages.

A close examination of table 6–26 shows that the forgone earnings of an incomplete paraplegic have been assumed representative of the forgone earnings of a non-SCI MAIS 5 case of similar age and sex. The rationale for this assumption derives partially, although not exclusively, from the precedent set during the analysis of direct costs. There several of the cost-component values for non-SCI patients were obtained from multiples of corresponding values for incomplete paraplegics. To justify the exact correspondence postulated here, however, we recall that the relative mortality rate estimated for non-SCI MAIS 5 patients is assumed roughly the same as the relative mortality rate for incomplete paraplegics (RMR = 1.81). The stream of survival probabilities used in the preceding earnings model thus would be the same for both groups of patients. In addition, the reader may remember that the type of injury considered most prevalent among MAIS 5 patients is severe head injury with resulting neurological complications. Data from Dresser et al. (1973) on the employment prospects of Korean War veterans who suffered head injuries suggest that the likelihood of an individual returning to work, given that he experiences significant neurological damage and complications, is slightly over 60 percent.[53] Although this is not a random sample, the veterans' employment history supports our belief that the reemployment rate for non-SCI MAIS 5 patients is close to that for incomplete paraplegics (66 percent). This, in turn, further substantiates our claim that forgone earnings for incomplete paraplegics serve as a good approximation of forgone earnings for non-spinal-cord-injured MAIS 5 cases.

Table 6–26
Present Value of Forgone Earnings per Person, by Age and Sex,
for MAIS 5 Nonfatalities, United States, 1975
(Dollars)

Age and Sex Group	Non-SCI Patients[a]	SCI Patients			
		Para Incomplete	*Para Complete*	*Quad Incomplete*	*Quad Complete*
Males					
0–14	35,517	35,517	53,547	52,117	98,436
15–24	75,052	75,052	102,405	102,567	173,368
25–34	94,568	94,568	123,169	122,603	194,694
35–44	81,109	81,109	109,023	104,508	168,034
45–54	54,744	54,744	76,562	70,254	115,943
55–64	21,620	21,620	30,270	26,373	45,358
65–74	2,723	2,723	3,967	2,969	5,290
75+	326	326	468	352	577
All males	64,326	72,910	98,580	87,511	143,923
Females					
0–14	25,581	25,581	33,878	36,354	63,741
15–24	55,437	55,437	68,209	72,981	113,662
25–34	60,687	60,687	73,886	77,041	116,120
35–44	53,138	53,138	65,785	66,502	100,084
45–54	39,819	39,819	49,676	48,748	72,133
55–64	19,286	19,286	24,854	23,446	34,791
65–74	5,422	5,422	7,801	6,833	10,780
75+	1,485	1,485	2,019	1,755	2,619
All females	49,031	49,160	60,664	54,833	85,916
Total nonfatalities	60,340	65,353	86,486	81,295	133,103

Note: Forgone earnings expressed in 1975 dollars, discounted at 6 percent.
[a]Equal to corresponding forgone-earnings estimate for paraplegic incompletes.

Total Forgone Earnings of Nonfatalities. Multiplying the average forgone-earnings values shown in tables 6–25 and 6–26 by corresponding nonfatal incidence estimates gives us estimates of total forgone earnings by age, sex, and injury-severity category; summing these results yields total forgone earnings for all nonfatalities. Table 6–27 presents aggregate earnings estimates with a total of $2.609 billion for all nonfatalities injured in 1975.

The total implies average forgone earnings per person of only $618. This is misleading, given the wide range of averages for the individual injury-severity groups: from average forgone earnings of only $35 and $255 for MAIS 1 and 2 cases, respectively, the average values increase significantly for MAIS 3 ($885) and MAIS 4 ($2360) cases; for the MAIS 5 cases (representing nearly 69 percent of total forgone earnings), the result jumps to

Table 6-27
Present Value of Total Forgone Earnings of Motor Vehicle Nonfatalities, by Age, Sex, and Injury-Severity Group, United States, 1975
(Thousands of Dollars)

Age and Sex Group	MAIS 1	MAIS 2	MAIS 3	MAIS 4	MAIS 5 Non-SCI Patients	MAIS 5 SCI Patients	Total Forgone Earnings
Males							
0–14	0	0	0	0	90,533	2,156	92,689
15–24	18,034	29,721	48,520	38,234	698,580	97,606	930,695
25–34	24,244	37,560	63,196	59,733	170,505	50,276	405,514
35–44	13,121	19,070	47,188	28,705	179,818	23,140	311,042
45–54	9,964	17,304	32,967	19,058	62,573	15,208	157,074
55–64	4,821	8,425	18,829	10,200	28,754	4,366	75,395
65–74	739	3,080	3,321	1,499	1,517	215	10,321
75+	38	158	171	74	82	13	536
All males	70,961	115,318	214,192	157,453	1,232,362	192,980	1,983,226
Females							
0–14	0	0	0	0	15,553	2,478	18,031
15–24	11,323	17,791	20,779	11,171	152,506	22,641	236,211
25–34	12,721	16,640	22,889	14,452	80,167	7,997	154,866
35–44	6,817	10,808	20,186	7,934	55,582	4,155	105,482
45–54	5,756	10,970	16,221	9,628	18,794	3,172	64,541
55–64	2,860	4,674	12,255	3,311	7,965	1,186	32,251
65–74	777	3,252	6,086	1,866	515	130	12,626
75+	124	520	973	298	73	24	2,012
All females	40,378	64,655	99,389	48,660	331,157	41,781	626,020
Total nonfatalities	$111,339	$179,973	$313,581	$206,113	$1,563,518	$234,762	$2,609,286

Note: All costs are in 1975 dollars, discounted at 6 percent.

$62,850. Differences in underlying assumptions, methodological approaches, and sample data prevent a meaningful comparison of our estimates with those of Faigin (1976) and Marsh et al. (1977). However, even a cursory appraisal suggests that our estimates of average forgone earnings and, hence, total forgone earnings are conservative.

Like male fatalities, male nonfatalities account for over 75 percent of total forgone earnings, and young men between the ages of 15 and 24 account for 36 percent of the total. In fact, if the losses suffered by both young men and young women in the 15 to 24 age group are combined, they constitute 45 percent of total earnings losses. This serves as a vivid reminder of the harsh human and economic burden suffered by people of this age injured in motor vehicle crashes, and correspondingly by the nation.

Because the forgone earnings of nonfatalities are estimated conservatively, they do not exceed direct costs: total direct costs for nonfatalities ($3.843 billion) are substantially greater than corresponding earnings losses. This contrasts markedly with motor vehicle fatality cases, where the magnitude of lost earnings makes the proportional contribution of direct costs to total economic costs insignificant.

Summary and Sensitivity Analysis

Direct, Indirect, and Total Costs

Tables 6–28, 6–29, and 6–30 present a summary of the direct, indirect, and total economic costs of motor vehicle injuries incident in 1975. Table 6–28 displays a breakdown by age, sex, and fatal versus nonfatal status; table 6–29 presents costs disaggregated by age and sex alone; and table 6–30 presents a breakdown by injury severity type.

In table 6–28 we see that the ratio of direct to indirect costs is strikingly different for fatalities and nonfatalities. For fatalities, the vast majority of total costs is due to forgone earnings (98 percent). For nonfatalities, direct costs are more important, representing 64 percent of the total. This division between direct and indirect costs is, however, not uniform for the different nonfatal groups. While table 6–30 indicates that individuals in the four less severely injury groups (MAIS 1 through 4) provide $3.353 billion in direct costs (81 percent of their total costs) compared with only $0.811 billion in forgone earnings, the most severely injured nonfatalities (the MAIS 5 group) show an opposite relationship: forgone earnings account for the majority of their costs, with $1.798 billion (59 percent) of a $3.042 billion total. (This despite the fact that the contribution of MAIS 5 patients to total direct costs still outranks that of any other injury-severity group.) Combining the fatal and nonfatal groups, we observe that motor vehicle injuries, like cancer

Table 6-28
Total Costs of Motor Vehicle Injuries, by Age and Sex, United States, 1975
(Millions of Dollars)

Age and Sex Group	Fatalities			Nonfatalities			
	Direct Costs		Indirect Costs	Direct Costs		Indirect Costs	
	Treatment-Related[a]	Legal and Court	Forgone Earnings	Treatment-Related[a]	Legal and Court	Forgone Earnings	Total Costs
Males							
0–14	3.3	8.0	378.2	232.0	45.6	92.7	759.8
15–24	13.4	33.8	2,768.4	1,087.9	186.4	930.7	5,020.6
25–34	6.5	16.6	1,491.4	437.6	89.6	405.5	2,447.2
35–44	3.6	8.8	658.8	249.4	45.8	311.0	1,277.4
45–54	3.5	8.0	395.3	172.9	34.6	157.1	771.4
55–64	2.9	6.5	123.6	132.5	25.6	75.4	366.5
65–74	2.8	5.1	10.7	94.0	14.1	10.3	137.0
75+	2.5	4.2	0.8	41.8	6.5	0.5	56.3
All males	38.5	91.2	5,827.3	2,448.0	447.9	1,983.3	10,836.2
Females							
0–14	1.7	4.6	154.4	131.7	32.8	18.0	343.2
15–24	3.7	9.5	538.7	481.1	103.2	236.2	1,372.4
25–34	1.9	4.4	245.6	235.1	54.3	154.9	696.2
35–44	1.2	2.9	133.2	156.3	34.2	105.5	433.3
45–54	1.2	3.0	95.0	133.5	31.0	64.5	328.2
55–64	1.4	3.0	43.2	100.8	24.5	32.3	205.2
65–74	1.5	3.0	12.6	101.3	16.6	12.6	147.6
75+	1.5	2.6	2.4	54.8	9.0	2.0	72.3
All females	14.2	33.0	1,225.2	1,394.5	305.6	626.0	3,598.5
Total population	52.7	124.2	7,052.5	3,842.5	753.5	2,609.3	14,434.7

Note: All costs are in 1975 dollars, discounted at 6 percent.
[a]Includes insurance administration costs.

Table 6–29

Present Value of Direct, Indirect, and Total Costs of Motor Vehicle Injuries, by Age and Sex, United States, 1975

(Millions of Dollars)

Age and Sex Group	Direct Costs	Indirect Costs	Total Costs
Males			
0–14	288.9	470.9	759.8
15–24	1,321.5	3,699.1	5,202.6
25–34	550.3	1,896.9	2,447.2
35–44	307.6	969.8	1,277.4
45–54	219.0	552.4	771.4
55–64	167.5	199.0	366.5
65–74	116.0	21.0	137.0
75+	55.0	1.3	56.3
All males	3,025.6	7,810.6	10,836.2
Females			
0–14	170.8	172.4	343.2
15–24	597.5	774.9	1,372.4
25–34	295.7	400.5	696.2
35–44	194.6	238.7	433.3
45–54	168.7	159.5	328.2
55–64	129.7	75.5	205.2
65–74	122.4	25.2	147.6
75+	67.9	4.4	72.3
All females	1,747.3	1,851.2	3,598.5
Total population	4,772.9	9,661.8	14,434.7

Note: All costs are in 1975 dollars, discounted at 6 percent.

Table 6–30

Direct, Indirect, and Total Costs of Motor Vehicle Injuries, by Severity Group

(Millions of Dollars)

Injury-Severity Group	Direct Costs	Indirect Costs	Total Costs
MAIS 1	922.0	111.4	1,033.4
MAIS 2	787.8	180.0	967.8
MAIS 3	969.6	313.6	1,283.2
MAIS 4	673.4	206.1	879.5
MAIS 5	1,243.2	1,798.3	3,041.5
Fatality	176.9	7,052.5	7,229.4
All MVI	4,772.9	9,661.8	14,434.7

Note: All costs in 1975 dollars, discounted at 6 percent.

cases, have substantial total direct costs ($4.773 billion), but that these are eclipsed by total indirect costs ($9.662 billion).

The age by sex breakdown of economic costs reveals the disproportionate burden placed on younger people as a result of crash-related sequelae. The 15 to 24 age group, which represented only 19 percent of the national population in 1975, comprised 39 percent of the MVI incidence population and accounted for 45 percent of total economic costs. Male adolescents and young men in this age group alone generated over one-third of total costs, even though they represented just one-tenth of the national population. In fact, male fatalities of that age, who comprised a mere 0.3 percent of total MVI incidence, accounted for approximately 29 percent of forgone earnings and 20 percent of all costs associated with motor vehicle crashes.

Although it is difficult to single out which factors are the most important in interpreting the various aftereffects of a disease or injury, certain factors are more obvious than others when evaluating the economic consequences of motor vehicle injuries. In addition to the disproportionate effects on younger people and, in particular, younger men mentioned earlier, men, in general, bear more of the economic costs related to crashes than women. Their large representation in the incidence population (63 percent) and the current wage structure that values the productivity of men more than that of women helps to explain why men account for fully 80 percent of all forgone earnings and 75 percent of all costs.

Certain classes of injuries have more disastrous human and economic effects than others. This is best demonstrated by fatalities and MAIS 5 nonfatalities, which represent the most critical of all MVI cases. Together these two subgroups comprise but 73,600 cases out of a total incidence of 4,270,400 in 1975. However, they account for over 70 percent of total MVI costs, with fatalities (45,000 cases) alone being responsible for half of all costs. The unusual influence that fatalities have on MVI costs is a good example of the important role that indirect costs play in determining the overall economic effects of any health impairment.

Sensitivity Analysis

We acknowledge, as for cancer, coronary heart disease, and stroke, the possibility of inaccuracies in our economic analysis of motor vehicle injuries. The multitude of data sources and the variety of assumptions necessary to complete the analysis suggest that certain elements of imprecision may exist. We address five major sources of potential error through sensitivity analyses covering incidence, mortality, direct costs, discounting, and indirect costs.

Incidence. Because of the manner in which we have estimated total economic costs resulting from motor vehicle injuries, one of the most important variables entering our calculations is the estimate of total incidence. In 1975, we estimated that 44,995 persons died in motor vehicle crashes. Data from the Fatal Accident Reporting System (FARS) adjusted by 1 percent to account for those fatalities succumbing more than 30 days but less than 1 year after injury served as our primary data base. Since the FARS data are most carefully gathered, we feel that any error in the incidence of fatalities is attributable to our adjustment factor of 1 percent. If this adjustment were, in fact, unnecessary (that is, virtually no fatalities in 1975 actually survived more than 30 days), we would have overestimated costs resulting from fatalities by approximately $70 million. This represents only a 0.5 percent error in our estimate of total costs.

A much more serious source of potential error exists in our estimation of the total incidence of nonfatalities. Recall that we chose to base our incidence estimate on data gathered by the National Center for Health Statistics, although three other possible, albeit less reliable, data sources existed. The range of conflicting estimates extended from 1,800,000 nonfatal cases (National Safety Council) to 2,810,000 cases (Federal Highway Administration) to 4,225,400 cases (NCHS) and finally, to 4,987,000 cases (Insurance Information Institute). It would be straightforward to calculate the impact of an error in nonfatal incidence on total costs if those costs were underestimated or overestimated in direct proportion to the error in incidence estimation. This, however, is not the case. Our estimate of the incidence of MAIS 5 SCI patients is independent of the nonfatality total and is considered to be quite accurate. Since SCI patients account for a proportion of economic costs that vastly exceeds their proportion of total incidence, the resulting errors in total costs as a result of an error in total incidence are less severe than might be expected.

If the incidence totals from the four data sources are each disaggregated by age, sex, and injury-severity level according to the guidelines of our analysis, and if per-patient costs remain unchanged, the total costs of nonfatalities would vary as follows:

Data Source	Total Costs of Nonfatalities (in $000,000)
National Safety Council	$4077
Federal Highway Administration	5380
NCHS (base case)	7205
Insurance Information Institute	8187

This indicates a possible range of estimates from 43 percent below to 14 percent above our base-case estimate. If the costs of fatalities (which are judged to be relatively insensitive to errors in incidence) are included, the range of errors in total costs is reduced dramatically—from 22 percent below to 7 percent above our initial results. If, for instance, the Federal Highway Administration's estimate of total nonfatalities were correct, the total costs of motor vehicle injuries would be $12.609 billion versus our estimate of $14.435 billion. This would represent an overestimation on our part of roughly $1.826 billion, or 13 percent.

Mortality. In our mortality analysis, we arrived at an injured person's survival expectations through the implementation of the relative-mortality-rate (RMR) concept. (Recall that an RMR of 1.00 indicates no excess mortality owing to injury and suggests a normal life expectancy.) Our estimated RMR of 1.00 for MAIS 1 through 4 patients is considered to be reasonably accurate. Without evidence to the contrary, we judge that Geisler's (1977) estimated RMRs for spinal cord patients (used in our analysis) are also accurate. We acknowledge, however, that the RMR of 1.81 applied to non-SCI MAIS 5 patients may be in error because of the relatively subjective process used to estimate it. An argument could be made tha the average RMR for such patients lies somewhere between a lower bound of 1.00 and an upper bound of 3.00. To test the sensitivity of total costs of these patients to the assigned RMR, we recomputed costs assuming a RMR of 1.00, 3.00, and 2.23 (same as that for an incomplete quadriplegic). The results are summarized below:

RMR	Direct Costs ($000,000)	Indirect Costs ($000,000)	Total Costs ($000,000)
1.00	$962	$1449	$2411
1.81 (base case)	931	1564	2495
2.23	918	1621	2539
3.00	894	1726	2620

Notice that direct and indirect costs move in opposite directions as the RMR is increased and then decreased in value. The net result is that the total costs of non-SCI MAIS 5 cases could vary from 3 percent below to 6 percent above our initial cost estimate. The effect on the total costs of all motor vehicle injuries is, of course, far less.

A sensitivity analysis also was performed on the implicit assumption that the RMR of non-SCI MAIS 5 patients remained at its initially higher level during each succeeding year past injury. The analysis indicated that even in the extreme situation where the RMR is assumed to return to 1.00 shortly after injury, total costs associated with this patient group would change by, at most, 3 percent. In general, total-cost estimates appear relatively insensitive to the precise choice of an RMR for injury cases in this group.

Direct Costs. We feel that large errors in the estimates of treatment costs of fatalities are possible. Potential sources of error exist in the estimation of the various cost parameters, any of which could be in error by a significant margin. In particular, our method of dividing fatalities into three "treatment" classes (DOAs, deaths in the emergency room, and deaths inhospital) is subject to reassessment. However, if any one of the treatment-related parameters or modeling assumptions is altered in such a way that all possible contingencies are taken into account, treatment costs of fatalities vary by, at most, 100 percent. Although a large proportional error, this translates into an absolute error of only $50 million and causes but a 0.3 percent adjustment in total economic costs.

Since nonfatalities generate about 99 percent of all treatment costs attributed to motor vehicle injuries, they require very close and detailed analysis. Possible errors in three major sets of cost components were considered: (1) those relating to emergency services, (2) those relating to hospitalization, and (3) those relating to physician and surgeon services. We also performed a sensitivity analysis on the assumption that the future costs of MAIS 5 non-SCI patients are proportional to those of a paraplegic incomplete.

Our analysis indicated that potential errors in the emergency-services components resulted in insignificant changes in total direct costs, but that errors in the hospital and physician/surgeon components could have significant cost effects. We judged that, on average, a 20 percent error was possible in the hospital length-of-stay estimates for MAIS 1 through 5 patients (excluding the spinal-cord-injured); in the extreme, this would mean an error of $480 million, or 10 percent, in total direct costs. We concluded that the data indicating that all severely and critically injured nonfatalities required hospitalization were correct. However, errors of up to 10 percent might exist in the case-hospitalization rates calculated for the less seriously injured patients (MAIS 1, 2, and 3 cases). This would result in a maximum error of 2.5 percent in total direct costs. Up to a 25 percent error is possible in the values derived for the proportion of time spent by a patient in intensive care and for the ratio of physician and surgeon fees to total hospitalization charges. In this eventuality, direct costs could vary from up to 2.5 to 3.5 percent above or below their value in the base case as a result of an error in one of those variables.

The ad hoc procedure used to estimate the costs of rehabilitation and annual follow-on care for a non-SCI MAIS 5 patient (essentially as a fixed proportion of corresponding costs for an incomplete paraplegic) suggests that these cost components may be in error by as much as 20 percent. If this were so, the direct costs of patients in this group would be misestimated by $113 million, or 12 percent. This would represent a misestimation of total direct costs of 2.4 percent and total economic costs of only 0.8 percent. If, for some reason, an error of 20 percent existed in *all* treatment-related costs incurred past the first year by nonfatalities (including the spinal-cord-injured), the result would be a misestimate of roughly $210 million in total direct costs. This would translate into a 1.5 percent error in total economic costs.

Legal and court costs represent a unique category of direct costs that was estimated only for motor vehicle injuries and not for the three diseases. The scantiness of the data and the very broad modeling approach adopted in our analysis leave open the possibility of error in these costs. If an across-the-board error of 15 percent existed in the per-case estimates of legal and court costs, this would mean an absolute error of $132 million in direct costs and a proportional error of 0.9 percent in total economic costs.

Discounting. The choice of discount rate affects the present valuation of all future costs. Table 6–31 displays the effects of discounting at 2 and at 10 percent—as well as at the 6 percent rate used in our base case—on the direct costs of MAIS 5 patients. The table shows that the greatest *proportional* change brought about by varying the discount rate occurs for the youngest

Table 6–31
Sensitivity to the Discount Rate of the Direct Costs of MAIS 5 Nonfatalities, by Age and Sex
(Millions of Dollars)

Age	2 Percent	6 Percent	10 Percent
Males			
0–14	169	100	76
15–24	702	450	349
25–34	161	112	89
35–44	127	95	79
45–54	66	53	47
55–64	53	46	42
65–74	16	16	14
75+	6	6	6
Total males	1300	879	702
Females			
0–14	57	32	24
15–24	234	141	107
25–34	92	59	45
35–44	60	42	34
45–54	28	21	17
55–64	19	16	14
65–74	4	4	2
75+	2	2	1
Total females	496	318	244
Total			
population	1796	1197	946

age group, whose future treatment costs will be discounted over the greatest number of years. The greatest *absolute* change occurs for young males between 15 and 24. Discounting at a rate of 2 percent (instead of at 6 percent) increases the direct costs of MAIS 5 cases by $599 million, or 50 percent, over their base-case value. Discounting at 10 percent decreases the estimated costs by 21 percent.

Table 6–32 shows the comparable effects of discounting on the indirect costs of fatalities. Again the table indicates that the greatest proportional change induced by varying the discount rate occurs for the youngest age group: if the discount rate is changed from 6 to 2 percent, the forgone earnings of children under 15 increase by over 200 percent; if the discount rate is increased to 10 percent, earnings decrease by 60 percent. The greatest absolute change again occurs for adolescents and young men between the ages of 15 and 24. Discounting at a rate of 2 rather than 6 percent increases the forgone earnings of all fatalities by 87 percent, while discounting at 10 percent decreases forgone earnings by 35 percent.

The same type of sensitivity has been performed for all direct and indirect costs associated with fatal and nonfatal injuries. The results are shown in

Table 6–32
**Sensitivity to the Discount Rate of the Indirect Costs of Fatalities,
by Age and Sex**
(Millions of Dollars)

Age	2 Percent	6 Percent	10 Percent
Males			
0–14	1,181	378	151
15–24	5,579	2,768	1,662
25–34	2,464	1,491	1,028
35–44	952	659	494
45–54	503	395	324
55–64	142	124	110
65–74	12	11	10
75+	1	1	1
Total males	10,833	5,827	3,779
Females			
0–14	469	154	64
15–24	1,063	539	336
25–34	416	246	168
35–44	200	133	98
45–54	127	95	76
55–64	53	43	36
65–74	15	13	11
75+	3	2	2
Total females	2,345	1,225	792
Total			
population	13,178	7,052	4,571

Table 6–33

Sensitivity to the Discount Rate of Direct, Indirect, and Total Costs of Motor Vehicle Injuries[a]

(Billions of Dollars)

		Fatalities	Nonfatalities	Total MVI
Direct costs	2%	0.18	5.29	5.47
Discounted at	6%	0.18	4.60	4.78
	10%	0.18	4.31	4.49
Indirect costs	2%	13.18	4.06	17.24
Discounted at	6%	7.05	2.61	9.66
	10%	4.57	2.04	6.61
Total costs	2%	13.36	9.35	22.71
Discounted at	6%	7.23	7.21	14.44
	10%	4.75	6.35	11.10

Note: All costs are in 1975 dollars.

table 6–33. Direct costs are only moderately sensitive to changes in the discount rate, increasing by 14 percent when a discount rate of 2 rather than 6 percent is used and decreasing by 6 percent when a rate of 10 percent is used. As one might expect, indirect costs are considerably more sensitive to the choice of discount rate. The value of indirect costs fluctuates from 78 percent above the base-case value to 32 percent below that value, depending on whether a 2 or a 10 percent rate is selected.

Indirect Costs. Our calculation of indirect costs presumed a discount rate of 6 percent, a productivity growth factor of 1 percent, and market valuation of household labor. Table 6–34 displays the results of altering these assumptions to allow for simultaneous changes in parameter values. We see in the table that indirect costs of motor vehicle injuries can be estimated as low as $6.1 billion and as high as $23.2 billion, depending on which set of analytical assumptions is applied. As we noted for each of the three diseases, the significance of this variation in costs is greater for each condition individually than it is on a comparative basis across conditions. If the assumptions are changed consistently across the four conditions, the relative economic ordering of the conditions will change only slightly.

Besides the analytical assumptions, certain other parameters were key determinants of forgone earnings. For both fatalities and nonfatalities, we rely on the assumption that values today for labor-force participation rates by age and sex and relative wage levels in the general population are good approximations of similar values in the future. Although this assumption can be challenged, it is commonly made and provides an important cornerstone for the calculation of forgone-earnings estimates in literally hundreds of studies. Closer to home, in our analysis of forgone earnings owing to

Table 6–34
Sensitivity of Indirect Costs of Motor Vehicle Injuries (MVI) to the Discount Rate, Productivity Growth Factor, and Mode of Valuing Household Labor
(Billions of Dollars)

			Productivity Growth Factor		
			0 Percent	*1 Percent*	*2 Percent*
Market-value approach	Discount rate	2%	14.5	17.2	20.8
		6%	8.6	9.7	10.9
		10%	6.1	6.6	7.2
Opportunity-cost approach	Discount rate	2%	16.0	19.1	23.2
		6%	9.4	10.6	12.0
		10%	6.6	7.2	7.8

Note: All costs are in 1975 dollars.

nonfatalities, an important parameter was the average number of days of restricted activity for MAIS 1, 2, 3, and 4 patients. For MAIS 5 patients, a parameter of equal import was the *ceiling* (or absolute) work rate.

In the first case, we ran a sensitivity analysis on the days of restricted activity. Recall that we constructed this parameter by assuming it was a sum of the following variables: average number of hospital days, average number of days of bed rest, and average number of days of other restricted activity. To correct for possible double counting by NCSS, however, we arbitrarily assumed that a certain percentage of the days of other restricted activity are actually days of bed rest. Our base-case estimate of this parameter was 20 percent. The parameter could be reasonably assumed to take any value ranging from 0 percent (no double counting) up to 40 percent. If the parameter is set to 40 percent, forgone earnings for MAIS 1 to 4 patients are estimated to be $691.7 million. If we assume no double counting, the forgone earnings increase to $929.8 million. Forgone earnings for MAIS 1 to 4 patients would then be in error by as much as 15 percent as a result of the misestimation of this double-counting parameter. Total costs, however, would be in error by only 0.8 percent.

In the case of the MAIS 5 patients, the *ceiling* work rate is the critical parameter. (Recall that we estimated ceiling work rates varying from 33 to 66 percent depending on the injury subtype.) If a 10 percent bias existed in our base-case estimates, table 6–35 presents the effect on forgone earnings. Note that forgone earnings could vary by 18 percent of the current estimate. This translates into a 2 percent bias in total economic costs.

One of the concepts used in our estimation of MAIS 5 forgone earnings that differed from those used in the cases of the three diseases studied was

Table 6–35
Changes in Forgone Earnings of MAIS 5 Cases Resulting from Variation in Ceiling Work Rates
(Millions of Dollars)

MAIS 5s	If 10 Percent Overestimate in Rates	If Correct As Is	If 10 Percent Underestimate in Rates
Non-SCI cases	1847	1564	1288
Para incompletes	58	49	40
Quad incompletes	62	56	50
Para completes	78	70	62
Quad completes	61	59	58
All MAIS 5 cases	2106	1798	1498

that of the ceiling work rate. This concept was initially put forth by Smart and Sanders to estimate the forgone earnings of SCI patients. We calculated the difference in our forgone-earnings estimates that would occur if we had instead treated these same ceiling rates as relative work rates. This would imply that instead of assuming that a patient has a ceiling on his employment rate, he has instead a proportional reduction in his employment rate compared with his peer in the general population. If we assume that this proportional reduction has the same value as our estimated ceiling rate, the forgone earnings of the MAIS 5 patients change. This is illustrated in the following table:

MAIS 5s	Current Results (Ceiling Rates) ($000,000)	Results Using Relative Work Rates ($000,000)
Non-SCI cases	$1564	$1884
Para incompletes	49	58
Quad incompletes	56	64
Para completes	70	78
Quad completes	59	61
All MAIS 5 cases	1798	2145

By using ceiling rates, we may have underestimated the forgone earnings of the MAIS 5 patients by 19 percent. This would translate into an error of about 2 percent in total costs.

Conclusions from the Sensitivity Analysis

While we have not exhaustively examined all possible sources of imprecision in our cost-estimation procedures, the sensitivity analysis has been useful in identifying the most important sources of error. These are, exclusive of the basis analytical assumptions concerning discount rate, productivity growth factor, and method of evaluating household labor:

1. Misestimation of nonfatal incidence. The entire analysis for nonfatalities is based on the assumption that the NCHS estimate of total incidence is the most accurate and therefore most reasonable one to use. If this is not the case, our total costs may be in error by as much as 22 percent, although an error between 7 and 13 percent would be more likely.

2. Direct costs. The literature and existing data bases on the direct costs of motor-vehicle-related trauma are limited, leaving open the possibility of significant estimation error. Even large errors in the estimation of direct costs for fatalities are not significant, but errors as high as 3 percent of total economic costs (roughly $480 million) are possible for nonfatalities if any one of such important parameters as length of hospital stay, proportion of patients' inhospital time spent in intensive care, and the costs of physician and surgeon services is incorrectly estimated.

3. Ceiling work rates of critically injured nonfatalities. The only data source located to estimate these rates for SCI patients and, by association, for non-SCI MAIS 5 patients is the Smart and Sanders (1976) study. Possible errors in the rates, owing to deficiencies in the data, might translate into 2 percent errors in total economic costs. Relative work rates may be the more appropriate method to model reduction in work capacity for MAIS 5 cases. In that eventuality, and if the values of the relative work rates are approximated well by our current ceiling-rate estimates, an error of 2 percent may exist in total costs.

In conclusion, we assume from the sensitivity analysis that the ultimate likely impact of possible errors does not cripple our study or its results. The largest potential error in total costs is theoretically 22 percent, but the likelihood of its existence is extremely small (for it derives from the least reliable of the four estimates of total nonfatal incidence). Errors owing to other variables are far less and certainly do not upset the economic ordering of motor vehicle injuries relative to the three disease conditions. On a scale with respect to economic costs, motor vehicle injuries are clearly below cancer, above stroke, and roughly equivalent to coronary heart disease.

Notes

1. U.S. Department of Transportation, Federal Highway Administration, *Fatal and Injury Accident Rates on Federal-Aid and Other Highway Systems, 1975*, p. v; U.S. Department of Health, Education and Welfare, National Center for Health Statistics, *Current Estimates from the Health Interview Survey, United States, 1975*, p. 20.

2. U.S. Department of Transportation, National Highway Traffic Safety Administration, *Fatal Accident Reporting System: 1975 Annual Report*, October 1976.

3. Interview with Marvin Stephens, Chief Statistician, National Center for Statistics and Analysis, National Highway Traffic Safety Administration, U.S. Department of Transportation, August 31, 1977.

4. U.S. Department of Transportation, National Highway Traffic Safety Administration, *Highway Safety Facts*, May 1978, p. 1.

5. Estimates developed from unpublished data for 1975, obtained from the Fatal Accident Reporting System, U.S. Department of Transportation.

6. U.S. Department of Transportation, National Highway Traffic Safety Administration, *Highway Safety Facts*, April 1979, p. 1; and June 1980, p. 1.

7. U.S. Department of Transportation, Federal Highway Administration, *Fatal and Injury Accident Rates on Federal-Aid and Other Highway Systems, 1975*, table ITT-1, p. 38; National Safety Council, *Accident Facts, 1976*, p. 40; phone interview with John D. Craigie, Vice President, Insurance Information Institute, September 2, 1977; and U.S. Department of Health, Education and Welfare, National Center for Health Statistics, unpublished data on moving motor vehicle traffic injuries (1975) obtained from the Health Interview Survey.

8. Estimates developed from unpublished data for 1975 obtained from the Fatal Accident Reporting System.

9. American Association for Automotive Medicine, *The Abbreviated Injury Scale (AIS)*, 1980 revision; Committee on Medical Aspects of Automotive Safety, Rating the severity of tissue damage. II: The comprehensive scale, *Journal of the American Medical Association* 220(May 1972):717–720; and Susan P. Baker, Brian O'Neill, William Haddon, Jr., and W.B. Long, The injury severity score: A method for describing patients with multiple injuries and evaluating emergency care, *Journal of Trauma* 14(1974):187–196.

10. See Susan C. Partyka, NCSS—The analyst's companion, National Center for Statistics and Analysis, National Highway Traffic Safety Administration, U.S. Department of Transportation, May 1980. The seven geographic areas surveyed in the NCSS include Erie County (less the city of Buffalo), New York; Washtenaw and Lenawee Counties, Michigan; sixteen counties in rural southwest Indiana; Miami, Florida; Lexington, Kentucky and seven surrounding counties; Bexar and Guadelupe Counties, including San Antonio, and thirteen counties in rural south Texas; and three police districts in central Los Angeles, California.

11. Unpublished data, National Crash Severity Study, National Highway Traffic Study Administration, U.S. Department of Transportation, May 1980 file.

12. Unpublished data, Restraint System Evaluation Project, National Highway Traffic Safety Administration, U.S. Department of Transportation, 1975.

13. Estimates of these values represent the authors' best subjective judgment based on a number of interviews with various emergency medical personnel in Massachusetts and nationally. We are especially indebted to Dr. Charles S. Lipson of the staff of the Newton-Wellesley Hospital, Newton, Massachusetts and Richard Potts of the Massachusetts Department of Public Health for their insights on this matter and their generous assistance.

14. Horace Wuerdemann and Hans C. Joksch, *National Indirect Costs of Motor Vehicle Accidents*, Center for the Environment and Man, Report 4114-494-B, June 1973, p. 54.

15. *Fatal Accident Reporting System: 1975 Annual Report*, pp. 22–23. Data from this source indicate that of those fatal crashes with known emergency medical service disposition, only 6 percent did not require some form of emergency medical attention. This 6 percent undoubtedly required coroner/medical services, including transportation, that paralleled emergency medical services in expense.

16. Based primarily on a survey of 1977 ambulance charges at the following private companies: Bay State Ambulance Service and Commonwealth Ambulance Service, Boston, Mass.; Newton-Wellesley Ambulance Service, Newton, Mass.; All Cape Ambulance Service, Hyannis, Mass.; Keith and Keith Ambulance Service, New York City; Somerset Ambulance Service, Skowhegan, Maine; and Delta Ambulance Service, Waterville, Maine.

17. Derived from data in *Fatal and Injury Acident Rates on Federal-Aid and Other Highway Systems/1975*, table FFT–1, p. 26.

18. Costs primarily from Boston City Hospital, Charge directory (11/12/75), computer printout, Boston, Mass. Original estimate of $50 in emergency medical charges multiplied by a deflation factor of 0.73 to yield national estimate of approximately $36. Deflation factor represents the ratio of United States to Massachusetts average hospital costs per patient in 1974 (assumed the same in 1975) as per U.S. Bureau of the Census, *Statistical Abstract of the United States, 1976*, p. 76.

19. Emergency room charges for non-DOA fatalities are based on survey of emergency-treatment procedures, level of care, and associated charges at the following Massachusetts hospitals: Somerville Hospital, Somerville; Sturdy Memorial Hospital, Attleboro; Newton-Wellesley Hospital, Newton; and Massachusetts General Hospital, Boston.

20. If we let x equal the time to death after 1 month for those fatalities surviving at least 30 days, the average value of x given a triangular probability distribution over the range 0 to 11 month is approximately 3.7

months. This means that the average time to death *following the crash* is $1 + 3.7 = 4.7$ months, or approximately 140 days, for fatalities in this group.

21. D.R. Boyd, B.A. Flashner, and C.M. Nyhus, Clinical and epidemiologic characteristic of non-surviving trauma victims in an urban environment, *Journal of the American Medical Association* 64(1):1–7, 1972.

22. Barbara M. Faigin, *1975 Societal Costs of Motor Vehicle Accidents* (U.S. Department of Transportation, National Highway Traffic Safety Administration, December 1975), p. 17. The value of 32 percent was derived by taking the ratio of average cost per patient of physician care ($315) and average cost per patient of hospital care ($990).

23. Ibid., p. 2. Estimate obtained by summing data from table 1.

24. Ibid., p. 18. Estimate of 5.9 percent hospitalized obtained from table 37.

25. Ibid., p. 18.

26. The average costs of police-related activities are estimated as MAIS 4, $70; MAIS 3, $50; MAIS 2, $35; and MAIS 1, $25. The progressively lower costs for less serious injuries reflect, in part, the fact that some of these injuries will occur in crashes involving more serious injuries and thus generate little in the way of additional marginal costs. Our estimate correspond well with similar estimates of the costs of accident-investigation activities developed by Faigin (1976), table 51, p. 23.

27. Derived from data in *Fatal and Injury Accident Rates on Federal-Aid and Other Highway Systems/1975*, table ITT–1, p. 38.

28. Charles N. Smart and Claudia R. Sanders, *The Costs of Motor Vehicle Related Spinal Cord Injuries* (Insurance Institute for Highway Safety, 1976), p. 50.

29. Emergency room charges for nonfatalities other than spinal cord patients are based on a survey of emergency-treatment procedures, level of care, and associated charges at the following Massachusetts hospitals: Somerville Hospital, Somerville; Sturdy Memorial Hospital, Attleboro; Newton-Wellesley Hospital, Newton; and Massachusetts General Hospital, Boston. The concensus among administrative staff interviewed at the hospitals was that in many cases patients are not charged for the full value of the resources and services provided to them in the emergency room. Because of this, the use of patient charge data as a surrogate for costs in this analysis should make the cost estimates necessarily conservative. Massachusetts charges in 1977 were deflated to conform with 1975 national cost levels.

30. All-Industry Research Advisory Committee, *Automobile Injuries and Their Compensation in the United States, vol. 1* (March 1979), p. 45.

31. Commission on Professional and Hospital Activity (CPHA), Ann Arbor, Michigan. Data on average length of stay have been obtained from a special study that used the CPHA, Professional Activities Survey (PAS) 7th Patient Sample. A subsample of approximately 21,100 patients were identi-

fied from within the 7th Patient Sample via a motor vehicle code. The data obtained in the special study are for calendar year 1973.

32. Smart and Sanders, *The Costs of Motor Vehicle Related Spinal Cord Injuries*, pp. 52–53.

33. John Z. DeLorean Corporation, *Automotive Occupant Protective Safety Air Cushion Expenditure/Benefit Study* (August 1975), p. 92 and figure C-4, p. 97.

34. A. Owens, At last: Hard figures on how fast fees have been climbing, *Medical Economics* (October 13, 1975):102.

35. Smart and Sanders, *The Costs of Motor Vehicle Related Spinal Cord Injuries*, p. 74, table 19. Estimates of annual costs of follow-on care have been inflated from 1974 to 1975 cost levels.

36. Ibid., pp. 54–56.

37. Ibid., pp. 56–58.

38. Faigin, *1975 Societal Costs of Motor Vehicle Accidents*, p. 2. Estimates obtained by summing data in table 1 for the average costs of accident investigation, hospitalization, physicians' and other medical services, and rehabilitation.

39. U.S. Department of Transportation, *Automobile Accident Litigation, A Report to the Federal Judicial Center*, April 1970, p. 8.

40. Wuerdemann and Joksch, *National Indirect Costs of Motor Vehicle Accidents*, pp. 60–61.

41. *Automobile Injuries and Their Compensations in the United States*, p. 62.

42. Derived in part from data in Faigin, *1975 Societal Costs of Motor Vehicle Accidents*, p. 20. Faigin has used the attorneys' expenses from *Automobile Accident Litigation* (p. 37) as her estimate of the cost of hiring an attorney without filing suit. Our estimate of $300 is more representative of the average cost of this service for all cases.

43. Ibid., p. 20.

44. Derived from information in *Automobile Accident Litigation* on the averge cost of defense attorneys in civil cases. Their estimate of $820 (1968 dollars) has been limited to the more severe case, those involving a fatality or a MAIS 4 or 5 nonfatality. We assume a lower figure of $450 (1968 dollars) applies to civil cases involving a MAIS 1, 2, or 3 nonfatality. Adjusting these estimates to 1975 levels (using *Index for Legal Services*, U.S. Bureau of Labor Statistics, 1968–1975), we have $1485 (that is, $820 × 1.81) for defense attorney fees in cases involving a fatality or a MAIS 4 or 5 nonfatality and $815 (that is, $450 × 1.81) for similar fees in cases involving a MAIS 1, 2, or 3 nonfatality.

45. Derived in part from estimates of civil court costs for motor vehicle crash cases found in *Automobile Accident Litigation*, p. 49—$4200 per state trial in 1968—and Wuerdemann and Joksch, *National Indirect Costs*,

p. 60—$5 to $200 per state and local case filed in 1969. Based on these sources, we estimate that in 1968 dollars the average court cost was roughly $3000 for a fatality or a MAIS 4 or 5 nonfatality and $1500 for a MAIS 1, 2, or 3 nonfatality. Adjusted to 1975 dollars (using data in *Government Employees' Salary Trends*, Bureau of Labor Statistics, 1977, p. 36), the estimates are $4830 (that is, $3000 × 1.61) for court costs for a fatality or MAIS 4 or 5 case and $2415 (that is, $1500 × 1.61) for court costs for a MAIS 1, 2, or 3 case.

46. Wuerdemann and Joksch, *National Indirect Costs*, p. 62. An adjustment factor of 1.42 (derived from information in *Government Employees' Salary Trends*, p. 36) was used to adjust costs of prosecutors' time from 1969 to 1975 price levels. For fatalities and MAIS 4 and 5 nonfatalities, the cost of this time is approximately $140 in 1975 (that is, $100 × 1.42, to the nearest $5), and for less severely injured persons, $65 (that is, $45 × 1.42, to the nearest $5).

47. From Wuerdemann and Joksch, *National Indirect Costs*, p. 60, criminal court costs ranged from $2 to $70 in 1969 dollars. We assigned an approximate cost of $30 to a MAIS 1, 2, or 3 nonfatality and $70 to a more severely injured case. Adjusted to 1975 dollars, these figures become $45 and $100, respectively (using an inflation factor of 1.42; see note 46).

48. Faigin, *1975 Societal Costs of Motor Vehicle Accidents*. Percentage for fatalities based on data both from Faigin and from *Economic Consequences of Automobile Accident Injuries* (Automobile Insurance and Compensation Study, U.S. Department of Transportation, April 1970), p. 50.

49. Faigin, *1975 Societal Costs of Motor Vehicle Accidents*, p. 20.

50. *Automobile Injuries and Their Compensation in the United States*, p. 14.

51. Percentages derived from data in Faigin, *1975 Societal Costs of Motor Vehicle Accidents*, of crashes involving certain types of injuries that lead to criminal action, and data in *Fatal and Injury Accident Rates on Federal-Aid and Other Highway Systems, 1975*, pp. 26 and 38, on the crash-to-injury case ratio for that group of motor vehicle crashes. For crashes involving MAIS 1, 2, or 3 injury cases only, we have 26.8 percent leading to criminal action with a crash-to-injury case ratio of approximately 0.66. Hence, about 17.7 percent (that is, 26.8 × 0.66) of all MAIS 1, 2, and 3 nonfatalities result in some form of criminal action. For crashes involving MAIS 4 or 5 nonfatalities or fatalities, the corresponding numbers are 24.8 percent and 0.88; thus the resulting 21.8 percent (that is, 24.8 × 0.88) of all cases leading to criminal prosecution.

52. Smart and Sanders, *The Costs of Motor Vehicle Related Spinal Cord Injuries*, pp. 86–87, and pp. 105–108 in Appendix B.

53. Derived from data in Astha C. Dresser, Arnold Meirowsky, George Weiss, Mildred McNeel, Gary Simon, and William Caveness, Gainful employment following injury, *Archives of Neurology* 29(August 1973):115. In our usage, the existence of "significant neurological damage and complications" is synonymous with the onset of epileptic seizures.

7 Summary Results and Applications

We bring together in this final chapter many of the results separately calculated for the four conditions: incidence, mortality; direct, indirect, and total costs; and sensitivity analyses. We note limitations and aspects of the methodology that should be kept in mind. With these understandings, we examine in a few simple instances how economic costs might be used in allocating societal resources.

Results

Incidence

Incidence of the four conditions studied, disaggregated by age and sex, is displayed in table 7–1. In terms of total numbers affected, motor vehicle injuries dominate, with more than 6 times the incidence of any of the three diseases. To some extent this is misleading, since most of these injuries are not life-threatening. The average incident cancer, in contrast, is much more serious in terms of both threats to life and costs.

The four health impairments, as table 7–1 shows, have distinct patterns of incidence by age. Motor vehicle injuries (MVI) peak at the earliest age—between 15 and 24 for both sexes. Most initial events of coronary heart disease (CHD) occur between 55 and 64; of cancer, between 65 and 74; and of stroke, after 75. The incidence of cancer is greater in males than in females for those under 25 and over 55. For the other three impairments, incidence among males exceeds that among females at younger ages and trails at older ages (although in each case the rate of incidence—incident events per 1000 population—remains higher for males). More males than females are stricken with coronary heart disease and stroke up to age 75; motor vehicle injuries among women begin to exceed those among men for the group aged 55 to 64. Among men, motor vehicle injuries are more numerous than any (indeed, all combined) of the three listed diseases at younger ages; coronary heart disease has the highest incidence of the four conditions for the 55 to 64 age group; cancers are more numerous than any of the other three conditions for males over 65. Among women, the incidence of coronary heart disease and of cancer does not surpass that of motor vehicle injuries except for the two groups aged over 65. Cancers have the highest incidence of the four conditions for women over 75.

Table 7-1
Annual Incidence of Cancer, Coronary Heart Disease, Motor Vehicle Injuries, and Stroke, by Age and Sex; United States, 1975

Age	U.S. General Population, 1975	Cancer	Coronary Heart Disease (CHD)	Motor Vehicle Injuries (MVI)	Stroke[a]
Males					
0–14	27,365,000	3,585	119	275,520	354
15–24	20,375,000	4,661	500	997,434	502
25–34	15,355,000	6,150	5,939	492,651	962
35–44	11,153,000	11,210	34,730	229,600	2,322
45–54	11,491,000	37,954	81,184	185,693	9,512
55–64	9,345,000	80,555	150,464	127,720	26,086
65–74	6,027,000	104,340	90,043	73,346	43,191
75+	3,145,000	83,366	47,269	34,188	47,589
Total males	104,238,000	331,821	410,248	2,416,152	130,518
Females					
0–14	26,284,000	2,944	23	227,905	206
15–24	19,913,000	4,502	99	657,827	274
25–34	15,580,000	10,876	1,218	342,609	564
35–44	11,671,000	22,888	7,345	196,149	1,353
45–54	12,280,000	54,891	28,514	179,422	3,805
55–64	10,435,000	73,974	82,082	131,884	22,837
65–74	7,847,000	80,312	77,261	76,430	33,348
75+	5,382,000	78,472	53,136	42,017	59,961
Total females	109,392,000	328,859	249,678	1,854,243	122,348
Total population	213,630,000	660,680	659,926	4,270,395	252,866

[a]Stroke incidence figures do not include transient ischemic attacks (TIAs).

Table 7–2

Estimated Incidence of Diseases and Injuries, Average Age at Incidence, and Proportion of Incidence that is Male, by Impairment Subcategories, United States, 1975

| Disease/Injury | Incidence | Average Age at Incidence | | | Proportion of Incidence That Is Male |
		Male	Female	Both Sexes	
Cancer					
Digestive system	168,411	66.8	68.6	67.7	0.522
Respiratory system	99,889	64.0	63.2	63.8	0.796
Buccal cavity	23,562	61.9	61.7	61.8	0.710
Reproductive system	214,758	69.9	59.8	62.7	0.283
Urinary system	43,577	65.7	66.3	65.9	0.698
Nervous system	10,570	48.5	48.0	48.3	0.548
Leukemias	21,293	58.4	60.6	59.3	0.568
Lymphomas	29,338	56.4	60.5	58.3	0.542
Other sites	49,282	58.3	57.7	58.0	0.460
All cancers	660,680	64.7	62.2	63.5	0.502
Coronary heart disease (CHD)					
Sudden death	68,967	59.1	68.4	62.2	0.671
MI	231,842	61.3	66.1	62.4	0.777
CI	75,151	56.9	64.0	59.7	0.610
APU	283,966	60.6	65.0	62.9	0.486
All CHD	659,926	60.3	65.5	62.3	0.622
Motor vehicle injuries (MVI)					
Fatalities	44,995	33.8	37.0	34.7	0.734
MAIS 1[a]	3,053,035	28.7	30.4	29.5	0.555
MAIS 2[a]	702,923	30.4	33.0	31.5	0.565
MAIS 3[a]	353,569	31.4	39.7	34.7	0.602
MAIS 4[a]	87,262	30.4	34.6	31.8	0.678
MAIS 5[a]	28,611	28.8	29.7	29.0	0.739
All MVI	4,270,395	29.3	31.6	30.3	0.566
Stroke					
Hemorrhage	35,485	61.3	63.7	62.5	0.518
Infarction	217,381	71.3	74.7	72.9	0.516
All stroke[b]	252,866	69.9	73.1	71.5	0.516

[a]MAIS 1 through MAIS 5 injuries that are nonfatalities.

[b]Stroke incidence figures do not include transient ischemic attacks (TIAs).

Disaggregation of the four impairments by subcategories, as shown in table 7–2, sheds further light on patterns of incidence. We see there that mean age at incidence is younger, by three decades, for motor vehicle injuries than for the three diseases. Males tend to get cancer at a somewhat older age than they first show coronary heart disease, while the reverse is true for females. For both sexes, the mean age of first stroke is, at close to 70 years, greater than that for the other conditions.

Among cancers, those of the nervous system tend to strike younger persons and those of the digestive system and the urinary tract to strike older persons. Average age at incidence for both sexes for cancers at other anatomic sites is between 58 and 64. The most striking difference in mean age at incidence between the sexes occurred for cancers of the reproductive system. The 10-year difference reflects largely the difference between the ages at incidence of cancers of the breast for women and of the prostate for men. Considerably less variation in age at incidence among subtypes of the impairment is found for coronary heart disease, motor vehicle injuries, and stroke.

The final column of table 7–2 indicates the breakdown between male and female incidence. Women tend to have vastly more cancers of the reproductive system owing largely to the inclusion of breast cancer in this category; they also have slightly more cancers of other sites and cases of APU. Male predominance is most marked among cancers of the respiratoy system, buccal cavity, and urinary tract, among all coronary heart disease but APU, and among motor vehicle fatalities and severely injured nonfatalities. Males have slightly more strokes than females.

Mortality

The indirect costs of a condition depend on the age at incidence and on its severity in terms of mortality or disabling morbidity. Mortality effects are displayed in table 7–3. The average life expectancies of persons with various impairments are—in the first two sets of columns—compared with those of age- and sex-matched persons of the general population. The differences are given in the third set of columns as the average number of life-years lost per patient. This shows that all groups of cancers are to be taken seriously, since the smallest decrease in life expectancy among the groups shown in table 7–3 is 4.2 years. Most life-years are lost per patient for cancers of the nervous system, leukemias, lymphomas, and cancers of the respiratory system. The average cancer is associated with an expected loss of 10.5 life-years. In contrast, initial events of CHD, stroke, and MVI are associated with expected losses of 9.1, 6.6, and 0.5 life-years, the last being more than an order of magnitude lower than each of the others because of the much lower MVI case fatality rate.

Multiplying the incidence by the expected loss of years per impaired person gives, in the last set of columns, the total life-years lost associated with incident events in 1975. Among cancers, the higher incidence of cancers in the digestive, respiratory, and reproductive systems means that a greater total loss of life-years is associated with them. For CHD and MVI, 35 and 90 percent, respectively, of the life-years lost are lost by those whose disease or injury first appears in an immediately fatal form: CHD sudden death and MVI fatalities. Forty-nine percent of the CHD life-years lost are for those who first have a myocardial infarction and 16 percent for those whose disease begins as coronary insufficiency.

Table 7–3 shows that among the four impairments, the total life-years lost by affected individuals is greatest for cancer: people with cancers incident in 1975 had 6.94 million fewer expected life-years than age- and sex-matched persons in the general population. The second greatest loss of life expectancy, 3.43 million years, was for persons with coronary heart disease; the third greatest, 2.01 million years, for MVI victims; and 1.68 million years of lost life expectancy were associated with stroke. Comparing these totals by sex, we see that there was a greater loss in life-years among women than among men with cancer, owing to the seriousness of cancers of the female reproductive system. Males with heart disease and motor vehicle injuries lost more than twice as many life-years as did females. Among persons sustaining strokes, women lost 14 percent more life-years than did men.

Indirect Costs

The economic significance of lost life-years depends on their productive potential: very young and very old life-years have less economic significance, although their noneconomic aspects may be important. Productive years lost well in the future are—owing to discounting—less valuable than those lost soon. In this perspective, lost life-years owing to stroke are relatively less valuable than years lost as a result of heart disease, since less productive years are involved. For motor vehicle injuries, conflicting effects are at work: the life-years lost are among the most productive, yet many are lost so far in the future that they have small present value because of the discounting effect.

These conditions are brought together in calculating the present value of expected postmorbid earnings (*PVPM*) for individuals with each of the four impairments. This is shown in table 7–4. There we see, for instance, in the first line, that a boy under 15 who gets cancer has a *PVPM* of only $40,542; if he gets heart disease, this value is $71,199; if a motor vehicle injury, $129,152; if a stroke, $48,660. Subtracting the *PVPM* of patients from the earnings expectations of the general population yields forgone earnings, which are presented in table 7–5—the expected future productivity lost when a person sustains a motor vehicle injury or acquires one of the three diseases. For the boy under 15 getting cancer, the average forgone earnings are thus $90,321 (that is, $130,863 − 40,542).

Table 7–5 combines all subcategories of the four impairments. Because

Table 7–3
Estimated Number of Lost Life-Years Associated with the Incidence of Cancer, Coronary Heart Disease, Motor Vehicle Injuries, and Stroke, United States, 1975

Disease/Injury	Average Life Expectancy if Free of Condition (in Years)			Average Life Expectancy with Condition (in Years)			Average Life-Years Lost per Patient			Total Lost Life-Years Associated with Condition (in thousands)		
	Male	Female	Both Sexes	Male	Female	Both Sexes	Male	Female	Both Sexes	Male	Female	Both Sexes
Cancer												
Digestive system	13.1	15.8	14.5	3.5	5.2	4.4	9.6	10.6	10.1	849	855	1704
Respiratory system	14.7	19.9	15.8	1.9	2.1	2.0	12.8	17.8	13.8	1019	363	1382
Buccal cavity	16.2	21.2	17.7	7.6	10.6	8.5	8.6	10.6	9.2	144	73	217
Reproductive system	11.5	22.5	19.4	7.3	12.2	10.8	4.2	10.3	8.6	256	1593	1849
Urinary system	14.1	17.8	15.2	7.0	8.5	7.4	7.1	9.3	7.8	216	122	338
Nervous system	26.9	33.0	29.7	5.9	8.9	7.3	21.0	24.1	22.4	122	115	237
Leukemias	20.3	23.1	21.5	2.0	2.3	2.1	18.3	20.8	19.4	221	191	412
Lymphomas	18.3	18.8	18.6	4.1	4.8	4.5	14.2	14.0	14.1	226	188	414
Other sites	22.4	29.7	26.6	14.0	22.2	18.7	8.4	7.5	7.9	191	201	391
All cancers	14.9	21.2	18.0	5.1	9.9	7.5	9.8	11.3	10.5	3242	3701	6943
Coronary heart disease												
Sudden death	17.8	15.9	17.1	0	0	0	17.8	15.9	17.1	823	360	1183
MI	16.7	17.6	16.9	9.9	8.5	9.6	6.8	9.1	7.3	1218	469	1687
CI	20.0	19.0	19.6	12.9	11.1	12.2	7.1	7.9	7.4	324	232	556
APU	16.8	18.3	17.6	*	*	*	*	*	*	*	*	*
All CHD[a]	17.4	17.6	17.5	8.7	7.4	8.4	8.7	10.2	9.1	2365	1061	3426

Motor Vehicle Injuries												
Fatalities	39.1	42.9	40.1	0[b]	0[b]	0[b]	39.1	42.9	40.1	1293	514	1807
MAIS 1	43.5	48.5	45.6	43.5	48.5	45.6	0	0	0	0	0	0
MAIS 2	41.9	46.1	43.7	41.9	46.1	43.7	0	0	0	0	0	0
MAIS 3	40.9	40.2	40.7	40.9	40.2	40.7	0	0	0	0	0	0
MAIS 4	41.7	44.8	42.7	41.7	44.8	42.7	0	0	0	0	0	0
MAIS 5	43.2	49.0	44.0	36.2	42.2	37.0	7.0	6.8	7.0	148	51	199
All MVI	42.7	47.4	44.7	42.1	47.1	44.2	0.6	0.3	0.5	1441	565	2006
Stroke												
Hemorrhage	17.4	20.3	18.8	6.4	7.1	6.7	11.0	13.2	12.1	202	226	428
Infarction	11.6	12.8	12.2	6.4	6.4	6.4	5.2	6.4	5.8	581	669	1251
TIA	12.7	13.4	13.0	*	*	*	*	*	*	*	*	*
All Stroke[b]	12.4	14.1	13.0	6.4	6.8	6.4	6.0	7.3	6.6	783	895	1678

*For analytical purposes, no life-years were assumed lost owing to either APU or TIA per se, although persons with those conditions were admittedly more susceptible to subsequent, more lethal cardiovascular conditions.

a Averages computed for all CHD and all stroke patients exclude APU and TIA cases, respectively.

b Average life expectancy for MVI fatalities is approximately 10 days.

Table 7-4
Expected Earnings per Person, by Age and Sex, for the General Population and People with Cancer, Coronary Heart Disease, Motor Vehicle Injuries, and Stroke, United States, 1975

Age	U.S. General Population, 1975	Cancer	Coronary Heart Disease (CHD)	Motor Vehicle Injuries (MVI)	Stroke[a]
Males					
0–14	130,863	40,542	71,199	129,152	48,660
15–24	225,992	84,585	137,392	222,283	67,028
25–34	247,881	105,409	159,745	224,030	71,686
35–44	205,687	68,631	138,765	201,463	59,994
45–54	135,972	42,685	95,428	132,997	41,596
55–64	52,199	19,421	33,517	50,641	17,610
65–74	5,754	2,450	3,092	5,468	1,658
75+	533	242	302	493	233
All males	157,030	16,327	46,138	188,464	9,170
Females					
0–14	92,241	36,433	61,806	91,484	30,591
15–24	156,059	76,983	113,635	154,881	40,366
25–34	153,131	83,951	112,326	151,962	38,415
35–44	126,642	67,165	93,762	125,425	31,890
45–54	87,150	46,582	64,312	86,129	24,285
55–64	39,950	21,158	31,440	39,378	12,635
65–74	11,682	6,091	7,698	11,352	3,244
75+	2,556	1,384	1,786	2,451	1,185
All females	97,016	23,183	23,800	119,196	5,250
All persons	126,299	19,740	37,687	158,387	7,274

Note: All earnings figures are in 1975 dollars, discounted at 6 percent.
[a]Excluding transient ischemic attacks (TIAs).

Table 7–5
Average Forgone Earnings per Person, by Age and Sex, for Cancer, Coronary Heart Disease, Motor Vehicle Injuries, and Stroke, United States, 1975
(Dollars)

Age	Cancer	Coronary Heart Disease (CHD)	Motor Vehicle Injuries (MVI)	Stroke[a]
Males				
0–14	90,321	59,664	1,711	82,203
15–24	141,407	88,600	3,709	158,964
25–34	142,472	88,136	3,851	176,195
35–44	137,056	66,922	4,224	145,693
45–54	93,287	40,544	2,975	94,376
55–64	32,778	18,682	1,558	34,589
65–74	3,304	2,662	286	4,096
75+	291	231	40	300
All males	29,972	22,557	3,233	19,981
Females				
0–14	55,808	30,435	757	61,650
15–24	79,076	42,424	1,178	115,693
25–34	69,180	40,805	1,169	114,716
35–44	59,477	32,880	1,217	94,752
45–54	40,568	22,838	1,021	62,865
55–64	18,792	8,510	572	27,315
65–74	5,591	3,684	330	8,438
75+	1,172	770	105	1,371
All females	20,654	7,895	998	11,964
All persons	25,334	17,010	2,263	16,102

Note: All earnings figures are in 1975 dollars, discounted at 6 percent.
[a]Excluding transient ischemic attacks (TIAs).

the many nonserious motor injuries are vastly more numerous than the more serious ones, the average forgone earnings of MVIs are a relatively low $2263 per injured person. Average earnings forgone per person amounted to $25,334 for cancer, $17,010 for heart disease, and $16,102 for stroke. The *PVPM* of the general population shows that future productivity is highest for those between 15 and 44 and higher for males than for females up to retirement age. The two phenomena (recalling that males have a generally younger age at incidence) imply that the forgone earnings for each condition are higher on average for males than for females.

Direct, Indirect, and Total Costs

Direct, indirect, and total costs, are shown in table 7–6. The first column shows the costs of treatment in the first year—primarily the costs of treating

Table 7-6
Estimated Direct and Indirect Costs Associated with the Incidence of Cancer, Coronary Heart Disease, Motor Vehicle Injuries, and Stroke, United States, 1975
(Millions of Dollars)

Disease/Injury	Direct Costs				Indirect Costs	
	Treatment During First Year	Future Treatment	Other[a]	Total Direct	Forgone Earnings	Total Costs
Cancer						
Digestive system	1,172	207	62	1,441	3,569	5,010
Respiratory system	690	102	36	828	3,760	4,588
Buccal cavity	182	93	12	287	593	880
Reproductive system	1,111	1,030	96	2,237	3,711	5,948
Urinary system	267	137	18	422	781	1,203
Nervous system	87	49	6	142	917	1,059
Leukemias	157	50	9	216	944	1,160
Lymphomas	198	133	15	346	1,383	1,729
Other sites	266	205	21	492	1,079	1,571
All cancers	4,130	2,005	276	6,411	16,737	23,148
Coronary heart disease (CHD)						
Sudden death	7	0	0	7	3,891	3,898
MI	974	459	64	1,497	5,369	6,866
CI	329	248	26	603	1,958	2,561
APU	77	290	17	384	7	391
All CHD	1,387	997	107	2,491	11,225	13,716
Motor vehicle injuries (MVI)						
Fatalities	50	0	126	176	7,062	7,228
MAIS 1	561	0	71	632	111	743
MAIS 2	674	0	123	797	180	977
MAIS 3	727	15	228	970	314	1,284
MAIS 4	434	122	109	665	206	871
MAIS 5	412	733	388	1,533	1,798	3,331
All MVI	2,858	870	1,045	4,773	9,662	14,435
Stroke						
Hemorrhage	165	64	10	239	1,470	1,709
Infarction	1,345	583	87	2,015	2,602	4,617
TIA	16	93	5	114	16	130
All strokes	1,526	740	102	2,368	4,088	6,456
All conditions	9,901	4,612	1,530	16,043	41,712	57,755

Note: All costs are in 1975 dollars, discounted at 6 percent.

[a]"Other" costs include insurance administration costs and, in the case of motor vehicle injuries, legal and court costs as well. For motor vehicle injuries, legal and court costs constitute $878 million of the $1.045 million in "other" costs.

the initial episode of that condition. Costs of subsequent treatment, present-valued at a discount rate of 6 percent, are given in the second column. Other costs—primarily insurance administration, but also, for motor vehicle injuries, legal and court costs—appear in the third column. The fourth column contains the sums of the three components of direct costs, while the fifth presents forgone earnings, seen earlier in table 7–5 on a per-person basis, but here broken down by totals per subcategory of condition. The sum of all direct and indirect costs is given in the final column of table 7–6 and is also presented graphically in figure 7–1.

Among cancers, the types leading to both greatest direct and indirect costs are those of the digestive, respiratory, and reproductive systems. This is primarily due to their greater incidence. Although both direct and indirect costs vary along with incidence, there are striking exceptions. Cancers of the respiratory system, for instance, have significantly lower incidence than

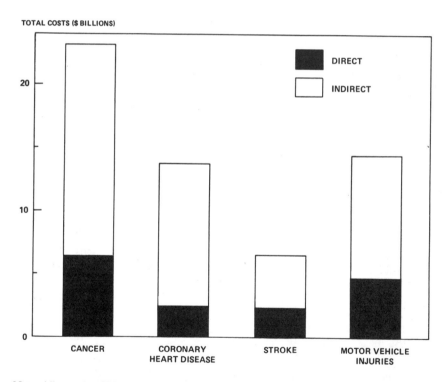

Note: All costs in 1975 dollars, discounted at 6 percent.

Figure 7–1. Total Economic Costs Associated with the Incidence of Cancer, Coronary Heart Disease, Stroke, and Motor Vehicle Injuries, United States, 1975

cancers of the digestive system, and therefore, they have lower direct costs. Since, however, respiratory system cancers strike at a somewhat younger age (see table 7–2) and occasion more lost years of life per person (see table 7–3), their forgone earnings exceed those of digestive system cancers. Similarly, cancers of the nervous system strike the young, are associated with a large loss of life expectancy per patient, and hence have total forgone earnings far beyond the proportion of their incidence—indeed greater than the forgone earnings of urinary system cancers, whose incidence is 4 times as large.

Similar phenomena are seen in the other impairments. Sudden death in coronary heart disease causes little direct cost but large forgone earnings. Since both APU and TIA are considered of themselves non-life-threatening, their indirect costs are incurred solely in earnings lost while seeking treatment or in recuperation. These are, accordingly, small. Among motor vehicle injuries, the four least severe categories (MAIS 1 to MAIS 4) account for 64 percent of all MVI direct costs but for only 8 percent of the indirect costs, indicating their responsibility for extensive short-term medical expenses, but their limited impact on long-term productivity. Critical but not immediately fatal injuries (MAIS 5) have greater direct costs than any other subcategory of MVI. Cancer, of the four conditions studied, poses the greatest economic burden to our society: $23.1 billion. Next highest costs are due to motor vehicle injuries and coronary heart disease: $14.4 billion and $13.7 billion, respectively.

Sensitivity Analysis

Table 7–7 displays for each disease the sensitivity of direct, indirect, and total costs to the choice of discount rate. This table shows, first, a result seen for each condition separately: that indirect costs are more sensitive than direct costs to the choice of discount rate. We see, second, that the costs of motor vehicle injuries are comparatively sensitive to the discount rate, while stroke costs are relatively insensitive. The costs of cancer and coronary heart disease exhibit intermediate sensitivity. If, for instance, we had discounted at 2 instead of at 6 percent, MVI costs would have risen by 57 percent, stroke costs by 22 percent, cancer costs by 38 percent, and CHD costs by 32 percent.The greater sensitivity of MVI costs to the discount rate is understandable: these injuries afflict a younger population and have economic repercussions over a greater number of years. Conversely, strokes are incident on a generally older population, have impact over shorter time horizons, and have total costs that are relatively insensitive to the choice of discount rate.

In table 7–8 we present a more extended comparative sensitivity analysis,

Table 7–7
Sensitivity of Direct, Indirect, and Total Costs of Each Health Impairment to the Discount Rate
(Billions of Dollars)

	Health Impairment	Discount Rate		
		2 Percent	*6 Percent*	*10 Percent*
Direct costs	Cancer	7.43	6.41	5.80
	Coronary heart disease (CHD)	2.96	2.49	2.23
	Motor vehicle injury (MVI)	5.47	4.77	4.24
	Stroke	2.51	2.37	2.29
	Total	18.37	16.04	14.56
Indirect costs	Cancer	24.53	16.74	12.75
	CHD	15.09	11.23	8.94
	MVI	17.24	9.66	6.61
	Stroke	5.36	4.09	3.36
	Total	62.22	41.72	31.66
Total costs	Cancer	31.96	23.15	18.55
	CHD	18.05	13.72	11.17
	MVI	22.71	14.43	10.85
	Stroke	7.87	6.46	5.65
	Total	80.59	57.76	46.22

Note: All costs are in 1975 dollars.

one that displays the sensitivity of indirect and total costs for the four conditions to the choice of discount rate, to the choice of productivity growth factor, and to the mode of valuing household labor. Direct costs are not included, since they are insensitive to the productivity growth factor and to the mode of valuing household labor and their sensitivity to the discount rate was presented in table 7–7.

Phenomena similar to those seen in table 7–7 are also presented in table 7–8. In general, the younger the average age of the persons involved, the greater is the sensitivity to both the discount rate and the productivity growth factor. We thus see that shifting from the 1 percent productivity growth factor to a 2 percent factor would increase total MVI costs by 9 percent but would increase stroke costs by only 3 percent. Cancer and CHD costs would increase by intermediate amounts of 7 and 6 percent, respectively. We note also that over this range of variability for the productivity growth factor (0 to 2 percent), sensitivity is far less than sensitivity to the discount rate, varying between 2 and 10 percent.

For the mode of valuing household labor, the general order of sensitivity across conditions is reversed. The older the persons involved, the more likely they are to be retired and to have extensive amounts of household labor

Table 7-8
Sensitivity of Indirect and Total Costs of Each Health Impairment to the Discount Rate, Productivity Growth Factor, and Mode of Valuing Household Labor

Market-Value Approach

Discount Rate/ Productivity Growth	Cancer			Coronary Heart Disease (CHD)			Stroke			Motor Vehicle Injury (MVI)		
	0%	1%	2%	0%	1%	2%	0%	1%	2%	0%	1%	2%
Indirect costs												
2%	21.9	24.5	27.7	13.9	15.1	16.5	4.9	5.4	5.8	14.5	17.2	20.8
6%	15.4	16.7	18.3	10.5	11.2	12.0	3.8	4.1	4.3	8.6	9.7	10.9
10%	12.0	12.8	13.6	8.5	8.9	9.5	3.2	3.4	3.5	6.1	6.6	7.2
Total costs												
2%	29.3	32.0	35.1	16.9	18.1	19.5	7.4	7.9	8.3	20.0	22.8	26.3
6%	21.8	23.1	24.7	13.0	13.7	14.5	6.2	6.5	6.7	13.4	14.4	15.7
10%	17.8	18.6	19.4	10.7	11.2	11.7	5.5	5.7	5.8	10.3	10.8	11.4

Opportunity-Cost Approach

Discount Rate/ Productivity Growth	Cancer			Coronary Heart Disease (CHD)			Stroke			Motor Vehicle Injury (MVI)		
	0%	1%	2%	0%	1%	2%	0%	1%	2%	0%	1%	2%
Indirect costs												
2%	27.9	31.3	35.5	17.2	18.7	20.5	6.8	7.4	8.0	16.0	19.1	23.2
6%	19.5	21.2	23.1	12.9	13.8	14.8	5.3	5.6	6.0	9.4	10.6	12.0
10%	15.0	16.0	17.1	10.4	11.0	11.6	4.4	4.6	4.8	6.6	7.2	7.8
Total costs												
2%	35.3	38.7	42.9	20.2	21.7	23.5	9.3	9.9	10.5	21.5	24.6	28.7
6%	25.9	27.6	29.5	15.4	16.3	17.3	7.8	8.1	8.5	14.2	15.4	16.8
10%	20.8	21.8	22.9	12.7	13.3	13.9	6.7	6.9	7.1	10.8	11.4	12.0

Note: All costs are in 1975 dollars.

affected in the near term. Accordingly, we find that total stroke costs are most sensitive in this regard, increasing by 25 percent if opportunity-cost valuation is substituted for market valuation. MVI total costs would rise by only 7 percent with this substitution, while cancer and CHD costs would both rise by 19 percent.

Importance of Sensitivity to Analytical Methods

The variation in illness costs arising from the choice of analytical methods is seen in table 7–8 to be considerable. Even for stroke, the least sensitive of the four conditions, the choice of methods can shift results by a factor of 2. The total costs of stroke might thus be found to be as low as $5.5 billion or as high as $10.5 billion.

Looking at the variability in cost estimates for one disease or injury overstates, however, the variability across conditions. This occurs because altering the analytical assumptions affects cost estimates for all conditions in the same direction. Lowering the discount rate, increasing the productivity growth factor, and using the opportunity-cost value of household labor all increase the estimated economic costs of any disease or injury. For impairments of comparable severity incident at similar ages, the intracondition variability (owing to analytical choices) may be greater, while the intercondition variability (expressed as the ratios of costs across conditions) may be limited. This can be seen in table 7–8, where both cancer and heart disease exhibit greater intracondition variability (more than a factor of 2 for each), while the total costs of CHD range only between 55 and 61 percent of those for cancer, whatever the methods used, as long as consistency is maintained. This observation underscores the need for analytical consistency in comparisons of different impairments to health.

For conditions incident at different ages, the intracondition sensitivity is still likely to exceed the intercondition sensitivity, but the latter may, nevertheless, be important. This can be seen in the comparison between heart disease and motor vehicle injuries. In our base case, MVI total costs exceed those of CHD by 5 percent. If, however, a discount rate of 10 percent had been used or if household labor were valued at its opportunity cost, then CHD total costs would become roughly 5 percent larger than MVI total costs.

Conclusions from Sensitivity Analysis

Our sensitivity analyses indicate that the current state of the art in estimating the economic costs of illness has limited numerical precision. For many decisions involving comparisons across health conditions, the numerical accuracy can be kept within acceptable bounds—provided that care is taken to maintain methodological consistency. For other decisions, useful guidance on the size of likely errors may be derived from sensitivity analyses. In this way, applications of economic-cost estimates can be restricted to those for which their precision is adequate.

Contrasting the Incidence and Prevalence Approaches

To estimate the impact of adopting the incidence approach rather than the prevalence approach, we compare our results with those calculated by Berk (1978) following the prevalence approach. Berk estimated the 1975 annual cost of stroke to be $6.84 billion—in contrast with our incidence-based estimate of $6.46 billion. For cancer, Berk calculated $22.36 billion in annual costs versus our figure of $23.15 billion. Berk did not obtain figures for CHD or for MVI. The discrepancy between the two approaches is close to that expected for stroke but puzzling for cancer. In the absence of dramatic trends in cancer costs, we would expect the prevalence-based figures to exceed the incidence-based numbers. This departure from the expected relationship most likely is due to subtle differences in the analytical methods used.

Limitations in Using Economic Costs of Disease and Injury

The numbers reported in this book pertain exclusively to the economic costs of disease and injury and do not reflect (1) pain and suffering, which was mentioned earlier; (2) research and detection costs; (3) prevention costs; and (4) societal values. Explicit consideration of research costs has normally not occurred in estimating the economic costs of disease or injury—with the noteworthy exception of Weisbrod's (1971) work on polio. They seem, in any case, more of a societal reaction to the perceived importance of a disease or injury rather than an intrinsic measure of importance. Detection and prevention costs have been even more neglected in the literature on costs of illness. This has occurred primarily because of the inadequacy of data and not because of any conceptual inappropriateness. A worthwhile extension of all current studies would be to calculate and to include these costs.

Societal values with regard to health impairment and lifesaving are difficult to formulate. Expected future earnings, as used earlier, remain the predominant way of valuing human lives. Nevertheless, many authors, notably Schelling (1968) and Mishan (1971), have pointed out the drawbacks of this methodology. This discrepancy between true societal values and expected future earnings is evident: our society simply does not agree that the average male between the ages of 25 and 34 is 1.6 times as valuable (as the earnings expectations indicate) as the average female of comparable age and that intervention programs should accordingly be targeted to save the life of the former in perference to the latter. The best way to proceed seems to be to use forgone earnings as a measure of the economic impact of lost lives, but not to perceive them as intrinsic or societally accepted life values.

The General Applicability of the Economic Costs of Disease and Injury

Notwithstanding the limitations noted for economic costs, their potential applicability in policymaking is great, as is evidenced by the proliferation of economic-cost studies and the growing use of them in public decisions. When their limitations are suitably recognized, economic costs can guide a variety of societal choices. Other things being equal (recognizing the possible biases in economic valuations and considering the comparative prospects for success of alternative programs), we should take economic costs into account in setting research priorities. In allocating funds to competing preventive and ameliorative programs, economic costs, along with comparative estimates of efficacy and other factors, are of unquestioned relevance. In seeking to justify public health expenditures, estimates of economic costs are invaluable in making the case that the expenditures will in the long run more than pay for themselves. For estimating the likely payoff for possible programs of prevention, treatment, or care, economic-cost estimates—calculated by the prevalence or incidence approaches—provide essential baseline data for subsequent analyses.

The Importance of Indirect Costs

The most common ways for conceptualizing the importance of illnesses have been through mortality figures and through estimates of current direct costs. A number of authors (for example, Fein, 1958; Mushkin, 1959; Weisbrod, 1961; Klarman, 1965; Rice, 1966; and Cooper and Rice, 1976) have, however, argued that this was not enough, and that the importance of the lives lost—as measured by the forfeited economic product—should also be taken into account. They contend that losing a young, potentially productive life is worse than losing an older life with few productive years remaining.

Comparing the direct and indirect costs calculated in this study provides graphic evidence in support of their argument.

Direct costs—money actually spent—and death are the most salient manifestations of disease or injury. Indirect costs—economic product not produced—are in comparison much less visible and often overlooked. Examining the four major conditions covered in our study, we find a variety of relationships between direct and indirect costs. For all four, indirect costs exceed direct costs. For heart disease, the discrepancy is greatest, with indirect costs equaling 4.5 times direct costs. For stroke, in contrast, indirect costs are 1.8 times direct costs. This occurs because stroke affects relatively fewer productive years. Cancer and motor vehicle injuries have indirect costs equal to 2.6 and 2.0 times their respective direct costs.

The importance of calculating indirect costs—and not simply assuming that they are proportional to incidence—can be seen in the breakdowns of the individual impairments. In the case of stroke, for example, it is seen in table 7–1 that males between 35 and 64 account for only 15 percent of all incidence. It was seen in table 4–22 (and can be calculated from tables 7–1 and 7–5) that this group incurs 53 percent of all forgone earnings for stroke. This finding might be used to justify preventive interventions for this population segment.

Application to Resource-Allocation Decisions

The economic costs of illness may be useful in many types of societal decisions: in allocating research funds, in designing preventive strategies, and in identifying targets for cost containment or retrenchment. The advantage of a comprehensive methodology such as ours is that all factors influencing the economic impact are appropriately reflected. One does not just point simplistically to incidence figures, prevalence numbers, hospital usage, or mortality data as measures of illness importance. Instead, one takes into account (1) the number of people affected (as in table 7–1), (2) the productivity of the life-years affected (tables 7–2 and 7–4), (3) the average numbers of years lost per impaired person (table 7–3), and (4) the treatment costs (table 7–6). The importance of all such factors is evident to common sense; yet common sense unaided cannot appropriately combine the factors to obtain an overall gauge of economic importance. Reliable analyses require quantification, aggregation, and comparison of effects—as provided in studies such as this.

Once, however, the full economic costs have been calculated, three important points must be borne in mind: first, that other factors besides economic impact determine the importance of a condition to society; second, that economic measures themselves have limited precision; third, that the efficacy of the possible programs is critical. We now briefly examine possible societal applications of economic-cost calculations.

Overall-Condition Estimates

One way to use the numbers obtained through this study would be to translate them proportionately into health-impairment allocations. For instance, our base-case estimates indicate that the economic costs of motor vehicle injuries exceed those of coronary heart disease by 5 percent. This could be construed to mean that 5 percent more funding should go to research and preventive programs addressed to MVI than for CHD.

Such reasoning is shortsighted for all the reasons cited earlier. First, the accuracy of economic-cost methods does not permit the confident assertion of a 5 percent difference. It would be more appropriate to conclude that CHD and MVI have the same approximate magnitudes of cost than to infer a precise, 5 percent difference. Second, either condition might be rendered more or less important to society by a variety of factors apart from the economic impact. These factors might include pain and suffering, perceptions of the noneconomic importance of life-years lost or impaired, or greater societal indifference toward conditions that are, to some extent, self-caused. Third, it would be wrong to allocate research moneys according to the economic impacts if one area of research—perhaps into low-cost therapies for CHD—were considered much more likely to be successful.

Given these pitfalls, a more appropriate conclusion to be drawn from our figures would be that, other things being equal, economic considerations indicate that roughly the same amounts of resources should be devoted to research and prevention activities for MVI and CHD. To the extent that other things are not equal—if, for instance, other factors affect societally perceived importance or if one type of preventive program is more or less effective—this societal conclusion should be appropriately modified.

Cerebral Infarctions and Respiratory System Cancers

The incidence of cerebral infarctions is 2.2 times that of respiratory system cancers. These cancers, however, occasion loss of (1) more life-years and (2) more productive life-years per incident case than do infarctions. These varied disease features all are reflected in the total economic costs of disease, which, as table 7–6 shows, are $4.6 billion for each condition. We would conclude that, other things being equal, purely economic considerations argue for devoting roughly the same amount of resources to respiratory cancers as to infarctions.

Critical Motor Vehicle Injuries and
Coronary Sudden Death

A society paring down its planned expenditures to satisfy budget constraints might force a tough decision between reductions in funding for research on ameliorating critical (MAIS 5) MVIs or for research on preventing sudden-death heart attacks. Comparisons between the programs are difficult and should take into account a number of observations: (1) that there are roughly 2.4 times as many sudden deaths as critical MVIs; (2) that sudden deaths occasion the loss of 5.9 times as many life-years; (3) that the life-years lost because of sudden death have lower average productivity; (4) that the direct costs of critical injuries are 200 times those of sudden deaths. The economic aspects of these varied elements all are reflected in our computations of the total costs of sudden deaths at $3.9 billion and of critical injuries at $3.3 billion. These figures provide good rough estimates of the economic importance of each condition. Suppose, furthermore, that (1) noneconomic considerations are roughly proportional to economic considerations, (2) that the sudden-death research might prevent one-fourth of the current economic loss, (3) that the critical-injury research might avoid two-thirds of the current economic loss, and (4) that the research programs are equally expensive and equally likely to be successful. In this case, a strong argument would be mustered for giving the critical-injury program (with potential annual benefits of $2.2 billion) priority over the sudden-death program (with potential annual benefits of $1 billion). (This scenario would be rendered less likely if the budgets were compartmentalized. That is, if moneys for heart-disease research were seen as different from MVI research funds and subject to a separate budget limit. It can be argued, however, that such compartmental-ization is suboptimal, that all programs extending or enhancing lives should be thought of as competing for the same resources, and that those with greatest expected benefit per unit of cost should be funded first—regardless of which budget heading they fall under.)

Recapitulation

The preceding examples are, to some extent, hypothetical, but the underlying principle is fundamental. Our society has limited resources that can be devoted to programs that enhance and extend lives. For any set amount of resources, we want to achieve as much societally perceived benefit as possible. To do this, we must take into account the potential economic effects, the noneconomic effects, and the likely success of alternative programs. Economic measures of disease and injury costs—such as those presented in this book—provide essential data for estimating the potential economic effects.

Public decisions—on support for research, prevention, and payments for health care—have often been based on dramatic but crude statistics. A more systematic and, in the long run, probably more fruitful approach would be based on carefully comparing different aspects of disease and injury. This book has sought to serve that purpose by consolidating and presenting the more quantifiable aspects: the economic costs. For programs addressed to the prevalence population of a chronic disease or of an injury sequela, prevalence-cost estimates will be more pertinent; for preventive programs, incidence-based costs of the type provided here should usefully assist decisions. Our analysis has indicated the importance of taking into account incidence rates, the age at incidence, the mortality rates, the rates of subsequent work, and the direct costs. Such calculations help to correct the many intuitive, but often false, impressions created by inexact, piecemeal measures of disease and injury effects.

Bibliography

Chapters 1, 2, and 7

Abbreviated Injury Scale (AIS). Joint Committee on Injury Scaling of the Amercian Medical Association, American Association for Automotive Medicine, and Society of Automotive Engineers, 1980 Revision.

Abt Associates Inc. and Boston University Cancer Research Center. *The Measurement of the Cost of Cancer Care. Task Two Report. Literature Review and Recommendations for Further Work*. Prepared for the National Cancer Institute, Division of Cancer Control and Rehabilitation, December 1976.

Acton, J.P. *Evaluating Public Programs to Save Lives: The Case of Heart Attacks*. Santa Monica, Calif.: The Rand Corporation, January 1973.

Amercian Cancer Society. *The Amercian Cancer Society—A Fact Book for the Medical and Related Professions*. New York, 1975.

Berk, A., Paringer, L., and Mushkin, S.J. The economic cost of illness, fiscal 1975. *Medical Care* 16:785–790, 1978.

Berry, R.E., and Boland, J.P. *The Economic Cost of Alcohol Abuse*. New York: Free Press, 1977.

Birnbaum, H. *The Cost of Catastrophic Illness*. Lexington, Mass.: Lexington Books, D.C. Heath and Company, 1978.

Blair, R.D., and Vogel, R.J. *The Cost of Health Insurance Administration*. Lexington, Mass.: Lexington Books, D.C. Heath and Company, 1975.

Brody, W.H. *Economic Value of a Housewife*. Research and Statistics Note 9, DHEW Publication No. SSA 75-11701. Washington: Social Security Administration, Office of Research and Statistics, August 28, 1975.

Conley, R., and Milunsky, A. The economics of prenatal genetic diagnosis. In A. Milunsky (ed.), *The Prevention of Genetic Disease and Mental Retardation*. Philadelphia: W.B. Sanders, 1975.

Commission on Professional and Hospital Activities. *Length of Stay in PAS Hospitals by Diagnosis, United States, 1975*. Ann Arbor, Michigan, 1976.

Cooper, B.S., and Rice, D.P. The economic cost of illness revisited. *Social Security Bulletin* 39(2):21–36, 1976.

Cutler, S.J., and Young, J.L., eds. *Third National Cancer Survey: Incidence Data*. National Cancer Institute Monograph 41. U.S. Department of Health, Education and Welfare, Public Health Services, National Institutes of Health, Publication No. (NIH) 75-787, 1975.

DeLorean Corporation. *Automotive Occupant Protective Safety Air Cushion Expenditure/Benefit Study*. Report prepared for the Allstate

Insurance Company, Northbrook, Ill., Bloomfield Hills, Michigan, August 1975.

Dresser, A., Meirowsky, A., Weiss, G., McNeel, M., Simon, G., and Caveness, W. Gainful employment following head injury. *Archives of Neurology* 29:111–116, 1973.

Emlet, H.E., Jr., Williamson, J.W., Dittmer, D.L., et al. *Estimated Health Benefits and Costs of Post-Onset Care for Stroke*. Falls Church, Va.: Analytic Services, Inc., 1973.

Faigin, B.M. *1975 Societal Costs of Motor Vehicle Accidents*. U.S. Department of Transportation, National Highway Traffic Safety Administration. Washington: U.S. Government Printing Office, December 1976.

Fein, R. *Economics of Mental Illness*. New York: Basic Books, 1958.

The Framingham Study—An Epidemilogical Investigation of Cardiovascular Disease, Sections 1 through 32. U.S. Department of Health, Education and Welfare, Public Health Service, and National Institutes of Health, Washington, 1977.

Furlan, A.J., et al. The decreasing incidence of primary intra-cerebral hemorrhage: A population study. *Annals of Neurology* 5:367–373, 1979.

Garraway, W.M., et al. The changing pattern of cerebral infarction: 1945–1974. *Stroke* 10:657–663, 1979*b*.

Geisler, W.D., Jousse, A.J., Wynne-Jones, M. Survival in traumatic transverse myelitis. *Paraplegia* 14:262–275, 1977.

Gresham, G.E., Fitzpatrick, T.E., Wolf, P.A., et al. Residual disability in survivors of stroke—The Framingham study. *New England Journal of Medicine* 293:954–956, 1975.

Hodgson, T. and Meiners, M. Guidelines for cost of illness studies in the public health service. Public Health Service Task Force on Cost of Illness Studies unpublished paper, May 1979.

Klarman, H.E. Syphilis control programs. In Robert Dorfman (ed.), *Measuring the Benefits of Government Investments*. Washington: Brookings Institution, 1965, pp. 367–414.

Luce, B.R., and Schweitzer, S.O. Smoking and alcohol abuse: A comparison of their economic consequences. *New England Journal of Medicine* 238: 569–571, 1978.

Matsumoto, N., Whisnant, J.P., Kurland, L.T., et al. Natural History of Stroke in Rochester, Minnesota, 1955–1969: An extension of a previous study, 1945–1954. *Stroke* 4:20–29, 1973.

Mills, E., and Thompson, M.S. The economic costs of stroke in Massachusetts. *New England Journal of Medicine* 299:415–418, 1978.

Mishan, E.J. Evaluation of life and limb: A theoretical approach. *Journal of Political Economy* (July/August 1971):687–705.

Mueller, M.S., and Gibson, R.M. National health expenditures, fiscal year 1975. *Social Security Bulletin* (February 1976):3–20.

Mueller, M.S. Private health insurance in 1975: coverage, enrollment, and financial experience. *Social Security Bulletin* (June 1977):3–21.

Mushkin, S.J., and Collings, E.A. Economic costs of disease and injury. *Public Health Reports* 74(a):795–809, 1959.

Mushkin, S.J. Health as an investment. *Journal of Political Economy* 70(5): 129–157, 1962.

National Center for Health Statistics. *The National Nursing Home Survey: 1977 Summary for the United States*. DHEW Publication No. (PHS) 79-1974, 1979b.

Prest, A.P., and Turvey, R. Cost benefit analysis: A survey. *Economic Journal* 75:683–735, 1965.

Rhoads, S.E. How much should we spend to save a life? *The Public Interest* 51:74–92, 1978.

Rice, D.P. *Estimating the Cost of Illness*.Health Economic Series No. 6, PHS Publication No. 947-6. Washington: U.S. Government Printing Office, May 1966.

Rufener, B.L., Rachal, J.V., and Cruze, A.M., Management effectiveness measure for NIDA drug abuse treatment programs. In *Cost to Society of Drug Abuse, Vol. II*. Washington: U.S. Government Printing Office, 1976, pp. 975–1016.

Schelling, T.C. The life you save may be your own, in Samuel B. Chase, Jr. (ed.), *Problems in Public Expenditure Analysis*. Washington: Brookings Institution, 1968, pp. 127–176.

Shepard, D.S., and Zeckhauser, R.J. Long-term effects of interventions to improve survival in mixed populations. *Journal of Chronic Diseases* 33: 413–433, 1980.

Shurtleff, D. *Some Characteristics Related to the Incidence of Cardiovascular Disease and Death: Framingham Study, 18-year Follow-up. The Framingham Study: An Epidemiological Investigation of Cardiovascular Disease*, Section 30. Washington: U.S. Government Printing Office, 1974.

Smart, C.N., and Sanders, C.R. *The Costs of Motor Vehicle Related Spinal Cord Injuries*. Washington: Insurance Institute for Highway Safety, 1976.

Thompson, M.S. *Benefit-Cost Analysis for Program Evaluation*. Beverly Hills and London: Sage Publications, 1980.

U.S. Department of Commerce, Bureau of the Census. Current population survey, May 1975. Unpublished data on U.S. mean full- and part-time earnings for 1975.

U.S. Department of Commerce, Bureau of the Census. *Statistical Abstract of the United States, 1979.* Washington: U.S. Government Printing Office, July 1979.

U.S. Department of Health, Education and Welfare, Health Resources Administration, National Center for Health Statistics. Current estimates from the health interview survey, United States, 1975. *Vital and Health Statistics* [10]115, March 1977.

U.S. Department of Health, Education and Welfare, National Center for Health Statistics. Life tables. *Vital Statistics of the United States II, 1977,* Vol. 2, Section 5. Washington: U.S. Government Printing Office, 1980.

U.S. Department of Health, Education and Welfare. *National Survey of Stroke.* NIH Publication No. 80-2069, 1980.

U.S. Department of Labor, Bureau of Labor Statistics. *Employment and Earnings* 22(7), January 1971 and January 1976.

U.S. Department of Transportation. *Automobile Accident Litigation.* A Report of the Federal Judicial Center to the Department of Transportation, April 1970 (from *Automobile Insurance and Compensation Study*).

U.S. Department of Transportation, National Highway Traffic Safety Administration. *Fatal Accident Reporting System: 1975 Annual Report.* Washington: U.S. Government Printing Office, October 1976.

U.S. Department of Transportation, National Highway Traffic Safety Administration. National crash severity study. Unpublished data on nonfatal motor vehicle injuries from the May 1980 data file.

U.S. Executive Office of the President, Office of Management and Budget. *Circular No. A-94 (Revised).* Washington, March 27, 1972.

Weinstein, M.C., and Stason, W.B. Foundations of cost-effectiveness analysis for health and medical pracices. *New England Journal of Medicine 296:716–721, 1977.*

Weisbrod, B.A. *Economics of Public Health.* Philadelphia: Univ. of Pennsylvania Press, 1961.

Weisbrod, B.A. Costs and benefits of medical research: A case study of poliomyelitis. *Journal of Political Economy* 79(3):527–544, 1971.

Wuerdemann, H., and Joksch, H.C. *National Indirect Costs of Motor Vehicle Accidents.* Center for the Environment and Man, Report No. 4114-494-B, Hartford, Conn., June 1973.

Young, J.L., Jr., Asire, A.J., and Polack, E.S. *SEER Program: Cancer Incidence and Mortality in the United States, 1973–1976.* U.S. Department of Health, Education and Welfare, National Cancer Institute, DHEW Publication No. (NIH) 78-1837, 1978.

Chapter 3

Acton, J.P. *Evaluating Public Programs to Save Lives: The Case of Heart Attacks*. Santa Monica, Calif.: Rand Corporation, January 1973.

Alderman, E.L., Matlof, H.J., Wexler, L. Shumway, N.E., and Harrison, D.C., Results of direct coronary-artery surgery for the treatment of angina pectoris. *New England Journal of Medicine* 288(11):535–539, 1973.

Altman, L.K. Coronary bypass patients found not outliving those using drugs. *New York Times*,September 22, 1977.

American Hospital Association. *Hospital Statistics*. Chicago, 1976.

Badger, G.F., Liebow, I.M., and Shirreffs, T.G. Myocardial infarctions in the practices of a group of private physicians. III:Causes of death among patients who have survived a myocaridal infarction. *Journal of Chronic Diseases* 21(1968):467–471.

Bainton, C., and Peterson, D.R. Deaths from coronary heart disease in persons fifty years of age and younger. A community-wide study. *New England Journal of Medicine* 268(11):569–575, 1963.

Bendor, D., and Fowkes, W. Sudden and unexpected death due to arterio-sclerotic heart disease—Implications for mobile coronary care units. *Circulation [Suppl. 3]* 40(4):III-43, 1969.

Berndt, T.B. Miller, D.C., Silverman, J.F., Stinson, E.B., Harrison, D.C., and Schroeder, J.S. Coronary by-pass surgery for unstable angina pectoris. Clinical follow-up and results of post-operative treadmill electrocardiograms. *American Journal of Medicine* 58(2):171–176, 1975.

Bloom, B.S., and Peterson, O.L. End results: Cost and productivity of coronary care units. *New England Journal of Medicine* 228(2):72–78, 1973.

Bloomfield, D.K., Slivka, J., Vossler, S., and Edelstein, J. Survival in acute myocardial infarction before and after the establishment of a coronary care unit. *Chest* 57(3):224–229, 1970.

Braunwald, E. Coronary-artery surgery at the crossroads. *New England Journal of Medicine* 297(12):661–663, 1977.

Bunker, J.P., Barnes, B.A., and Mosteller, F. *Costs, Risks, and Benefits of Surgery*. New York: Oxford Univ. Press, 1977.

Cady, L.D., Jr., Epidemiology of coronary heart disease. *American Journal of Cardiology* 20(5):692–702, 1967.

Carveth, S., Olson, D., and Bechtel, J. Emergency medical care system. *Archives of Surgery* 108:528–530, 1974.

Cassel, J. Summary of major findings of the Evans county cardiovascular studies. *Archives of Internal Medicine* 128:887–889, 1971.

Cassel, J., Heyden, S., Bartel, A.G., Kaplan, B.H., Tyroler, H.A., Cornoni, J.C., and Hames, C.G. Incidence of coronary heart disease by ethnic group, social class, and sex. *Archives of Internal Medicine* 128(6): 901–906, 1971.

Cassel, J., Heyden, S., Bartel, A.G., Kaplan, B.H., Tyroler, H.A., Cornoni, J.C., and Hames, C.G. Occupation and physical activity and coronary heart disease. *Archives of Internal Medicine* 128(6):920–928, 1971.

Chapman, J.M., Goerke, L.S., Dixon, W., Loveland, D.B., and Phillips, E. The clinical status of a population group in Los Angeles under observation for 2 to 3 years. *American Journal of Public Health* 47(Suppl.):33–52, 1957.

Commission on Professional and Hospital Activities. *Length of Stay in PAS Hospitals by Diagnosis, United States, 1975*. Ann Arbor, Michigan, 1976.

Conti, C.R., Brawley, R.K., Griffith, L.S., Pitt, B., Humphries, J. O'N., Gott, V.L., and Ross, R.S. Unstable angina pectoris: Morbidity and mortality in 57 consecutive patients evaluated angiographically. *American Journal of Cardiology* 32(6):745–750, 1973.

Costas, R., Jr., Garcia-Palmieri, M.R., and Feliberti, M. Morbidity and mortality surveillance in a prospective epidemiological study of coronary heart disease. *Puerto Rico* 61(6):207–211, 1969.

Cretin, S. A model of the risk of death from myocardial infarction. Innovative Resource Planning in Urban Public Safety Systems, Technical Report No. 09–74, Massachusetts Institute of Technology, 1974.

Cretin, S. Cost/benefit analysis of treatment and prevention of myocardial infarction. *Health Services Research* (Summer 1977):174–187.

Cretin, S. Modeling the impact of treatment strategies on death from myocardial infarction. In T.R. Willemain and R.C. Larson (eds.), *Emergency Medical Systems Analysis*. Lexington, Mass.: Lexington Books, D.C. Heath and Co., 1977.

Dawber, T.R., and Kannel, W.B. Susceptibility to coronary heart disease. *Modern Concepts of Cardiovascular Disease* 30(7):671–676, 1961.

Dawber, T.R., Moore, F.E., and Mann, G.V. Coronary heart disease in the Framingham study. *American Journal of Public Health* 47(Suppl):4–24, 1957.

Dawber, T.R., Kannel, W.B., Gordon, T. Coffee and cardiovascular Disease: Observations from the Framingham study. *New England Journal of Medicine* 291(17):871–874, 1974.

Dewar, H.A., McCollum, J.P.K., and Floyd, M. A years's expereince with a mobile coronary resuscitation unit. *British Journal of Medicine* 4(677): 226–229, 1969.

Doyle, J.T., Heslin, A.S., Hilleboe, H.E., Formel, P.F., and Korns, R.F. A prospective study of degenerative cardiovascular disease in Albany: Report of three years experience. I: Ischemic heart disease. *American Journal of Public Health* 47(Suppl.):25–32, 1957.

Drake, R.M., Buechley, R.W., and Breslow, L. An epidemiological investigation of coronary heart disease in the California health survey population. *American Journal of Public Health* 47(Suppl.):43–63,1957.

Eisenberg, H., Feltner, W.R., Payne, G.H., and Haddad, C.A. The epidemiology of coronary heart disease in Middlesex County, Connecticut. *Journal of Chronic Diseases* 14(2):221–235, 1961.

Epstein, F.H. The epidemiology of coronary heart disease. *Journal of Chronic Diseases* 18:735–775, 1965.

Epstein, F.H., Ostrander, L.D., Jr., Johnson, B.C., Payne, M.W., Hayner, N.S., Keller, J.B., and Thomas, F., Jr. Epidemiological studies of Cardiovascular disease in a total community—Tecumseh, Michigan. *Annals of Internal Medicine* 62:1170, 1965.

Epstein, F.H., Francis, T., Jr., Hayner, N.S., Johnson, B.C., Kjelsberg, M.O., Napier, J.A., Ostrander, L.D., Jr., Payne, M.W., and Dodge, H.J. Prevalence of chronic diseases and distribution of selected physiologic variables in a total community, Tecumseh, Michigan. *American Journal of Epidemiology* 87:307–322, 1965.

Fagan, I.D., and Anadiah, K.M. The coronary care unit and mortality from myocardial infarction: A continued evaluation. *Journal of the American Geriatrics Society* 19(8):675–686, 1971.

Feinleib, M., Kannel, W.B., Garrison, R.J., McNamara, P.M., and Castelli, W.P. The Framingham offspring study: Design and preliminary data. *Journal of Preventive Medicine* 4(4):518–525, 1975.

Framingham Heart Study. Unpublished data.

The Framingham Study—An Epidemiological Investigation of Cardiovascular Disease, Sections 1 through 32. U.S. Department of Health, Education and Welfare, Public Health Service, and National Institutes of Health.

Frank, C.W., Weinblatt, E., and Shapiro, S. Angina pectoris in men. Prognostic significance of selected medical factors. *Circulation* 47:509, 1973.

Friedman, G.D., Kannel, W.B., Dawber, T.R., and McNamara, P.M. Comparison of prevalence, case history and incidence data in assessing the potency of risk factors in coronary heart disease. *American Journal of Epidemiology* 83(2):366–378, 1966.

Friedman, G.D., Klatsky, A.L., Siegelaub, A.B., and McCarthy, N.

Kaiser-Permanente epidemiologic study of myocardial infarction—Study design and results for standard risk factors. *American Journal of Epidemiology* 99(2):101–116, 1974.

Fulton, M., Julian, D.G., and Oliver, M.F. Sudden death and myocardial infarction. *Circulation* 39 and 40 (Suppl. IV):IV-181–IV-193, 1949.

Gordon, T., Garcia-Palmieri, M., Kagan, A., Kannel, W., and Schiffman, J. Differences in coronary heart disease in Framingham, Honolulu, and Puerto Rico. *Journal of Chronic Diseases* 27:329–344, 1974.

Gordon, T., and Kannel, W. Premature mortality from coronary heart disease. *Journal of the American Medical Association* 215:1617–1625, 1971.

Graf, W.S., Polin, S.S., and Paegel, B.L. A community program for emergency cardiac care. A three year coronary ambulance-paramedic evaluation. *Journal of the American Medical Association* 226(2): 156–160, 1973.

Hagstrom, R.M., Federspiel, C.F., Ho, Yaw Chin. Incidence of myocardial infarction and sudden death from coronary heart disease in Nashville, Tennessee. *Circulation* 44:884–890, 1971.

Hammermeister, K.E., DeRouen, T.A., English, M.T., and Dodge, H.T. Effect of surgical versus medical therapy on return to work in patients with coronary artery disease. *American Journal of Cardiology* 44:105–110, 1979.

Hill, J.D., Hampton, J.R., and Mitchell, J.R.A. Home or hospital for myocardial infarction—Who cares? (editorial). *American Heart Journal* 98:545–547, 1979.

Hirshman, J.C., Nussenfield, S.R., and Nagel, E.L. Mobile physician command: A new dimension in civilian telemetry-rescue systems. *Journal of the American Medical Association* 230(2):255–258, 1974.

Hood, W.B., Jr., Madias, J.E., and Pozen, M.W. *Operational Plans for the Boston City Hospital Coronary Care Unit and Progressive Care Unit*, 4th ed. Boston, August 15, 1976, amended May 1, 1977.

Kahn, H.A. The relationship of reported coronary heart disease mortality to physical activity of work. *American Journal of Public Health* 53(7): 1058–1967, 1963.

Kannel, W.B. *The Natural History of Myocardial Infarction: The Framingham Study*. Leiden, Germany: Leiden Univ. Press, 1973.

Kannel, W.B. Prevention of heart disease in the young coronary candiate. *Primary Care* 4(2):229–243, 1977.

Kannel, W.B. Some lessons in cardiovascular epidemiology from Framingham. *American Journal of Cardiology* 37:269–282, 1976.

Kannel, W.B., and Castelli, W.P. The Framingham study of coronary heart disease in women. *Medical Times* 100(5):173–184, 1972.

Kannel, W.B., Castelli, W.P., and McNamara, P.M. The coronary profile: 12 year follow-up in the Framingham study. *Journal of Occupational Medicine* 9(12):611–619, 1967.

Kannel, W.B., Doyle, J.T., McNamara, P.M., Quickenton, P., and Gordon, T. Precursors of sudden coronary death. Factors related to the incidence of sudden death. *Circulation* 51(4):606–613, 1975.

Kannel, W.B., and Feinleib, M.M. The natural history of angina pectoris in the Framingham study: Prognosis and survival. *American Journal of Cardiology* 29:154–163, 1972.

Kannel, W.B., Skinner, J.J., Jr., Schwartz, M.J., and Shurtleff, D. Intermittent claudication: Incidence in the Framingham study. *Circulation* 41:875–883, 1970.

Kannel, W.B., and Thom, T.J. Implications of the recent decline in cardiovascular mortality. *Cardiovascular Medicine* 4:983–997, 1979.

Kolata, G.N. Coronary bypass surgery: Debate over its benefits. *Science* 194:1263–1265, 1976.

Kuller, L. Sudden death in arteriosclerotic heart disease. *American Journal of Cardiology* 24:617–628, 1969.

Kuller, L., Cooper, M., Perper, J., and Fisher, R. Myocardial infarction and sudden death in an urban community. *Bulletin of the New York Academy of Medicine* 49(6):532–543, 1973.

Kuller, L.A., Lilienfeld, A., and Fisher, R. Epidemiological study of sudden and unexpected deaths due to arteriosclerotic heart disease. *Circulation* 34:1056–1068, 1966.

Kuller, L., Perper, J., and Cooper, M. Demographic characteristics and trends in arteriosclerotic heart disease mortality: Sudden death and myocardial infarction. *Circulation* 52(6):1–11, 1975.

Lawrie, D.M., Goddard, M., Greenwood, T.W., Harvey, A.C., Donald, K.W., Julian, D.C., and Oliver, M.F. A coronary care unit. *Lancet* 2: 109, 1967.

Little, J.A., Shanoff, H.M., Csima, A. (with technical assistance of Ruth Yano). Studies of male survivors of myocardial infarcting. IX: Mortality experience and insurability. *Canadian Medical Association Journal* 96: 1204–1207, 1967.

Lown, B. Are mobile coronary care units the answer? (editorial). *Hospital Practice* (August 1969).

Lown, B., Fakhro, A.M., Hood, W.B., Jr., and Thorn, G.W. The coronary care unit. New perspectives and directions. *Journal of the American Medical Association* 199(3):156–166, 1967.

Lown, B., Klein, M.D., and Herschberg, P.I. Coronary and precoronary care. *American Journal of Medicine* 46:705–724, 1969.

Lown, B., and Ruberman, W. The concept of precoronary care. *Modern*

Concepts of Cardiovascular Disease 39(5):97–102, 1970.

Lown, B., and Wolf, M. Approaches to sudden death from coronary heart disease. *Circulation* 44(1):130–142, 1971.

Margolis, J.R., Kannel, W.B., Feinleib, M., Dawber, T.R., and McNamara, P.M. Clinical features of unrecognized myocardial infarction—Silent and symptomatic. *American Journal of Cardiology* 32:1–7, 1973.

Margolis, J.R., Gillum, R.F., Feinleib, M., Brasch, R.C., and Fabsitz, R.R. Community surveillance for coronary heart disease: The Framingham cardiovascular disease survey. Comparisons with the Framingham heart study and previous short-term studies. *American Journal of Cardiology* 37(1):61–67, 1976.

Margolis, J.R., Gillum, R.F., Feinleib, M., Brasch, R.C., and Fabsitz, R.R. Community surveillance for coronary heart disease: The Framingham cardiovascular disease survey. Methods and preliminary results. *American Journal of Epidemiology* 100(6):425–426, 1974.

McDonough, J.R., Hames, C.G., Stulb, S.C., and Garrison, G.E. Coronary heart disease among Negroes and whites in Evans County, Georgia. Journal of Chronic Diseases 18:443–468, 1965.

McNeer, J.F., Wallace, A.G., Wagner, G.S., Starmer, C.F., and Rosati, R.A. The course of acute myocardial infarction feasibility of early discharge of the uncomplicated patient. *Circulation* 51(3):410–413, 1975.

Medalie, J.H., Kahn, H.A., Neufeld, H.N., Riss, E., Goldbourt, U., Perlstein, T., and Oron, D. Myocardial infarction over a five-year period. I: Prevalence, incidence and mortality experience. *Journal of Chronic Diseases* 26(2):63–84, 1973.

Mortality from heart disease—All forms. *Statistical Bulletin of the Metropolitan Life Insurance Company* (November 1972):2–5.

Mundth, E.D., and Austen, G.W. Surgical measures for coronary heart disease. *New England Journal of Medicine* 293(3):124–130, 1975.

National Center for Health Statistics. Advance report: Final mortality statistics, 1976. *Monthly Vital Statistics Report.* DHEW Publication No. (PHS) 78-1120, Vol. 26, No. 12, Supplement 2, 1978.

Owens, A. At last: Hard figures on how fast fees have been climbing. *Medical Economics* (October 13, 1975):98–126.

Pell, S., and D'Alonzo, C.A. Immediate mortality and five-year survival of employed men with first myocardial infarction. *New England Journal of Medicine* 270(18):915–922, 1964.

Recent trends in mortality from heart disease. *Statistical Bulletin of the Metropolitan Life Insurance Company* (June 1975).

Reeves, T.J., Oberman, A., Jones, W.B., and Sheffield, L.T. Natural history of angina pectoris. *American Journal of Cardiology* 33(423):423–430, 1974.

Regional variations in mortality from heart disease. *Statistical Bulletin of the Metropolitan Life Insurance Company* (November 1972).

Rice, D. *Economic Costs of Cardiovascular Diseases and Cancer, 1962*. U.S. Department of Health, Education and Welfare, Health Economics Series, No. 5, 1965.

Sampson, J.J., and Hyatt, K.H. Management of the patient with severe angina pectoris. An internist's point of view. *Circulation* 46:1185–1196, 1972.

Shapiro, S., Weinblatt, E., and Frank, C.W. The HIP study of incidence and prognosis of coronary heart disease. *HIP News* 1(1):10–16, 1970.

Shapiro, S., Weinblatt, E., and Frank, C.W. Return to work after first myocardial infarction. *Archives of Environmental Health* 24(1):17–26, 1972.

Shapiro, S., Weinblatt, E., Frank, C.W., and Sager, R.V. Incidence of coronary heart disease in a population insured for medical care (HIP). Part II. *American Journal of Public Health* 59(6):1–101, 1969.

Shurtleff, D. *Some Characteristics Related to the Incidence of Cardiovascular Disease and Death: Framingham Study, 18-Year Follow-up. The Framingham Study: An Epidemiological Investigation of Cardiovascular Disease*, Section 30, Washington: U.S. Government Printing Office, 1974.

Sidel, V.W., Action, J., and Lown, B. Models for the evaluation of prehospital coronary care. *American Journal of Cardiology* 24(5):674–688, 1969.

Singer, R.B. Insurance mortality experience in coronary heart disease. *Transactions of the Association of Life Insurance Medical Directors of America* 52:94–114, 1968.

Singer, R.B. Mortality in 966 life insurance applicants with bundle branch block or wide QRS. *Transactions of the Association of Life Insurance Medical Directors of America* 52:94–114, 1968.

Stamler, J., Lindberg, H.A., Berkson, D.M., Shaffer, A., Miller, W., and Poindexter, A., Prevalence and incidence of coronary heart disease in strata of the labor force of a Chicago industrial corporation. *Journal of Chronic Diseases* 11:405–419, 1960.

Stern, M.P. The recent decline in ischemic heart disease mortality. *Annals of Internal Medicine* 91:630–640, 1979.

Survival among metropolitan employees with coronary heart disease. *Statistical Bulletin of the Metropolitan Life Insurance Company* (August 1973):7–9.

Survival among metropolitan policyholders with coronary heart disease. *Statistical Bulletin of the Metropolitan Life Insurance Company* 54:5–7, 1973.

Trueh, J., and Sorlie, P. Changes in successive measurements and the development of disease: The Framingham study. *Journal of Chronic Diseases* 24(6):349–361, 1971.

United States Department of Health, Education and Welfare. *Handbook of Heart Terms.* Publication Number (NIH) 76-131, reprinted in 1975.

Walker, W.J. Coronary mortality: What is going on? *Journal of the American Medical Association* 227(9):1045–1046, 1974.

Weinblatt, E., Shapiro, S., Frank, C.W., and Sager, R.V. Prognosis of men after first myocardiac infarction: Mortality and first recurrence in relation to selected parameters. *American Journal of Chronic Diseases* 21:231–245, 1968.

Weinblatt, E., Shapiro, S., Frank, C.W., and Sager, R.V. Prognosis factors in angina pectoris—A prospective study. *Journal of Chronic Diseases* 21:231–245, 1968.

Weinblatt, E., Shapiro, S., Frank, C.W., and Sager, R.V. Return to work and work status following first myocardial infarction. *American Journal of Public Health* 56(2):169–185, 1966.

Weinstein, B.J., Epstein, F.H., and the Working Subcommittee on Criteria and Methods, Committee on Epidemiological Studies, American Heart Association. Comparability of criteria and methods in the epidemiology of cardiovascular disease: Report of a survey. *Circulation* 30:443–468, 1969.

Weinstein, M.C., Pliskin, J.S., and Stason, W.B. Coronary artery bypass surgery: Decision and policy analysis. In J.P. Bunker, B.A. Barnes, and F. Mosteller (eds.), *Costs, Risks, and Benefits of Surgery.* New York: Oxford Univ. Press, 1977, pp. 342–371.

Wheatley, G.M. What do the heart disease mortality statistics tell us? (editorial). *American Heart Journal* 89(6):683–685, 1975.

Wilder, C.S. Prevalence of chronic circulatory conditions—U.S. 1972. *Vital and Health Statistics* [10] 94, 1974.

Wisoff, B.G., Fogel, R., Voleti, C., Weisz, D., Harstein, M.L., Aintablian, A., and Hamby, R.I. Survival after coronary surgery. *Journal of Thoracic and Cardiovascular Surgery* 76:108–110, 1978.

Yames, T.N. Sudden death related to myocardial infarction. *Circulation* 45: 1972.

Yater, W.M., Traum, A.H., Brown, W.G., Fitzgerald, R.P., Geisler, M.A., Wilcox, B.B. Coronary artery disease in men eighteen to thirty-nine years of age. *American Heart Journal* 36(3):334–372, 1948; 36(4):481–524, 1948; 36(5):683–721, 1948.

Zuckel, W.J., Lewis, R.H., Enterline, P.E., Painter, R.C., Ralston, L.S., Fawcett, R.M., Meredith, A.P., and Peerson, B. A short-term community study of the epidemiology of coronary heart disease. *American Journal of Public Health* 49(12):1630–1639, 1959.

Zucker, R. Social security medical reports for patients with heart disease. *Journal of the Medical Society of New Jersey* 63(1):8–10, 1966.

Chapter 4
Stroke

Acheson, J., and Hutchinson, E.C. Natural history of "focal cerebral vascular disease." *Quarterly Journal of Medicine* 40:15–23, 1971.

Acheson, J., and Hutchinson, E.C. Observations on the natural history of transient cerebral ischemia. *Lancet* 2:871–874, 1964.

Acheson, R.M., and Fairbairn, A.S. Record linkage in studies of cerebrovascular disease in Oxford, England. *Stroke* 2:48–57, 1971.

Adams, G.F., and Merrett, J.D. Prognosis and survival in the aftermath of hemiplegia. *British Medical Journal* 1:309–314, 1961.

Aho, K., and Fogelholm, R. Incidence and early prognosis of stroke in Espoo-Kauniainen Area, Finland, in 1972. *Stroke* 5:658–661, 1974.

Alter, M., Christoferson, L., Resch, J., et al. Cerebrovascular disease. Frequency and population selectivity in an upper midwestern community. *Stroke* 1:454–465, 1970.

Baker, R.N. Prognosis among survivors of ischemic stroke. *Neurology* 18: 933–941, 1968.

Baker, R.N. Prospective study of transient ischemic attacks. In J. Moossy and R. Janeway (eds.), *Cerebral Vascular Diseases: Seventh Conference*. New York: Grune and Stratton, 1971.

Baker, R.N., Ramseyer, J.C., and Schwartz, W.S. Prognosis in patients with transient cerebral ischemic attacks. *Neurology* 18:1157–1165, 1968.

Borhani, N.O. Differences among hospitals in case fatality ratios of cerebrovascular disease. *Annals of Internal Medicine* 72:953–955, 1970.

Borhani, N.O., and Meyer, J.S., eds. *Medical Basis for Comprehensive Community Stroke Programs*. Bethesda, Md.: National Institutes of Health, 1968.

Bryant, N.H., Candland, L., and Lowenstein, R. Comparison of care and cost outcomes for stroke patients with and without home care. *Stroke* 5: 54–59, 1974.

Californial Medical Association. *1974 Revision of the 1969 California Relative Value Studies*, 1974.

Carpenter, R.R., Rogers, K.D., and Reed, D.E. The use of medical facilities for cerebrovascular disease patients in western Pennsylvania. *Stroke* 3: 759–763, 1972.

Carroll, D. The disability in hemiplegia caused by cerebrovascular disease:

Serial studies of 98 cases. *Journal of Chronic Diseases* 15:179–188, 1962.

Carstairs, V. Stroke: Resource consumption and the cost to the community. in F.J. Gillingham, C. Mawdsley, and A.E. Williams, (eds.), *Stroke.* Edinburgh: Churchill Livingstone, 1976.

Carter, A.B. Prognosis of cerebral embolism. *Lancet* 2:514–519, 1965.

Center for Health Services Research and Development, American Medical Association. *Profile of Medical Practice.* Chicago: 1978.

Commission on Professional and Hospital Activities. *Length of Stay in PAS Hospitals by Diagnosis: United States, 1975.* Ann Arbor, Michigan, 1976.

Conant, R.G., Perkins, J.A., and Ainley, A.B. Stroke: Morbidity, mortality and rehabilitative potential. *Journal of Chronic Diseases* 18:397–403, 1965.

Cooper, B.S., and Rice, D.P. The economic cost of illness revisited. *Social Security Bulletin* 39:21–36, 1976.

David, N.J., and Heyman, A. Factors influencing the prognosis of cerebral thrombosis and infarction due to atherosclerosis. *Journal of Chronic Diseases* 11:394–404, 1960.

Dyken, M.L. Precipitating factors, prognosis and demography of cerebrovascular disease in an Indiana community: A review of all patients hospitalized from 1963–1965 with neurological examination of survivors. *Stroke* 1:261–269, 1970.

Dyken, M.L., Conneally, P.M., Haerer, A.F., et al. Cooperative study of hospital frequency and character of transient ischemic attacks. I: Background, organization, and clinical survey. *Journal of the American Medical Association* 237:882–886, 1977.

Eckstrom, P.T., Brand, F.R., Edlavitch, S.A., et al. Epidemiology of stroke in a rural area: Second year of the mid-Missouri stroke survey. *Public Health Reports* 84:878–882, 1969.

Eisenberg, H., Morrison, J.T., Sullivan, P., et al. CVAs. Incidence and survival rates in a defined population, Middlesex County, Connecticut. *Journal of the American Medical Association* 189:883–888, 1964.

Emlet, H.E., Jr., Williamson, J.W., Dittmer, D.L., et al. *Estimated Health Benefits and Costs of Post-Onset Care for Stroke.* Falls Church, Va.: Analytic Services, Inc., 1973.

Falk, L.A., Zimmerman, J.P., and Bisdee, C.H. Stroke among a coal mining population. *John Hopkins Medical Journal* 120:380–392, 1967.

Florey, C., Senter, M., and Acheson, R. A study of the validity of the diagnosis of stroke on mortality data. *Yale Journal of Biology and Medicine* 40:148–163, 1967.

Ford, A.B., and Katz, S. Prognosis after strokes. I: A critical review. *Medicine* 45:223–236, 1966.

Framingham Heart Study, unpublished data.

The Framingham Study: An Epidemiological Investigation of Cardiovascular Disease. Survival Following Certain Cardiovascular Events, Section 25. Washington: U.S. Government Printing Office, 1970.

Friedman, G.D., Wilson, W.S., Mosier, J.M., et al. Transient ischemic attacks in a community. *Journal of the American Medical Association* 210:1428–1434, 1969.

Furlan, A.H., et al. The decreasing incidence of primary intra-cerebral hemorrhage: A population study. *Annals of Neurology* 5:367–373, 1979.

Garraway, W.M., et al. The declining incidence of stroke. *New England Journal of Medicine* 300:449–452, 1979*a*.

Garraway, W.M., et al. The changing pattern of cerebral infarction: 1945–1974. *Stroke* 10:657–663, 1979*b*.

Gillingham, F.J., Mawdsley, C., and Williams, A.E., eds. *Stroke*. Edinburgh: Churchill Livingston, 1976.

Goldner, J.C., Payne, G.H., Watson, F.R., et al. Prognosis for survival after stroke. *American Journal of the Medical Sciences* 253:129–133, 1967.

Goldner, J.C., Whisnant, J.P., and Taylor, W.F. Long-term prognosis of transient cerebral ischemic attacks. *Stroke* 2:160–167, 1971.

Gresham, G.E., Fitzpatrick, T.E., Wolf, P.A., et al. Residual disability in survivors of stroke—The Framingham study. *New England Journal of Medicine* 293:954–956, 1975.

Grindal, A.B., Cohen, R.J., Saul, R.F., et al. Cerebral infarction in young adults. *Stroke* 9:39–41, 1978.

Gudmundsson, G., and Benedikz, J.E.G. Epidemiological investigation of cerebrovascular disease in Iceland, 1958–1968 (ages 0–35 years). *Stroke* 8:329–331, 1977.

Haerer, A.F., Smith, R.R., and Currier, R.D. The Mississippi RMP stroke unit: Critique and follow-up of the first 200 patients admitted. *Southern Medical Journal* 64:951–955, 1971.

Haerer, A.F., and Woosley, P.C. Prognosis and quality of survival in a hospitalized stroke population from the south. *Stroke* 6:543–548, 1975.

Heather, A.J. A two-year follow-up study of the patients admitted to the rehabilitation center of the hospital of the University of Pennsylvania. *American Journal of Physical Medicine* 37:237–255, 1968.

Heyman, A., Karp, H.R., Heyden, S., et al. Cerebrovascular disease in the bi-racial population of Evans County, Georgia. *Stroke* 2:209–518, 1971.

Howard, F.A., Cohen, P., Hickler, R.B., et al. Survival following stroke. *Journal of the American Medical Association* 183:921–925, 1963.

Hutchinson, E.C., and Acheson, J. *Strokes. Natural History, Pathology and Surgical Treatment*. London: W.B. Saunders, 1975.

Kannel, W.B. An evaluation of the epidemiology of ABI. *Milbank Memorial Fund Quarterly* 53:405–448, 1975.

Kannel, W.B., Dawber, T.R., Cohen, M.E., et al. Vascular disease of the brain—epidemiological aspects: The Framingham study. *American Journal of Public Health* 55:1355–1366, 1965.

Karp, H.R., Heyman, A., Heyden, S., et al. Transient cerebral ischemia. Prevalence and prognosis in a biracial rural community. *Journal of the American Medical Association* 225:125–128, 1973.

Katz, S., Ford, A.B., and Chinn, A.B. Prognosis after strokes. II: Long-term course of 159 patients. *Medicine* 45:236–246, 1966.

Kuller, L., Anderson, H., Peterson, D., et al. Nationwide cerebrovascular disease morbidity study. *Stroke* 1:86–99, 1970.

Kuller, L., Bolker, A., Saslaw, M., et al. Nationwide cerebrovascular disease mortality study. I: Methods and analysis of death certificates. *American Journal of Epidemiology* 90:536–544, 1969.

Kuller, L., Bolker, A., Saslaw, M., et al. Nationwide cerebrovascular disease mortality study. II: Comparison of clinical records and death certificates. *American Journal of Epidemiology* 90:545–555, 1969.

Kuller, L., Bolker, A., Saslaw, M., et al. Nationwide cerebrovascular disease mortality study. IV: Comparison of the different clinical types of cerebrovascular disease. *American Journal of Epidemiology* 90:567–578, 1969.

Kurtzke, J.F. *Epidemiology of Cerebrovascular Disease.* New York: Springer-Verlag, 1969.

Kurtzke, J.F. Epidemiology of cerebrovascular disease. In R.G. Siekert (ed.), *Cerebrovascular Survey Report for Joint Council Subcommittee on Cerebrovascular Disease.* Rochester, Minn.: Whiting Press, 1976.

Lehmann, J.F., DeLateur, B.J., Fowler, R.S., et al. Stroke: Does rehabilitation affect outcome? *Archives of Physical Medicine and Rehabilitation* 56:375–382, 1975.

Licht, S., ed. *Stroke and Its Rehabilitation.* Baltimore, MD.: Waverly Press, 1975.

Locksley, H.B. Hemorrhagic strokes: Principal causes, natural history, and treatment. *Medical Clinics of North America* 52:1193–1212, 1968.

Marquardsen, J. The natural history of acute cerebrovascular disease. A retrospective study of 769 patients. *Acta Neurologica Scandinavia* 45 (Suppl. 38): 1969.

Marshall, J. The natural history of transient ischemic cerebrovascular attacks. *Quarterly Journal of Medicine* 33:309–324, 1964.

Marshall, J., and Kaeser, A.C. Survival after non-hemorrhagic CVAs. A prospective study. *British Medical Journal* 2:73–77, 1961.

Matsumoto, N., Whisnant, J.P., Kurland, L.T., et al. Natural history stroke in Rochester, Minnesota, 1955–1969: An extension of a previous study, 1945–1954. *Stroke* 4:20–29, 1973.

Mills, E., and Thompson, M. The economic costs of stroke in Massachusetts. *New England Journal of Medicine* 299:415–418, 1978.

Minter, S.A., and Scovell, M.E. *Medicaid Fee Schedule—Service and Procedure Codes Effective January 1, 1974.* Massachusetts Department of Public Welfare, 1974.

Moossy, J., and Janeway, R., eds. *Cerebral Vascular Diseases. Seventh Conference.* New York: Grune and Stratton, 1971.

Moskowitz, E. Long-term follow-up of the poststroke patient. *Archives of Physical Medicine and Rehabilitation* 53:167–172, 1972.

National Center for Health Statistics. Advance report: Final mortality statistics, 1975. *Monthly Vital Statistics Report.* DHEW Publication No. (PHS) 78-1120, Vol. 26, No. 12, Supplement 2, 1977.

National Center for Health Statistics. Advance report: Final Mortality statistics, 1977. *Monthly Vital Statistics Report.* DHEW Publication No. (PHS) 79-1120, Vol. 28, No. 1, Supplement, 1979*a.*

National Center for Health Statistics. *The National Nursing Home Survey: 1977 Summary for the United States.* DHEW Publication No. (PHS) 79-1794, 1979*b.*

National Center for Health Statistics. Provisional statistics: Annual summary for the United States, 1978: Births, deaths, marriages, and divorce. *Monthly Vital Statistics Report.* DHEW Publication No. (PHS) 79-1120, Vol. 27, No. 13, 1979*c.*

Oh, S.H. Cerebral vascular diseases in negroes. *Journal of the National Medical Association* 63:93–98, 1971.

Ostfield, A.M., Shekelle, R.B., and Klawans, H.L. Transient ischemic attacks and risk of stroke in an elderly poor population. *Stroke* 4:980–986, 1973.

Pincock, J. Natural history of cerebral thrombosis. *Annals of Internal Medicine* 46:925–930, 1957.

Recent trends in mortality from cerebrovascular disease. *Statistical Bulletin of the Metropolitan Life Insurance Company* 56:2–4, 1975.

Rice, D.P. *Estimating the Cost of Illness.* Health Economics Series No. 6, PHS Publication No. 947-6. Washington: U.S. Government Printing Office, May 1966.

Robinson, R.W., Cohen, W.D., Higano, N., et al. Life-table analysis of survival after cerebral thrombosis—10 year experience. *Journal of the American Medical Association* 169:1149–1152, 1959.

Robinson, R.W., Demirel, M., and LeBeau, R.J. Natural history of cerebral thrombosis: 9–19 year follow-up. *Journal of Chronic Diseases* 21:221–230, 1968.

Sahs, A.L., Hartman, E.C., and Aronson, S.M., eds. *Guidelines for Stroke Care*. DHEW Publication No. (HRA) 76-14017. Washington: U.S. Government Printing Office, 1976.

Sahs, A.L., Perret, G.E., Locksley, H.B., et al., eds. *Intracranial Aneurysms and SAH: A Cooperative Study*. Philadelphia: J.B. Lippincott, 1969.

Schoenberg, B.S., Mellinger, J.F., and Schoenberg, D.G. Perinatal intracranial hemorrhage. *Archives of Neurology* 34:570–573, 1977.

Schoenberg, B.S., Mellinger, J.F., and Schoenberg, D.G. Cerebrovascular disease in infants and children: A study of incidence, clinical features, and survival. *Neurology* 28:763–768, 1978.

Shafer, S.Q., Bruun, B., and Richter, R.W. The outcome of stroke at hospital discharge in New York City blacks. *Stroke* 4:782–786, 1973.

Shurtleff, D. *Some Characteristics Related to the Incidence of Cardiovascular Disease and Death: Framingham Study, 18-Year Follow-Up. The Framingham Study: An Epidemiological Investigation of Cardiovascular Disease*, Section 30. Washington: U.S. Government Printing Office, 1974.

Soltero, I., et al. Trends in mortality from cerebrovascular diseases in the United States, 1960 to 1975. *Stroke* 9:549–555, 1978.

Stallones, R.A. Epidemiology of cerebrovascular disease. A review. *Journal of Chronic Diseases* 18:859–872, 1965.

Stallones, R.A., Dyken, M.L., Fang, H.C.H., et al. Epidemiology for stroke facilities planning. *Stroke* 3:351–371, 1972.

Swanson, P.D., Calanchini, P.R., Dyken, M.L., et al. A cooperative study of hospital frequency and character of transient ischemic attacks. II: Performance of angiography among six centers. *Journal of the American Medical Association* 237:2202–2206, 1979.

Thompson, R.A., and Green, J.R., eds. *Advances in Neurology Vol. 16: Stroke*. New York: Raven Press, 1977.

Toole, J.F. Management of TIAs and acute cerebral infarction. In R.A. Thompson and J.R. Green (eds.), *Advances in Neurology*. Vol. 16 *Stroke*. New York: Raven Press, 1977.

Toole, J.F., Janeway, R., Choi, K., et al. TIAs due to atherosclerosis. A prospective study of 160 patients. *Archives of Neurology* 32:5–12, 1975.

Toole, J.F., and Patel, A.N. *Cerebrovascular Disorders*, 2d ed. New York: McGraw-Hill, 1974.

U.S. Department of Health, Education and Welfare, National Center for Health Statistics. *Vital Statistics of the United States*, Vol. 2, Sec. 7, 1974.

U.S. Department of Health, Education and Welfare, Public Health Service.

Cerebrovascular disease epidemiology: A workshop. *Public Health Monographs* 76, 1966.

U.S. Department of Health, Education and Welfare, Public Health Service. *Economic Costs of Cardiovascular Disease and Cancer, 1962.* Health Economics Series 5, 1965.

U.S. Department of Health, Education and Welfare. *National Survey of Stroke.* NIH Publication No. 80-2069, 1980.

Wallace, D.C. A study of the natural history of cerebral vascular disease. *Medical Journal of Australia* 1:90–95, 1967.

Whisnant, J.P. Epidemiology of stroke: Emphasis on transient cerebral ischemic attacks and hypertension. *Stroke* 5:68–80, 1974.

Whisnant, J.P. A population study of stroke and TIA: Rochester, Minnesota. In F.J. Gillingham, C. Mawdsley, and A.E. Williams (eds.), *Stroke.* Edinburgh: Churchill Livingstone, 1976.

Whisnant, J.P., Fizgibbons, J.P. Kurland, L.T., et al. Natural History of stroke in Rochester, Minnesota, 1945 through 1954. *Stroke* 2:11–22, 1971.

Whisnant, J.P., Goldner, J.C., and Taylor, W.F. Cerebral vascular insufficiency (TIA): Natural history of transient ischemic attacks. In J. Moossy and R. Janeway (eds.) *Cerebral Vascular Diseases. Seventh Conference.* New York: Grune and Stratton, 1971.

Wolf, P.A., Dawber, T.R., Thomas, H.E., et al. Epidemiology of stroke. In R.A. Thompson and J.R. Green (eds.), *Advances in Neurology.* Vol. 16: *Stroke.* New York: Raven Press, 1977.

Wylie, C.M. An administrative view of stroke control: Current use and future organization of health resources and facilities. In A.L. Sahs, E.C. Hartman, and S.M. Aronson (eds.) *Guidelines for Stroke Care.* Washington: U.S. Government Printing Office, 1976.

Wylie, C.M. Age and long-term hospital care following cerebrovascular accidents. *Journal of the American Geriatrics Society* 12:763–770, 1964.

Wylie, C.M. Evaluating the stroke effort in regional medical programs. *American Journal of Public Health* 59:974–980, 1969.

Wylie, C.M. Rehabilitative care of stroke patients. *Journal of the American Medical Assocation* 196:1117–1120, 1966.

Zankel, H.T., Cobb, J.B., and Huskey, F.E. The rehabilitation of 500 stroke patients. *Journal of the American Geriatrics Society* 14:1177–1185, 1966.

Ziegler, D.K., and Hassanein, R.S. Prognosis for patients with TIAs. *Stroke* 4:666–673, 1973.

Zupping, R., and Roose, M. Epidemiology of cerebrovascular disease in Tartu, Estonia, USSR, 1970 through 1973. *Stroke* 7:187–190, 1976.

Chapter 5
Cancer

Abt Associates Inc. and Boston University Cancer Research Center. *The Measurement of the Cost of Cancer Care. Task Two Report. Literature Review and Recommendations for Further Work*. Prepared for the National Cancer Institute, Division of Cancer Control and Rehabilitation, December 1976.

Abt, C.C. The social costs of cancer. *Social Indicators Research* 2:175–190, 1975.

American Cancer Society. *The American Cancer Society—A Fact Book for the Medical and Related Professions*. New York, 1975.

American Cancer Society. Cancer statistics, 1975—25 year cancer survey. Reprinted from *Ca—A Cancer Journal for Clinicians* 25:2–21, 1975.

American Cancer Society. *A Cancer Source Book for Nurses*. New York, 1975.

American Cancer Society. *1977 Cancer Facts and Figures*. New York, 1976.

American Cancer Society. Proceedings of the American Cancer Society national conference on childhood cancer. Reprinted from *Cancer* 35:863–1026, 1975.

American Cancer Society. *Proceedings of the American Cancer Society's National Conference on Human Values and Cancer*. Atlanta, Ga., 1973.

American Cancer Society and National Cancer Institute. Proceedings of the national conference on advances in cancer management. II: Detection and diagnosis. Reprinted from *Cancer* 37 (Suppl.):417–617, 1976.

Axtell, L.M., Cutler, S.J., and Myers, M.H., eds. *End Results in Cancer. Report No. 4*. U.S. Department of Health, Education and Welfare, Public Health Service, National Institute of Health, National Cancer Institute, Publication No. (NIH) 73-272, 1972.

Axtell, L.M., and Myers, M.H., eds. *Recent Trends in the Survival of Cancer Patients* 1960–1971. U.S. Department of Health, Education and Welfare, Publication No. (NIH) 75-767, 1974.

Barckley, V. Families facing cancer. Reprinted from *Cancer News* (Spring/Summer 1970).

Birnbaum, H. *The Cost of Catastrophic Illness*. Lexington, Mass.: Lexington Books, D.C. Heath and Co., 1978.

Black, H. Cancer death rate takes a small dip. *Boston Globe* (April 10, 1977).

Cairns, J. The cancer problem. *Scientific American* 233:64–68, 1975.

Cancer in California. California Tumor Registry, State of California Department of Public Health, 1964.

Cancer mortality declines in 1975. *Statistical Bulletin of the Metropolitan Life Insurance Company* (December 1976).

Cancer survival among men. *Statistical Bulletin of the Metropolitan Life Insurance Company* (June 1974).

Cutler, S.J. Report on the third national cancer survey. *Proceedings of the Seventh National Cancer Conference* 7:639–645, 1973.

Cutler, S.J., and Ederer, F., eds. *End Results and Mortality Trends in Cancer*. U.S. Department of Health, Education and Welfare, National Cancer Institute Monograph No. 6, September 1961.

Cutler, S.J., Scotto, J., Devesco, S.S., and Connelly, R.R. Third national cancer survey—An overview of available information *Journal of the National Cancer Institute* 53(6):1565–1575, 1974.

Cutler, S.J., and Young, J.L., eds. *Third National Cancer Survey: Incidence Data*. National Cancer Institute Monograph 41. U.S. Department of Health, Education and Welfare, Public Health Services, National Institute of Health, Publication No. (NIH) 75-787, 1975.

Employing the cancer patient. *Statistical Bulletin of the Metropolitan Life Insurance Company* (June 1973).

Ferber, B., Handy, V.H., Gerhardt, P.R., and Solomon, M. *Cancer in New York State, Exclusive of New York City, 1941–1960*. Bureau of Cancer Control, New York State Department of Health, 1962.

Hodgson, T.A., Jr. The economic costs of cancer. In David Shottenfeld (ed.), *Cancer Epidemiology and Prevention*. Springfield, Ill.: Charles C. Thomas, 1975.

Holland, J.F. Prediction of time of death in patients with advanced cancer. *Annals of the New York Academy of Sciences* 164:678–686, 1969.

Impact. Costs and Consequences of Catastrophic Illness on Patients and Families. New York: Cancer Care, Inc., 1973.

Mabuchi, K., and Maruchi, N. The major causes of death in the United States and Japan. *Preventive Medicine* 1(1):252–254, 1972.

Mortality from cancer. *Statistical Bulletin of the Metropolitan Life Insurance Company* (June 1976).

Pekar, P.P., Jr. Costs analysis and consequences of the national cancer plan. *Federation Proceedings* 33(11):2225–2230, 1974.

Regional variations in mortality from cancer. *Statistical Bulletin of the Metropolitan Life Insurance Company* (February 1973).

Rice, D.P. *Economic Costs of Cardiovascular Diseases and Cancer, 1962*. U.S. Department of Health, Education and Welfare, Health Economics Series No. 5, 1965.

Robbins, G.F. The cost of cancer. *Proceedings of the Seventh National Cancer Conference* 7:859–861, 1973.

Scotto, J., and Chiazze, L., Jr. *Third National Cancer Survey: Hospitalizations and Payments to Hospitals. Part A: Summary*. U.S. Department of Health, Education and Welfare, Publication No. (NIH) 76-1094, March 1976.

Silverberg, E. *Gynecological Cancer: Statistical and Epidemiological Information.* New York: American Cancer Society, 1975.

Silverberg, E. *Urologic Cancer. Statistical and Epidemiological Information.* New York: American Cancer Society, 1975.

Spratt, J.S., Jr. Cost effectiveness in the post-treatment follow-up of cancer patients. *Journal of Surgical Oncology* 3:393–400, 1971.

Spratt, J.S., Jr. The physician's role in minimizing the economic morbidity of cancer. *Seminars in Oncology* 2(4):411–417, 1975.

Trends in cancer incidence. *Statistical Bulletin of the Metropolitan Life Insurance Company* (June 1976).

Trends in Cancer Mortality California 1910–1965. California Tumor Registry, State of California Department of Public Health, 1968.

U.S. Department of Health, Education and Welfare. *End Results and Mortality Trends in Cancer.* National Cancer Institute, Monograph No. 6, September 1961.

Wetherington, R. The crippling curses of cancer. *Sunday News* (August 19, 1973).

Young, J.L., Jr., Asire, A.J., and Pollack, E.S. *SEER Program: Cancer Incidence and Mortality in the United States, 1973–1976.* U.S. Department of Health, Education and Welfare, National Cancer Institute, DHEW Publication No. (NIH) 78-1837, 1978.

Zimmerer, E.G., Chancellor, L.E., and Wise, M.R. *A Study of Cancer Mortality in Iowa.* Iowa State Department of Health, American Cancer Society, Iowa Division, Mason City, Iowa, 1954.

Zinman, D. The war on cancer: Are we winning it? *Newsday* (January 1977).

Chapter 6
Motor Vehicle Injuries

Abbreviated Injury Scale (AIS). Joint Committee on Injury Scaling of the American Medical Association, American Association for Automotive Medicine, and Society for Automotive Engineers, 1980 Revision.

All-Industry Research Advisory Committee. *Automobile Injuries and Their Compensation in the United States*, Vols. I and II. Chicago, March 1979.

American Hospital. Association. *Hospital Statistics.* Chicago, 1976.

Baker, S.P., and O'Neill, B. The injury severity score: An update. *Journal of Trauma* 16(11):882–885, 1976.

Baker, S.P., O'Neill, B., Haddon, W., Jr., and Long, W.B. The injury severity score: A method for describing patients with multiple injuries and evaluating emergency care. *Journal of Trauma* 14:187–196, 1974.

Bennett, D.E., and Cherry, J.K. The natural history of traumatic aneurysms of the aorta. *Surgery* 61:516–523, 1967.

Boston City Hospital. Charge directory (11/12/75). Computer printout, Boston, Mass., 1975.

Boyd, D.R., Flashner, B.A., and Nyhus, C.M. Clinical and epidemiologic characteristics of non-surviving trauma vicitims in an urban enrivonment. *Journal of the American Medical Association* 64(1):1–7, 1972.

Brody, W.H. *Economic Value of a Housewife*. Research and Statistics Note 9, DHEW Publication No. SSA 75-11701. Washington, D.C.: Social Security Administration, Office of Research and Statistics, August 28, 1975.

Burney, R.E., and Robson, M.C. Measuring the emergency surgical care of auto accident patients. *Proceedings of the 18th Conference of the American Association for Automotive Medicine*. Toronto, Canada, 1974.

Caveness, W.F., Mierowsky, A.M., Rish, B.L., Mohr, J.P., Kistler, J.P., Dillon, J.D., and Weiss, G.H. The nature of posttraumatic epilepsy. *Journal of Neurosurgery* (1979).

Caveness, W.F., Walker, A.E., and Ascroft, P.B. Incidence of posttraumatic epilepsy in Korean veterans as compared with those from World War I and World War II. *Journal of Neurosurgery* 19:122–129, 1962.

Commission on Professional and Hospital Activities. Unpublished data for 1973 from the Professional Activities Survey, 7th Patient Sample, Ann Arbor, Michigan, 1973.

Committee on Medical Aspects of Automotive Safety. Rating the severity of tissue damage. II: The comprehensive scale. *Journal of the American Medical Association* 220:717–720, 1972.

Cowley, R.A., Hudson, F., Scanlan, E., Gill, W., Lally, R.J., Long, W., and Kahn, A.D. An economical and proved heliocopter program for transporting the emergency critically ill and injured patient in Maryland. *Journal of Trauma* 13(12):1029–1038, 1973.

Cretin, S. Cost/benefit analysis of treatment and prevention of myocardial infarction. *Health Services Research* (Summer 1977):174–187.

Cumulative Regulatory Effects on the Cost of Automotive Transportation: Final Report to the Ad Hoc Committee. Prepared for the Office of Science and Technology, Washington, February 28, 1972.

DeLorean Corporation. *Automotive Occupant Protective Safety Air Cushion Expenditure/Benefit Study*. Report prepared for the Allstate Insurance Company, Northbrook, Ill., Bloomfield Hills, Michigan, August 1975.

Donovan, A.J., Turrill, F., and Berne, C.J. Injuries of the pancreas from blunt trauma. *Surgical Clinics of North America* 52:649–665, 1972.

Dresser, A., Mierowsky, A., Weiss, G., McNeel, M., Simon, G., and Caveness, W. Gainful employment following head injury. *Archives of Neurology* 29:111–116, 1973.

Economics of road safety. *Lancet* 2(518):709, 1967.

Eraklis, A.J., Kevy, S.V., Diamond, L.K., et al. Hazard of overwhelming infection after splenectomy in childhood. *New England Journal of Medicine* 276(22):1225–1229, 1967.

Faigin, B.M. *1975 Societal Costs of Motor Vehicle Accidents*. U.S. Department of Transportation, National Highway Traffic Safety Administration. Washington: U.S. Government Printing Office, December 1976.

Flora, D., Bailey, J., and O'Day, J. The financial consequences of auto accidents. *HIT Lab Reports*, 5(10):1–7, 1975.

Geisler, W.D., Jousse, A.J., and Wynne-Jones, M. Survival in traumatic transverse myelitis. *Paraplegia* 14:262–275, 1977.

Gissane, W., Bull, J., and Roberts, B. Sequelae of road injuries: A review of one year's admissions to an accident hospital. *Injury* 1(3):195–203, 1970.

Grant, R.P., Gifford, R.W., Pudvan, W.R., Meaney, T.F., et al. Renal trauma and hypertension. *The American Journal of Cardiology* 27:173–176, 1971.

Haddon, W.,1 Jr. Options for prevention of motor vehicle crash injury. Keynote address: Conference on Options for Prevention of Motor Vehicle Injury, Beer Sheva, Israel. *Israel Journal of Medical Science* 16(1):45–65, 1980.

Haddon, W., Jr., Advances in the epidemiology of injuries as a basis for public policy. *Public Health Reports* 95:411–421, 1980.

Haddon, W., Jr., and Baker, S.P. Injury Control, in D. Clark and B. MacMahon (eds.) *Preventive and Community Medicine*, 2d ed. Boston: Little, Brown, in press 1980.

Hall, R.G. *Factbook: A Summary of Information About Towaway Accidents Involving 1973–75 Model Cars,* Vol. II. National Technical Information Service, Springfield, Va., September 1976.

Haller, J.A., and Jones, E.L. Effect of splenectomy on immunity and resistance to major infections in early childhood. *Annals of Surgery* 163:902–908, 1966.

Henle, J. Rehabilitation of auto accident victims. In *Automobile Accident and Compensation Study*. U.S. Department of Transportation, August 1970.

Holmes, R.A. On the economic welfare of victims of automobile accidents. *American Economic Review* 60(1): 143–152.

Insurance Information Institute. *Insurance Facts*. New York, 1975.

International trends in motor vehicle fatalities. *Statistical Bulletin of the Metropolitan Life Insurance Companay* (October 1973).

Jennet, W.B. *Epilepsy after Non-Missile Head Injuries*. Chicago: Year Book Publishers, 1975.

Jousse, A.T., Wynne-Jones, M., and Breithaupt, D.J. A follow-up study of life expectancy and mortality in traumatic transverse myelitis. *Canadian Medical Association Journal* 98:770–772, 1968.

Joyce, J.W., Fairbairn, J.F., Kincaid, O.W., and Juergens, J.L. Aneurysms of the thoracic aorta: A clinical study with special reference to prognosis. *Circulation* 29:176–181, 1964.

Kahane, C.J., Lee, S.N., and Smith, R.A. A program to evaluate active restraint system effectiveness. In *Proceedings of the Fourth International Congress on Automotive Safety*. Washington: U.S. Government Printing Office, 1975.

Kannel, W.B. Role of blood pressure in cardiovascular morbidity and mortality. *Progress in Cardiovascular Diseases* 17:5–24, 1974.

Marsh, J.C., Kaplan, R.J., Kornfield, S.M. *Financial Consequences of Serious Injury*. Final Report, University of Michigan Highway Safety Research Institute, December 1977.

Massachusetts General Hospital, Boston, Mass. Unpublished information on emergency medical procedures and financial charges, 1977.

Mitchell, H.H. *Emergency Medical Care and Traffic Fatalities*. Prepared for the National Highway Safety Bureau, Federal Highway Administration, by the Rand Corporation, April 1968.

Motor vehicle accident fatalities at peak at younger ages. *Statistical Bulletin of the Metropolitan Life Insurance Company* 52:5–8, 1971.

Mungerast, J.S., and Kahane, C.J. *Restraint Systems Evaluation Program Codebook*. National Highway Traffic Safety Administration Technical Note, DOT HS-802-285, U.S. Department of Transportation, March, 1977.

National Safety Council. *Accident Facts*. Chicago, 1976.

Newton-Wellesly Hospital, Newton, Mass. Unpublished information on emergency medical procedures and financial charges, circa 1977.

Nineteen seventy-five AMA-SAE-AAAM revision of the abbreviated injury scale (AIS). In Donald F. Huelke (ed.) *Proceedings of the 19th Conference of the American Association for Automotive Medicine*. San Diego, Calif., November 20–22, 1975.

OECD Road Research Group. *Road Research: Young Driver Accidents*. Organization for Economic Cooperation and Development, Paris, March 1975.

Owens, A. At last: Hard figures on how fast fees have been climbing. *Medical Ecnomics* (October 13, 1975):98–126.

Partyka, S. *NCSS—The Analyst's Companion*. National Center for Statistics and Analysis, National Highway Traffic Safety Administration, U.S. Department of Transportation, May, 1980.

Pedestrian fatalities continue to increase. *Statistical Bulletin of the Metropolitan Life Insurance Company* 50:6–7, 1969.

Pittman, M.A., and Loutzheiser, R.C. *A Study of Accident Investigation Sites on the Gulf Freeway*. Texas Highway Department Report 165-1, Texas Transportation Institute, August 1972.

Quattlebaum, J.K. Massive resection of the liver. *Annals of Surgery* 137:787–796, 1953.

Reinfurt, D.W., Silva, C.Z., and Siela, A.F. *A Statistical Analysis of Seat Belt Effectiveness in 1973–75 Model Cars Involved in Towaway Crashes*, Vol. I. Prepared for the National Highway Traffic Safety Administration by the Highway Safety Research Center, University of North Carolina, Chapel Hill, N.C., September 1976.

Reinfurt, D.W., Stewart, J.R., Hall, R.G., Dutt, A.K., Li, L.K., and Stutts, J.C. *Injury Scaling Research: An Interim Report*. Highway Safety Research Center, University of North Carolina, Chapel Hill, N.C., November 1977.

Rice, D.P. *Estimating the Cost of Illness*. Health Economics Series No. 6, PHS Publication No. 947-6. Washington: U.S. Government Printing Office, May, 1966.

Schlueter, C.F. Some economic dimensions of traumatic injuries. *Journal of Trauma* 10(1): 915–920, 1970.

Smart, C.N., and Sanders, C.R. *The Costs of Motor Vehicle Related Spinal Cord Injuries*. Washington: The Insurance Institute for Highway Safety, 1976.

Somerville Hospital, Somerville, Mass. Unpublished information on emergency medical procedures and financial charges, circa 1977.

Struble, D. *Societal Costs and Their Reduction by Safety Systems*. Minicars, Inc., Galeta, CA., July 1975.

Sturdy Memorial Hospital, Attleboro, Mass. Unpublished information on emergency medical procedures and financial charges, circa 1977.

Thorson, J. *Long-Term Effects of Traffic Accidents*. Lund, Sweden: Hakan Ohlssons Farlag, 1975.

U.S. Department of Commerce, Bureau of the Census, *Current Population Reports: Population Estimates and Projections*. Series P-25, No. 614, 1975.

U.S. Department of Commerce, Bureau of the Census. *Statistical Abstract of the United States 1976*. Washington: U.S. Government Printing Office, July 1976.

U.S. Department of Health, Education and Welfare, Health Resources Administration, National Center for Health Statistics. Current estimates from the health interview survey, United States 1975. *Vital and Health Statistics* [10]115, 1977.

U.S. Department of Health, Education and Welfare, Health Resources Administration, National Center for Health Statistics. Unpublished data on moving motor vehicle traffic injuries in 1975 obtained from the Health Interview Survey.

U.S. Department of Health, Education and Welfare, National Center for Health Statistics. Life tables. *Vital Statistics of the United States II, 1977*, Vol. 2, Section 5. Washington: U.S. Government Printing Office, 1980.

U.S. Department of Justice, Law Enforcement Assistance, Administration of U.S. Bureau of Census. *Expenditure and Employment Data for Criminal Justice System: 1975*. Washington: U.S. Government Printing Office, 1977.

U.S. Department of Labor, Bureau of Labor Statistics. *Government Employees Salary Trends*. Washington, U.S. Government Printing Office, 1977.

U.S. Department of Transportation. *Automobile Accident Litigation*. A Report of the Federal Judicial Center to the Department of Transportation, April 1970 (from *Automobile Insurance and Compensation Study*).

U.S. Department of Transportation. *Economic Consequences of Automobile Accidents*, Vols. I and II. From *Automobile Insurance and Compensation Study*. Washington: U.S. Government Printing Office, April 1970.

U.S. Department of Transportation, Federal Highway Administration. *Fatal and Injury Accident Rates on Federal-Aid and Other Highway Systems, 1975*. Washington: Superintendent of Documents.

U.S. Department of Transportation, National Highway Traffic Safety Administration. *Design for NASS: A National Accident Sampling System*, Vol. I. Prepared by the University of Michigan Highway Safety Research Institute, Ann Arbor, Michigan, May 1976.

U.S. Department of Transportation, National Highway Traffic Safety Administration. *Fatal Accident Reporting System: 1975 Annual Report*. Washington: U.S. Government Printing Office, October 1976.

U.S. Department of Transportation, National Highway Traffic Safety Administration. Fatal accident reporting system. Unpublished data for 1975 on the incidence and time-to-death of U.S. motor vehicle fatalities.

U.S. Department of Transportation, National Highway Traffic Safety Administration. *Highway Safety Facts*. Washington: U.S. Government Printing Office, May 1978, April 1979, and June 1980.

U.S. Department of Transportation, National Highway Traffic Safety Administration, National Center for Statistics and Analysis. Data reported from selected states on the incidence in 1975 of nonfatal motor vehicle injuries.

U.S. Department of Transportation, National Highway Traffic Safety Administration. National crash severity study. Unpublished data on nonfatal motor vehicle injuries from the May 1980, data file.

U.S. Department of Transportation, National Highway Traffic Safety Administration. *Preliminary Findings from the National Crash Severity Study*. Contract No. DOT HS-804-188, Washington, April 1979.

U.S. Department of Transportation, National Highway Traffic Safety Administration. Restraint systems evaluation program. Unpublished data on nonfatal motor vehicle injuries, 1975.

U.S. Department of Transportation. *The Secretary's Decision Concerning Motor Vehicle Occupant Crash Protection*. Washington: U.S. Government Printing Office, December 6, 1976.

Walker, A.E. Prognosis in posttraumatic epilepsy: A ten-year follow-up of craniocerebral injuries of World War II. *Journal of the American Medical Association* 164(15):1636–1641, 1957.

Walker, A.E., and Joblon, S. A follow-up of head-injured men of World War II. *Journal of Neurosurgery* 16:600–610, 1959.

Walker, A.E., Leuchs, H.K., Lechtape-Gruter, H., Caveness, W.F., and Kretschman, C. Life expectancy of head-injured men with and without epilepsy. *Archives of Neurology* 24:95–100, 1971.

Wuerdemann, H., and Joksch, H.C. *National Indirect Costs of Motor Vehicle Accidents*. Center for the Environment and Man, Report No. 4114-494-B, Hartford, Conn., June 1973.

Interviews

Chapter 3
Coronary Heart Disease

Castelli, William P., M.D., Public Health Officer with Framingham Heart Study Framingham, Mass., March through June 1977.

Chobanian, Aram V., M.D., Director, Cardio-Vascular Institute, Boston University Medical Center, Boston, Mass., March 16, 1977.

Cohn, Peter, M.D., Member, Department of Cardiology, Peter Bent Brigham Hospital, Boston, Mass., June 19, 1977.

Crocket, Charlotte, Director of Program Development, The American Heart Association, Brookline, Mass., April 11, 1977.

Feldman, Jacob, Ph.D., Associate Director, Statistics, the National Center for Health Statistics, Washington, D.C., March 9, 1977.

Hooley, Michael, Unit Manager, Emergency Department, Massachusetts General Hospital, Boston, Mass., July 21, 1977.

Jenkins, C. David, Ph.D., Professor of Psychiatry and Chairperson of Behavioral Epidemiology at Boston University Medical Center, Boston, Mass., April 15, 1977.

Kuller, Lewis, Ph.D., Professor at the University of Pittsburg School of Public Health, Pittsburg, Pennsylvania, April 15, 1977.

Levine, Paul, M.D., Cardiologist with Boston University Hospital, Boston, Mass., October 6, 1977.

Place, Erma, R.N., Staff Nurse, Outpatient Clinic at Massachusetts General Hospital, Boston, Mass., July 21, 1977.

Potts, Richard, Program Manager of Information Services, Office of Emergency Medical Services, Massachusetts Department of Public Health, Boston, Mass., July 18, 1977.

Pozen, Michael, M.D., Cardiologist with Boston University Medical Center, Boston, Mass., July 7, 1977.

Sorlie, Paul, Health Statistician, Biometrics Research Branch, National Heart, Lung, and Blood Institute, U.S. Department of Health, Education and Welfare, Bethesda, Maryland, January 13, 1978.

Stanton, Babette, Research Associate, Professor of Community Health, Boston University Medical School, Boston, Mass., June 1, 1977.

Urchak, Peter, M.D., Cardiac Unit, Massachusetts General Hospital, Boston, Mass., August 25, 1977.

Chapter 5
Cancer

Cromwell, Jerry, Ph.D., Senior Economist, Abt Associates, Cambridge, Mass., May 4, 1977.

Feldman, Jacob J., Ph.D., Associate Director, National Center for Health Statistics, Washington, D.C., March 9, 1977.

Friedman, Robert, M.D., Researcher/Clinician, Boston University Medical School, Boston, Mass., April 20, 1977.

Goldberg, Peter D., D.M.D., Massachusetts Eye and Ear Infirmary, Boston, Mass., May 6, 1977.

Goodman, Max, M.D., Pathologist, Massachusetts General Hospital, Boston, Mass., June 7, 1977.

Korn, Allen, M.D., Clinical Oncologist, Evansville, Ind., April 11, 1977.

Leffert, Robert, M.D., Massachusetts General Hospital, Boston, Mass., May 20, 1977.

Mankowitch, Ralph, M.D., General Surgeon, Waltham Hospital, Waltham, Mass., April 27, 1977.

May, George A., M.D., Surgeon, Newton-Wellesley Hospital, Newton, Mass., May 23, 1977.

Miller, Harry, M.D., Associate Professor of Surgery, New England Medical Center Hospital, Boston, Mass., May 16, 1977.

Newton, Robert A., Chairman, Research Investigation Committee, Newton-Wellesley Hospital, Newton, Mass., June 1, 1977.

Ojemann, Robert, M.D., Neurosurgeon, Massachusetts General Hospital, Boston, Mass., June 14, 1977.

Parker, John S., M.D., Surgeon, Newton-Wellesley Hospital, Newton, Mass., May 23, 1977.

Radley, Francis, Chief Accountant, Sidney Farber Cancer Institute, Boston, Mass., May 31, 1977.

Schottenfeld, David, M.D., Clinical Epidemiologist, Memorial Sloan-Kettering Hospital, New York, N.Y., March 8, 1977.

Scotto, Joseph, M.S., National Institutes of Health, March 4, 1977.

Stonberg, Marion, Social Worker, Sidney Farber Cancer Institute, Boston, Mass., March 2, 1977.

Vanderschmidt, G. Frederick, Ph.D., Vice President, Abt Associates, Cambridge, Mass., March 4, 1977.

Vernon, James K., M.D., Surgeon, Newton-Wellesley Hospital, Newton, Mass., May 23, 1977.

Weymuller, Ernest, M.D., Surgeon, Massachusetts Eye and Ear Infirmary, Boston, Mass., June 24, 1977.

Yerganian, George, M.D., Researcher, Sidney Farber Cancer Institute, Boston, Mass., March 1, 1977.

Young, John, Ph.D., Biostatistician, National Cancer Institute, Bethesda, Md., December 5, 1977.

Zinman, David, Medical/Science Reporter, *Newsday*, Long Island, N.Y., March 2, 1977.

Chapter 6
Motor Vehicle Injuries

All Cape Ambulance Service, Hyannis, Mass., July 1977.

Amsbough, William, Patient Accounts Manager, Newton-Wellesley Hospital, Newton, Mass., August 8, 1977.

Barren, Steven, Assistant Administrator, Newton-Wellesley Hospital, Newton, Mass, August 4, 1977.

Bay State Ambulance Service, Boston, Mass., July 1977.

Bentkover, Stuart, M.D., Surgical Resident, Massachusetts Eye and Ear Infirmary, Boston, Mass., September 2, 1977.

Bray, James, Department of Health and Hospitals, City of Boston, Boston, Mass., June 7, 1977.

Commonwealth Ambulance Service, Boston, Mass., July 1977.

Craigie, John D., Vice-President, Insurance Information Institute, New York, N.Y., September 2, 1977.

Dart, Barbara, R.N., Head Nurse, Emergency Department, Newton-Wellesley Hospital, Newton, Mass., August 8, 1977.

Delta Ambulance Service, Waterville, Maine, July 1977.

Hedlund, James, Ph.D., National Center for Statistics and Analysis, National Highway Traffic Safety Administration, U.S. Department of Transportation, Washington, D.C., August 1977 through August 1979.

Hooley, Michael, Unit Manager, Emergency Department, Massachusetts General Hospital, Boston, Mass., July 21, 1977.

Keith and Keith Ambulance Service, New York, N.Y., July 1977.

Lipson, Charles, S., M.D., Member, Surgical and Emergency Medical Staffs, Newton-Wellesley Hospital, Newton, Mass., September 6, 1977.

Newton-Wellesley Ambulance Service, Newton, Mass., July 1977.

Place, Erma, R.N., Staff Nurse, Outpatient Clinic at Massachusetts General Hospital, Boston, Mass., July 21, 1977.

Potts, Richard, Program Manager of Management Information Services, Office of Emergency Medical Services, Massachusetts Department of Public Health, Boston, Mass., July 1977.

Snyder, Lucinda, Director of the Hospital Section, Office of Emergency Medical Services, Massachusetts Department of Public Health, Boston, Mass., July 14, 1977.

Somerset Ambulance Service, Skowhegan, Maine, July 1977.

Stephens, Marvin, Chief Statistician, National Center for Statistics and Analysis, National Highway Safety Administration, U.S. Department of Transportation, Washington, D.C., August 31, 1977.

List of Abbreviations

AIS	Abbreviated Injury Scale
ALE	average life expectancy
ARP	annual reduction in productivity (per person)
AS	annual salary
ATC	annual treatment costs (per person)
CAS	carotid artery system TIA
CCU	coronary care unit
CHD	coronary heart disease
CI	coronary insufficiency
CIS	Comprehensive Injury Scale
CPI	Consumer Price Index
CVA	cerebrovascular accident
CVD	cerebrovascular disease
DC	direct cost(s)
DOA	dead on arrival
FARS	Fatal Accident Reporting System
FHS	Framingham Heart Study
FHWA	Federal Highway Administration
HIS	Health Interview Survey
IA	incidence approach
ICDA	International Classification of Diseases Adapted Code
ICU	intensive care unit
ISS	Injury Severity Score
MAIS	Maximum Abbreviated Injury Scale
MCCU	mobile coronary care unit
MI	myocardial infarction
MTC	mortality component of indirect costs
MVI	motor vehicle injuries
NASS	National Accident Sampling System
NCHS	National Center for Health Statistics
NCI	National Cancer Institute
NCSS	National Crash Severity Study
NHTSA	National Highway Traffic Safety Administration
NSC	National Safety Council
PA	prevalence approach
PAS	Professional Activities Survey
PIB	Patient Interview Book
PVC	present valued costs
PVFE	present value of expected forgone earnings
PVPM	present value of postmorbid earnings
RIND	reversible ischemic neurological deficit

RMR	relative mortality rate
RSEP	Restraint Systems Evaluation Program
RSR	relative survival rate
SEER	Surveillance, Epidemiology, and End Results Project
SCI	spinal cord injury
TIA	transient ischemic attack
TNCS	Third National Cancer Survey
VBS	vertebral-basilar TIA
VDR	value of a day of restricted activity

Index

Abbreviated Injury Scale, 261, 263–264

allocation decisions. *See* resource allocation

angina pectoris uncomplicated, 69, 73, 75–76, 93, 121; diagnosis, 75; direct costs, 100–102, 105–106, 111–113; forgone earnings, 117–119, 368; incidence, 80–81, 84; life expectancy, 92, 94, 117; mortality, 117; survival, 86, 92–93, 123; treatment, 97, 104–105. *See also* coronary heart disease; coronary insufficiency; myocardial infarction; sudden death

cancer, 19, 128, 193; bone, 210, 221; buccal cavity, 207, 360; data base, 65–66, 203, 219; digestive system, 193, 197, 199, 205, 216, 221, 235, 241, 243–244, 360, 367–368; direct costs, 195, 197, 219–221, 224–230, 232, 241–243, 245–247, 250–251, 339, 368, 374; End Results Group, 28, 203–204; epidemiology, 193–194; forgone earnings, 238, 241–242, 245, 250–251, 361, 365, Hodgkins' disease, 194, 216; incidence, 18, 193, 195–197, 199–201, 219, 230, 235, 241, 244–245, 250–251, 357, 359–360, 375; indirect costs, 195, 235, 241–243, 248–249, 368, 374; leukemias, 210, 221, 241, 360; life expectancy, 201, 215–216, 219, 245; lymphomas, 194–195, 210, 221, 232, 241, 360; metastasis, 193–194, 204; mortality, 193, 195, 201–204, 219, 245, 360–361; National Cancer Institute, 196, 203; nervous system, 207, 232, 360, 368; Patient Interview Book, 219, 224, 226, 235; postmorbid earnings, 235, 237–238, 334; reproductive system, 193, 195–196, 199, 207, 216, 221, 235, 241, 243, 360–361, 367; respir-

atory system, 28, 193, 199, 205, 207, 215–216, 221, 229–230, 234, 237–238, 241, 243–244, 246–248, 250, 360, 367–368, 375; SEER project, 203, 244, 251; skin, 197, 211, 216; staging, 194; survival, 28, 202–205, 207, 210, 214–216, 219, 232, 245; Third National Cancer Survey, 64, 195–197, 199–201, 219, 244–246, 250–251; treatment, 194–195, 219; urinary system, 207, 216, 221, 360, 368

cardiovascular diseases. *See* angina pectoris uncomplicated; coronary heart disease; coronary insufficiency; myocardial infarction; stroke; transient ischemic attack

cerebrovascular diseases. *See* angina pectoris uncomplicated; stroke; transient ischemic attack

coronary artery disease. *See* coronary heart disease

coronary heart disease, 4, 19, 69, 92, 137; arrythmia, 69–71, 74; atherogenic variables, 73, atherosclerosis, 69; coronary artery bypass graft, 70, 104, 123; coronary care unit, 90, 101–104; data base, 64–65, 71–72, 76–77; defined, 69, 73; direct costs, 65, 96–97, 102, 108–109, 111–113, 121, 123–124, 127, 369, 374; epidemiology, 76–78, 83–85, 89; etiology, 69–70, 73; forgone earnings, 117–120, 334, 361, 365, 368; Framingham Heart Study, 64, 72–73, 76–79, 86, 90, 137–138 incidence, 64, 70, 72–73, 78–80, 82–84, 119, 121–122, 127, 200, 357, 259, 260; indirect costs, 65, 113, 119–122, 125–127, 361, 374; life expectancy, 84–85; mobile coronary care unit, 71, 100; mortality, 64, 78–80, 84–85, 122, 360–361; recurrence, 64, 122, 127; treatment, 70, 96–97, 127;

About the Authors

Nelson S. Hartunian is a general partner in the consulting firm of Smart and Hartunian, Belmont, Massachusetts, and an assistant professor at Bentley College. He was previously a senior research associate at Policy Analysis, Inc., Brookline, Massachusetts. He received the Ph.D. in physics from Brandeis University and has completed postgraduate studies in economics and operations research as a CASE Fellow at the Massachusetts Institute of Technology. His research has focused on the economic costs of illness, evaluation methodology, and the development of computer-based algorithms for the solution of health-systems problems. He is coauthor of articles on various public health, astrophysical, and operations-research topics.

Charles N. Smart is a general partner in the consulting firm of Smart and Hartunian, Belmont, Massachusetts. He was previously a senior associate at Policy Analysis, Inc., Brookline, Massachusetts, and a management consultant at SRI International, Menlo Park, California. He received the A.M. in applied mathematics from Harvard University and the M.B.A. in finance and applied economics from the Sloan School of Management at the Massachusetts Institute of Technology. His research has focused on the economic costs of illness and the application of decision-analytic and financial-analytic techniques to major policy/management decisions. His works include *The Costs of Motor Vehicle Related Spinal Cord Injuries* (coauthor with Claudia Sanders) and various other publications on public health, applied economic, and policy decision-making issues.

Mark S. Thompson is an assistant professor of health services and a research associate in the Center for the Analysis of Health Practices at the Harvard School of Public Health. He was previously assistant to the director and research scholar at the International Institute for Applied Systems Analysis in Laxenburg, Austria. He received the Ph.D. in public policy from the John F. Kennedy School of Government at Harvard University. His research has focused on the application of decision-analytic, economic, and evaluative techniques to policy analysis. His previous works include *Evaluation for Decision in Social Programs*, *Systems Aspects of Health Planning* (coeditor with Norman Bailey), and *Benefit-Cost Analysis for Program Evaluation*.

About the Institute

The **Insurance Institute for Highway Safety** is an independent, nonprofit, scientific, and educational organization. It is dedicated to reducing the losses—deaths, injuries, and property damage—resulting from crashes on the nation's highways. The Institute is supported by the American Insurance Highway Safety Association, the American Insurers Highway Safety Alliance, the National Association of Independent Insurers Safety Association, and several individual insurance companies.